Introduction to the Cellular
and Molecular Biology of Cancer

Introduction to the Cellular and Molecular Biology of Cancer

Edited by

L. M. FRANKS and N. M. TEICH

Imperial Cancer Research Fund,
London

Oxford New York Tokyo
OXFORD UNIVERSITY PRESS
1986

Oxford University Press, Walton Street, Oxford OX2 6DP
Oxford New York Toronto
Delhi Bombay Calcutta Madras Karachi
Petaling Jaya Singapore Hong Kong Tokyo
Nairobi Dar es Salaam Cape Town
Melbourne Auckland
and associated companies in
Beirut Berlin Ibadan Nicosia

Oxford is a trade mark of Oxford University Press

Published in the United States
by Oxford University Press, New York

British Library Cataloguing in Publication Data
Introduction to the cellular and molecular
biology of cancer.
1. Cancer
I. Franks, L. M.   II. Teich, N.
616.99'4   RC261
ISBN 0-19-854169-4
ISBN 0-19-854168-6 Pbk

Library of Congress Cataloging in Publication Data
Introduction to the cellular and molecular biology of cancer.
Includes bibliographies and index.
1. Cancer.   2. Carcinogenesis.   3. Pathology,
Molecular. I. Franks, L. M. (Leonard Maurice)
II. Teich, N. (Natalie)   [DNLM: 1. Cytology.
2. Molecular Biology.   3. Neoplasms.   QZ 200 I6186]
RC261.I58   1986   616.99'4   86-5288
ISBN 0-19-854169-4
ISBN 0-19-854168-6 (pbk.)

Set by Cotswold Typesetting Ltd, Cheltenham
Printed in Great Britain by
Butler & Tanner Ltd,
Frome, Somerset

Preface

Cancer holds a strange place in modern mythology. Although it is a common disease and it is true to say that one person in five will die of cancer, it is equally true to say that four out of five die of some other disease. Heart disease, for example, a much more common cause of death, does not seem to carry with it the gloomy overtones, not always justifiable, of a diagnosis of cancer. This seems to stem largely from the fact that we had so little knowledge of the cause of a disease which seemed to appear almost at random and proceed inexorably. At the turn of the century, when the ICRF was founded (in 1902), the clinical behaviour and pathology of the more common tumours was known but little else. Over the years clinicians, laboratory scientists and epidemiologists established a firm database. The behaviour patterns of many tumours, and in some cases even the causal agents, were known but how these agents transformed normal cells and influenced tumour cell behaviour remained a mystery.

The development of molecular biology opened up a major new approach to the molecular analysis of normal and tumour cells. We can now ask and begin to answer questions particularly about the genetic control of cell growth and behaviour, that have a bearing on our understanding not only of the family of diseases that we know as cancer but of the whole process of life itself. It is this, as much as finding a cause and cure for the disease, that gives cancer research its importance.

The initiating event which ultimately led to the publication of this book was the realization that many graduate students and research fellows who came to work in our Institute, although highly specialized in their own fields, had relatively little knowledge of cancer and there were few suitable text books to which they could be referred. Consequently, regular introductory courses were organized for new staff members at which 'experts' were asked to give a general introduction to their particular field of study. The talks were designed to give a background for the non-expert, as for example, molecular biology for the morphologist or cell biology for the protein chemist. The courses proved to be very popular. This book follows a similar pattern and has many of the same contributors—hence the fact that most are, or have been, connected with the Imperial Cancer Research Fund.

After a general introduction describing the pathology and natural history of the disease, each section gives a more detailed, but nevertheless general, survey of its particular area. We have tried to present principles rather than a mass of information, but inevitably some chapters are more detailed than others. Each chapter gives a short list of recommended reading which provides a source for seekers of further knowledge.

The topics covered have been selected with some care. Although some, particularly those concerned with treatment, may not at first glance appear to be directly related to cell and molecular biology, we feel that a knowledge of the methods used must give a wider understanding of the practical problems which may ultimately prove to be solvable by the application of modern scientific technology. On the other hand, knowledge of inherent cell behaviour (e.g. radiosensitivity, cell cycling, development of drug resistance, etc.) is important for the design of novel therapeutic approaches that rely less on empirical considerations.

Despite differences in the levels of technical details presented in some chapters, we hope that all are comprehensible. We have provided a fairly comprehensive glossary so that if some terms are not explained adequately in the text, do try the glossary. Finally, the editors would appreciate any comments, suggestions or corrections should a second edition prove desirable.

London   L.M.F.
December 1985   N.M.T.

Acknowledgements

Many people, as well as the named authors, have contributed to this book. It would be impossible to name all except to say that we are particularly grateful to colleagues and friends who read many of the Chapters and made helpful comments.

Our special thanks are due to Miss Vivienne Griffin who was responsible for the final organization and processing of the typescript, without complaint in spite of unexpected problems, and Mrs Audrey Symons and Mr Gerald Leach who were responsible for most of the artwork.

Contents

Contributors

G. E. Adams	MRC Radiology Unit, Harwell, Didcot, Oxon
Peter Beverley	ICRF Human Tumour Immunology Section, University College Hospital Medical School, London
W. F. Bodmer	Imperial Cancer Research Fund, London
I. S. Fentiman	ICRF Unit, Guy's Hospital, London
L. M. Franks	Imperial Cancer Research Fund, London
Melvyn F. Greaves	The Leukaemia Research Fund Centre, Institute of Cancer Research, London
Beverly E. Griffin	Department of Virology, Royal Postgraduate Medical School, Hammersmith Hospital, London
I. R. Hart	Imperial Cancer Research Fund, London
W. I. P. Mainwaring	Department of Biochemistry, The University of Leeds, Leeds
J. S. Malpas	ICRF Medical Oncology Unit, St Bartholomew's Hospital, London
M. C. Pike	ICRF Cancer Epidemiology and Clinical Trials Unit, Radcliffe Infirmary, Oxford
J. M. Polak and S. R. Bloom	Department of Histochemistry, Royal Postgraduate Medical School, Hammersmith Hospital, London
D. Sheer	Imperial Cancer Research Fund, London
Natalie M. Teich	Imperial Cancer Research Fund, London
Philip E. Thorpe	Imperial Cancer Research Fund, London
M. D. Waterfield	Imperial Cancer Research Fund, London
Edward J. Wawrzynczak	Imperial Cancer Research Fund, London
Robin A. Weiss	Institute of Cancer Research, London
Caroline Wigley	Department of Anatomy, Guy's Hospital, London
J. A. Wyke	ICRF Tumour Virology Laboratory, St Bartholomew's Hospital, London

1

What is cancer?

L. M. FRANKS

1.1 Introduction

Cancer has been known since human societies first learnt to record their activities. It was well known to the ancient Egyptians and to succeeding civilizations but, as we shall see, most cancers develop late in life so that until the expectation of life began to increase from the middle of the 19th century onwards, the number of people surviving into the 'cancer age' was relatively small. Now that the common diseases of childhood and infectious diseases, the major causes of death in the past, have been controlled by improvements in public health and medical care, the proportion of older people at risk has increased dramatically. Although diseases of the heart and blood vessels are still the main cause of death in our ageing population, cancer is a major problem. At least one in five will develop cancer and for this reason alone its control, or even better, prevention, are important. But cancer research has an even wider significance. Cancer is not confined to man and the higher mammals but may affect almost all multicellular organisms, plant as well as animal. Since it involves disturbances in cell growth and development, a knowledge of the processes underlying the disease will help us to understand the basic mechanisms concerned with life itself.

About 140 years ago a German microscopist, Johannes Mueller, showed that cancers were made up of cells, a discovery which began the search for changes which would help to pinpoint the specific differences between normal and cancer cells. Although we know a great deal about the structure and behaviour of tumour cells, the main questions remain unanswered. The rapid advances in biological technology, particularly in cell and molecular biology, now allow us to try to answer questions which even 10 years ago could not be approached. But even the most advanced technology is of no value if it is not applied to the appropriate area. The cancer biologist must ask the right questions and to do this he must be aware of the biological background of the disease process he is studying. In this book we try to provide a brief background to the epidemiology and clinical aspects of the group of diseases we describe as 'cancer', and try to interpret changes in structure and behaviour of normal and tumour cells at the biological and molecular levels, against this background. We also try to indicate the areas in which new and exciting discoveries are being made. This introductory chapter provides a brief account of the general biology, cellular pathology and aetiology of cancer and some general definitions. The succeeding chapters deal with specific aspects in more detail.

Cancer is a disorder of cells and, although it usually appears as a tumour (a swelling) made up of a mass of cells, the visible tumour is the end result of a whole series of changes which may have taken many years to develop. In this Chapter I discuss what is known about the changes which take place during the process of tumour development and consider tumour diagnosis and nomenclature. To understand this, we need to know a little about the structure of normal cells and tissues and the mechanisms which control their growth.

1.2 Normal cells and tissues

The tissues of the body can be divided into four main groups; the general supporting tissues collectively known as mesenchyme; the tissue specific cells—epithelium; the 'defence' cells—the reticuloendothelial system; and the nervous system. The mesenchyme consists of connective tissue, fibroblasts which make collagen fibres and associated proteins, bone, cartilage, muscle, blood vessels, and lymphatics. The epithelial cells are the specific cells of the different organs, e.g. skin, intestine, liver, glands, etc. The reticuloendothelial system consists of a wide group of cells, mostly derived from precursor cells in the bone marrow, which give rise to all the red and white blood cells; in addition some of the cells (lymphocytes and macrophages) are distributed throughout the body either as free cells or as fixed constituents of other organs, e.g. in the liver, or as separate organs such as the spleen and lymph nodes. Lymph nodes are specialized nodules of lymphoid cells which are distributed throughout the body and act as filters for cells, bacteria, and other foreign matter. The nervous system is made up of the central nervous system (the brain and spinal cord and their coverings), and the peripheral nervous system of nerves leading from these central structures. Thus each tissue has its own specific cells, usually several different types, which maintain the structure and function of the individual tissue. Bone, for example, has one group of cells responsible for bone formation and a second group responsible for bone resorption when the need arises, as in the repair of fractures. The intestinal tract has many different epithelial cell types responsible for the different functions of the bowel, and so on.

The specific cells are grouped in organs which have a standard pattern (Fig. 1.1). There is a layer of epithelium, the tissue specific cells,

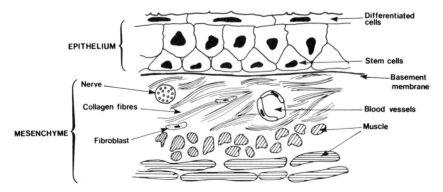

Fig. 1.1 A typical tissue showing epithelial and mesenchymal components.

separated from the supporting mesenchyme by a basement membrane. The supporting tissues (or stroma) are made up of connective tissue (collagen fibres) and fibroblasts (which make collagen), which may be supported on a layer of muscle and/or bone depending on the organ. Blood vessels, lymphatic vessels and nerves pass through the connective tissue and provide nutrients and nervous control among other things for the specific tissue cells. In some instances, e.g. the skin and intestinal tract, the epithelium, which may be one or more cells thick depending on the tissue, covers surfaces. In others it may form a system of tubes (e.g. in the lung or kidney), or solid cords (e.g. liver), but the basic pattern remains the same. Different organs differ in structure only in the nature of the specific cells and the arrangement and distribution of the supporting mesenchyme.

1.3 Control of growth in normal cells

The mechanism of growth control is one of the most important and least understood areas in biology. In normal development and growth, there is a very precise mechanism which allows individual organs to reach a specific size which, for all practical purposes, is never exceeded. If a tissue is injured, the surviving cells in most organs begin to grow and replace the damaged cells. When this has been completed, the process stops, i.e. the normal growth controlling mechanism persists throughout life. Although most cells in the embryo can proliferate (increase in number), not all adult cells do retain this ability. In most organs there are special reserve or stem cells which are capable of growing in response to a stimulus, e.g. an injury, and developing into the organ specific cells. The more highly differentiated (developed) a cell is, e.g. muscle or nerve, the more likely it is to have lost its capacity to grow. In some organs, particularly the brain, the most highly differentiated cells, the nerve cells, can only proliferate in the embryo, although the special supporting cells in the brain continue to be able to grow. A consequence of this, as we shall see later, is that tumours of nerve cells are only found in the very young and tumours of the brain in adults are almost invariably derived from the supporting cells.

From what little is known about growth control, it would appear that there are stimulating and inhibiting factors which are normally in balance until a growth stimulus is required, either for repair or because extra work is required from a particular organ. These objectives may be achieved by hypertrophy, i.e. an increase in size of individual components, usually of structures which do not normally divide. An example is the increase in size of particular muscles in athletes. The alternative is the increase in number of the cells of the organ involved—hyperplasia.

This may be in response to a physiological stimulus, e.g. some hormones, or in repair. These processes are all subject to normal growth control. When the stimulus is removed the situation returns to the status quo.

We now know that there is a close relationship between growth factor production and tumour growth and that their production may be controlled by some genes (protooncogenes) which are genetically similar to some tumour-producing viruses. These findings have opened up whole new areas in cancer research. They are discussed in Chapters 9, 10, 11, and 12.

1.4 The cell cycle

The method by which cells increase in number is similar in all somatic cells, and involves the growth of all cell components leading eventually to division of the cell into two new cells. Although the structural changes which take place have been known for many years, our knowledge of the molecular basis to the process is far from complete. Four stages are usually recognized: $G1 \rightarrow S \rightarrow G2 \rightarrow M$; G1 is a gap or pause after stimulation where little seems to be happening although there is some biochemical activity; S is the phase of synthesis, particularly of DNA, to double the normal amount, although other components also increase; G2 is a second gap period; and M is the stage of mitosis (see Chapter 11) in which the nucleus breaks down to form chromosomes which in the normal cell separate into two identical groups, the nuclear membranes reform about each group, and the whole cell then divides into two identical cells. Cells may be blocked at particular stages in the cycle by drugs (see Chapter 17) or by physiological agents, or they may move out of the division cycle into a resting phase known as G0. Other more complicated patterns of the cell cycle have been described but the one given here is sufficient for the purposes of this book.

1.5 Tumour growth or neoplasia

It is not possible to define a tumour cell in absolute terms. Tumours are usually recognized by the fact that the cells have shown abnormal growth, so that a reasonably acceptable definition is that tumour cells differ from normal cells in that they are no longer responsive to normal growth controlling mechanisms. Since there are almost certainly many different factors involved, the altered cells may still respond to some but not to others. A further complication (see on) is that some tumour cells, especially soon after the cells have been transformed from the normal, may not be growing at all. In the present state of knowledge any definition must be 'operational'.

Given these qualifications we can classify tumours into three main groups

1. *Benign tumours* may arise in any tissue, grow locally and may cause damage by local pressure or obstruction. However, the common feature is that they do not spread to distant sites.

2. *In situ tumours* usually develop in epithelium and are usually, but not invariably, small. The cells have the morphological appearances of cancer cells (see on) but remain in the epithelial layer. They do not invade the basement membrane and supporting mesenchyme. Some authorities recognize a stage of dysplasia-epithelial irregularity but not absolutely identifiable as cancer *in situ* which may sometimes precede cancer *in situ*. Theoretically, *in situ* cancers may arise in mesenchymal, reticuloendothelial or nervous tissue but they have not been recognized.

3. *Cancers* are fully developed (malignant) tumours with a specific capacity to invade and destroy the underlying mesenchyme—local invasion. The tumour cells need nutrients that are provided in normal tissues through the blood stream. Some tumour cells have been shown to produce a substance, tumour angiogenesis factor (TAF), that stimulates the growth of blood vessels into the tumour, thus allowing continuous growth to occur. The new vessels are not very well formed and are easily damaged so that the invading tumour cells may penetrate these and lymphatic vessels. Tumour fragments may be carried in these vessels to local lymph nodes or to distant organs where they may produce secondary tumours (metastases). Cancers may arise in any tissue. Although there may be a progression from benign to malignant, this is far from invariable. Many benign tumours never become malignant.

Some of these problems of definition may be more easily understood if we consider the whole process of tumour induction and development (carcinogenesis)—see Chapters 6–12 for a further discussion.

1.6 The process of carcinogenesis

Carcinogenesis is a multistage process (Fig. 1.2). The application of a cancer producing agent (carcinogen) does not lead to the immediate production of a tumour. There are a series of changes after the initiation step induced by the carcinogen. The subsequent stages—tumour promotion—may be produced by the carcinogen or by other substances (promoting agents) which do not themselves produce tumours. Initiation, which is the primary and essential step in the process, is very rapid but once the initial change has taken place the initiated cells may persist for a considerable time, perhaps the lifespan of the individual. The most likely

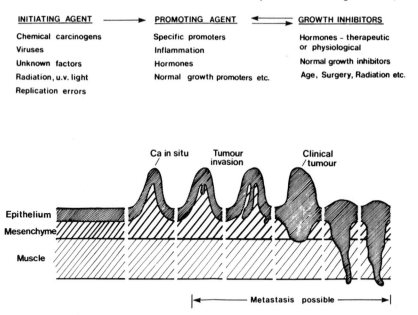

Fig. 1.2 Factors influencing tumour development showing progression from normal to invasive tumour.

site for the primary event is in the genetic material (DNA), although there are other possibilities. The carcinogen is thought to damage or destroy specific genes probably in the DNA of cells from the stem cell population of the tissue involved (see Cairns 1975 for review).

Initiated cells remain latent until acted upon by promoting agents. Many of these 'transformed' cells may not grow at all or grow very slowly. It is at this stage that the influence of growth appears. Promoting agents are not carcinogenic in themselves but they do induce cells to divide in an initiated tissue. Many agents will induce cell division, but only promoters will induce tumour development, so that although cell growth is necessary for tumour development there must also be other factors involved. The suggestion is that promoting agents may interfere with the process of differentiation which normally takes place when cells move from the dividing stem cell population into functioning and usually non-dividing cells. Even though these growth promoting stimuli are acting on the cells, they may still be sensitive to the normal growth inhibiting factors in the body so that the final outcome depends on the balance between the factors and the extent of the changes in the initiated cells. This explains why preneoplastic or even apparently fully transformed tumours can be found but do not appear to be growing, and sometimes even regress.

The whole sequence of events in the process of tumour formation is almost certainly a consequence of gene changes although gene expression may be influenced by the host. We are now beginning to understand some of these changes although there are still many problems unsolved. The discovery that oncogenes of tumour producing viruses are related to genes (protooncogenes) (see Chapter 10) in normal, as well as some tumour, cells has led to intensive research into the relationship of these genes to normal and tumour growth and development. Some of these genes have been localized to specific chromosomes and to sites of chromosome abnormalities (see Chapter 11) in tumours. Much speculation now centres on the question whether the initiation, progression and maintenance of some tumours depends on over-expression through gene amplification (an increase in number of a particular gene), or inappropriate expression (i.e. the wrong time) of normal genes or whether mutations in a critical region of a gene are necessary. A possible hypothesis is that a mutation may be necessary for the initiation event but that some or all of the later stages may depend on over- or inappropriate expression. These possibilities are discussed in the sections on carcinogenesis (Chapters 6–12).

Another major and unexplained area is concerned with the time scale of carcinogenesis. The latent period between initiation and the appearance of tumours is one of the least understood aspects of tumour development. After exposure to industrial carcinogens it may take over 20 years before tumours develop. Even in animals given massive doses, it may take up to a quarter or more of the total lifespan before tumours appear. Yet another unexplained fact is that only a very small number of cells 'initiated' by a carcinogen will eventually produce tumours—perhaps only one or two from many millions of treated cells.

1.7 Factors influencing the development of cancers

Many different factors are involved in the development of tumours. A cancer producing agent or carcinogen, and presumably promoting agents, must be present. Carcinogens may be chemical or physical, e.g. radiation or ultraviolet light which causes skin cancer in Caucasians exposed to tropical sunlight but rarely in coloured races. Identified chemical carcinogens include hydrocarbon carcinogens present in coal tar and a series of chemicals used in the rubber industry. Animal experiments suggest that viruses may be associated with the initiation of some cancers—mainly the leukaemic group; viruses also seem to be associated with some types of human cancer. The role of oncogenes has already been mentioned. This question is discussed in detail in Chapters 9–12. In other cases, such as with cigarette smoking, no single agent has been isolated but cigarette smoke is a very complex mixture of chemicals many of which may contribute to the carcinogenic effect of smoking. We know that cigarette smoking leads to the development of lung cancer and that the more an individual smokes the greater his (or her) chance of developing lung cancer, but all cigarette smokers do not develop lung cancer. There is considerable individual variation in response (see on). We know from animal experiments and epidemiological studies (see Chapters 4 and 5) that there is a genetic, i.e. DNA associated, basis for this. Analysis of these changes are now being done at a cellular (chromosomes) and molecular level (see Chapters 10 and 11). Some genetically homogeneous inbred strains of mice are particularly susceptible to tumour induction by particular viruses or chemicals and some species are more susceptible than others to particular chemicals. In human populations some families and some races are more prone to develop certain cancers. This may be due to genetic or environmental factors. The chance of a particular individual developing cancer depends on the balance between the various factors concerned. For example, exposure to a massive dose of a carcinogen may override inherent genetic resistance or, in others, genetic susceptibility may be so high that the development of specific tumours is invariable. With some tumours, particularly lung cancer and some industrial cancers, exposure to the carcinogen alone is sufficient to almost override other factors, but for the so-called spontaneous tumours, i.e. those which develop without a so far recognizable cause, we have little idea of the relative importance of the various factors. Some of these factors are considered in more detail in Chapters 4, 5, and 7.

Another factor which influences the type of cancer which develops is age. One of the few definite facts we have about cancer is that there is an age associated, organ specific tumour incidence. Most cancers in man and experimental animals can be divided into three main groups depending on their age incidence

1. Embryonic, e.g. neuroblastoma (tumours of embryonic nerve cells), embryonal tumours of kidney (Wilms' tumours), etc.
2. Those predominantly in the young, e.g. some leukaemias, tumours of the bone, testis, etc.
3. Those with an increasing incidence with age, e.g. tumours of prostate, colon, bladder, skin, salivary gland, etc.

The incidence of human tumours is considered in more detail in Chapter 4. There are at least three possible explanations for this last group of age associated tumours which includes the most frequently occurring human tumours. (i) There is a continuous exposure throughout life to low levels of a cumulative carcinogen. (ii) With age there are humoral changes induced, i.e. in the cellular environment, by alterations in the immune or hormonal systems which allow or encourage neoplastic change to take place. (iii) There are age associated changes in some cells which increase their susceptibility to neoplastic transformation.

We still do not know which of these explanations is correct or whether more than one process is involved.

1.8 The natural history of cancer or tumour progression

A series of changes takes place after a tissue cell is 'initiated' but the rate at which this occurs depends on changes in the cell and on changes in the host. Most chemical and physical cancer inducing agents are very highly reactive and when they react with DNA in the affected cell they usually damage many other sites as well as the relatively few which are thought to control neoplastic transformation. Thus the same agent may produce tumours in a given organ which differ greatly from each other, depending on the specific genes which have been altered or lost. At one extreme, if only the 'transforming' sites have been altered, the resulting tumour cells will still retain much of the normal differentiated structure and function of the cell from which they have arisen. In the skin, for example, it will still resemble a skin cell (Fig. 1.3) and may still produce normal skin products and be responsive to normal growth controlling factors. If the genes responsible for normal structure are more severely damaged, the resulting tumour cells have fewer normal properties. At the other extreme, the cells may have lost almost all the normal properties of the cell from which they have arisen. The loss of normal characteristics is known as dedifferentiation or anaplasia. The pathologist can grade tumours by making an approximate assessment of the degree of structural dedifferentiation by examining sections of tumours under the microscope. As a rule, there is an approximate correlation between the tumour grade and growth rate. The most differentiated tumours (low grade, i.e. Grade I) tend to be more slow growing, and the most anaplastic (high Grade III or IV) the more rapidly growing. Unfortunately this relationship is not absolute but it does give a useful guide to tumour behaviour. Human breast cancers have been graded in this way and it has been shown that about 80 per cent of patients with well differentiated Grade I breast cancers will be alive and well at five years (and much longer), but only 20 per cent of patients with Grade IV tumours will survive for this time. It is of course equally obvious from these figures that although 80 per cent of patients with Grade I cancers survive, 20 per cent with the same structural type of tumour do not; hence tumour

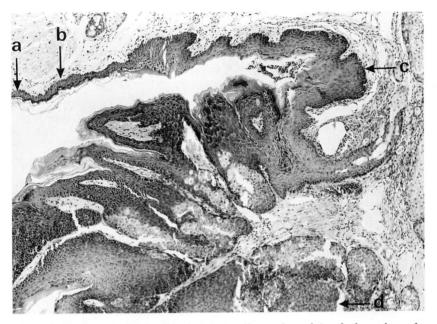

Fig. 1.3 Section (stained with haemotoxylin and eosin) of the edge of a squamous carcinoma of skin, with normal skin (a) on the left and increasing dysplasia (b) and (c) leading into the main mass of the tumour (d) below. (×50)

growth is influenced by factors other than tumour structure, particularly the reaction by the patient's own defence mechanisms. Unfortunately we have few ideas about the nature of these mechanisms. In hormone responsive tissues such as the breast, the tumour cells may still retain some of the normal responsiveness to hormones (see Chapters 12 and 14). The pathologist's assessment of tumour grade is based only on alterations in structure and these are not invariably related to changes in function. Some cells may have lost their specific structural characters but still retain differentiated biochemical characters, and others may still appear structurally differentiated but have lost many normal function attributes.

Another practical problem in the assessment of tumours is that tumours are not homogeneous (see Chapter 2 for fuller discussion) and some may contain areas with more than one tumour grade (Figs 1.3 and 1.4). Note that in the tumour shown in Figures 1.3 and 1.4, there is a progression from benign to malignant resembling that illustrated in Figure 1.2, but the progression is in space rather than necessarily in time. It used to be thought that tumours arose from a single altered cell, i.e. were clonal in origin, but there is now some evidence to suggest that this

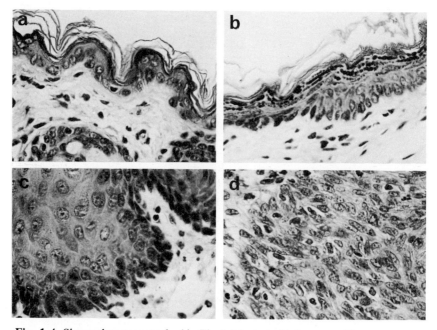

Fig. 1.4 Shows the areas marked in Fig. 1.3 but at a higher magnification.

(a) normal skin (compare with Fig. 1.1) showing mesenchyme below, covered by normal epithelium with basal cells and more differentiated superficial cells, covered by layers of keratin formed from the superficial cells. (× 360)

(b) an area of dysplastic skin. There is an increase of the basal cells, which are more irregular than the normal and there is a disturbance in the formation of keratin which is clumped into an irregular dark mass in the surface layer instead of the normal flattened sheets seen in Fig. 1.4(a), i.e. differentiation is disturbed. (× 360)

(c) in this area there is much overgrowth of cells. The cells themselves are abnormal; they vary in shape and size, the nuclei are much larger than normal and some are more deeply stained. The usually distinct separation between epithelium and stroma is not seen, suggesting that invasion may be taking place. The cells are still recognizable as skin cells. This would be diagnosed as a moderately well differentiated squamous carcinoma. (× 360)

(d) This area from the centre of tumour is made up of a mass of irregular spindle shaped cells with no recognizable skin features. This would be diagnosed as an anaplastic (undifferentiated) carcinoma. (× 360)

may not be invariably true. But even if it were true, there is no doubt that by the time a tumour is detectable clinically, whether it has arisen from one or many cells, it has been present for a long time and the cells have had to go through a large number of cell divisions so that variation and selection of different cell populations have occurred. A tumour about 0.5 cm in diameter, which is just detectable, may contain over 500 million cells. The developed tumour usually consists of a mixed population of cells, which may differ in structure, function, growth potential, resistance to drugs or X-rays, and ability to invade and metastasize. Many of these characters may not be stable and may be influenced by the host response or by treatment. An obvious example is the destruction of X-ray sensitive cells by X-ray treatment. If the tumour also contains X-ray resistant cells, the cancer cells which are left after treatment will be X-ray resistant. Any individual character may vary independently.

Tumour progression is the development by a tumour of changes in one or more characters in its constituent cells. Although progression is usually towards greater malignancy, this is not invariably so. There are a number of cases—unfortunately small—in which rapidly growing tumours have ceased to grow or even disappeared completely. Although we do not yet have any explanation for this, it does show that there are natural mechanisms still to be discovered which will eventually allow us to control tumour growth.

1.9 The diagnosis of tumours

There are no absolute methods for diagnosing and assessing the degree of malignancy of tumours. Although many laboratories are trying to establish methods for doing this, none are entirely satisfactory. Microscopic examination of tissue is still the most reliable method for routine use. The function of the pathologist is to decide whether the structure of the cells in the tissue is sufficiently removed from the normal to allow a diagnosis of neoplasia to be made and, if so, whether the tumour is likely to be benign or malignant, its probable cell of origin, its degree of malignancy and its extent of spread. For practical purposes the two techniques used are tumour grading and tumour staging. Tumour grading attempts to measure the degree of dedifferentiation in tumours and is based on histological and cytological criteria (Figs 1.3 and 1.4). Histological differentiation is concerned with alterations in the structure of the tissue, i.e. the relationship of cells to each other and to their underlying stroma. Cytological grading is based on the application of similar criteria to the structure of the specific tumour cells. Tumour staging assesses the extent of spread of tumours (see on). Many investigators in the laboratory and the clinic have tried to find absolute markers of malignancy but, as I have already indicated, carcinogenesis is a multistage process. We should like to have markers for each stage of the process but, unfortunately, apart from histology which as we have seen is not entirely satisfactory, we do not have such markers. This is a major deficiency in studying cancer. Many workers are now trying to identify tumour specific or tumour associated proteins, either by direct measurement or by developing specific antibodies to these proteins. This seems to be a promising approach not only in diagnosis (see Chapters 3 and 15), but also as a method for carrying drugs or other agents which destroy cancer cells to their specific targets (see Chapter 18).

For the moment the most commonly used method of diagnosis depends on histology.

Many millions of words have been written on tumour diagnosis and the World Health Organization has so far published 21 volumes on the structure and classification of tumours by an international panel of tumour pathologists. The following brief survey will only give a guide. I have chosen some of the examples, not because they are common, but because they illustrate some points more clearly than the more common tumours.

1.9.1 *Benign tumours*

Benign tumours usually resemble their tissue of origin but every tissue component need not be involved, and the cells may or may not be in their normal relationship. Benign tumours arise in most tissues, increase in size, but do not invade. They are usually separated from the surrounding normal tissue by a capsule of connective tissue. Cytologically the specific tumour cells do not differ substantially from the structure of the normal organ cells. Benign tumours of bone or cartilage may produce nodules of bone or cartilage indistinguishable from normal tissues. In epithelial tissues, groups of cells may also form local benign tumours made up of all tissue components. The covering or lining tissues of skin, intestinal tract, bladder, etc. may produce wart–like outgrowths containing all the tissue components, but closely packed to form a solid nodule. The common wart is a local outgrowth of all skin components. In other situations only one constituent cell may give rise to a benign tumour. The pituitary, for example, is a small gland at the base of the brain which produces many different hormones, each produced by a different type of cell, arranged in solid cords. Benign tumours of one cell type may develop and these tumours may then produce an excess of the particular hormone normally produced by that cell. Other benign tumours of the pituitary may contain more than one cell type, or produce more than one hormone, and some may be derived from non-hormone producing cells. The cells in all these tumours are arranged in solid cords as in the normal gland. The benign tumours do not invade the surrounding tissue but, if they increase in size, they may press on and damage the remaining normal cells or overlying nervous tissue or press on the optic nerves which pass nearby and lead to increasing blindness. So that although the tumours themselves are benign they may cause serious disturbances by local pressure, or they may continue to produce excessive amounts of their normal product, which may in itself cause severe symptoms. Benign tumours of any other hormone producing gland such as the thyroid, adrenal, etc. may have similar effects. Alternatively benign tumours may damage the remaining normal cells and cause a loss of normal function.

Benign epithelial tumours arise in many other organs. There is a different pattern of tumour growth in organs with a tubular structure. Both the kidney and breast, for example, are made up of tubular structures with the epithelial tubules lined by several different epithelial cell types and surrounded by connective tissue. Benign tumours in these organs are made up of tubules usually with one, or less commonly two, different epithelial cell types, together with a variable amount of connective tissue.

1.9.2 *Malignant tumours*

Malignant tumours show two characteristic features—cellular abnormalities (sometimes slight) and invasion of surrounding tissues. When both are present diagnosis is easy. The standard cellular criteria are a local increase in cell number, loss of the normal regular arrangement of cells, variation in cell shape and size, increase in nuclear size and density of staining (both of which reflect an increase in total DNA), an increase in mitotic activity (increased cell division) and the presence of abnormal mitoses and chromosomes (see Chapter 11). The diagnosis of carcinomas *in situ* depends on the recognition of these cellular changes in an area of epithelium, usually on a surface, the cervix of the uterus or skin, but it may occur in the bladder or other organs. The changes only involve the epithelium and there is no invasion of underlying tissues, i.e. the neoplastic cells remain where they began—*in situ*. The only definite evidence of malignancy is invasion of underlying tissues. In most cases this is easily recognized as the tumour cells destroy and replace the normal tissues. Sometimes tumour cells may be found invading blood or lymphatic vessels. The tumour cells may then be carried to other parts of the body in blood or lymph and develop into secondary tumours (metastases) in these distant sites. This type of spread is characteristic of malignant tumours and is the major problem in treatment since a tumour that remains localized to its site of origin can usually be removed surgically or destroyed by radiation. The problem of metastasis is discussed in Chapter 2. Malignant tumours have no well-defined capsule and the tumour cells grow in a much more disorganized form than is found in benign tumours. The same criteria apply to all malignant tumours, whatever their tissue of origin.

1.10 The names of tumours (nomenclature) and the need for tissue diagnosis

Although the precise naming of tumours may seem to be an academic exercise, it is of great practical importance in deciding on treatment of each individual patient (see Chapters 16 and 17). Obviously it is important for each pathologist and surgeon to use the same name for the same type of tumour. Even after many years of effort by international organizations, there is still some confusion about names although fortunately more or less agreed versions are now coming into general use. But an even more important point is that a knowledge of the type of tumour cell and the extent of spread are essential in planning treatment. Some tumours are known to be sensitive to drugs, hormones or X-rays but others are resistant. Knowing the extent of spread will help to define the area for treatment by radiation or surgery or even whether surgery is possible. For these reasons, the surgeon will usually remove a piece, or the whole tumour if it is readily accessible, for examination by a pathologist. The tissue removed (a biopsy) is preserved by a chemical fixative and thin sections are prepared for examination under an optical or electron microscope.

Although the names given to tumours seem to be confusing, there is a simple logical basis to tumour nomenclature. The terms tumour, growth or neoplasm can be used to describe a malignant tumour. Tumours are described by a generic name which specifies the general tissue of origin, i.e. mesenchyme, epithelium or reticuloendothelial, and whether the tumour is benign or malignant. This generic name is qualified by the specific tissue of origin, e.g. kidney, breast, and this too may be qualified by further terms describing the cell of origin (if identifiable) and the pattern of growth. Some examples will make this clearer. A list is given in Table 1.1.

1.10.1 *Tumours of epithelium*

Benign tumours. Benign tumours of epithelium are usually described by their growth pattern and their tissue of origin. Benign tumours of skin may be papillary (a warty outgrowth or papilloma) or solid. A benign skin tumour derived from squamous epithelium could be described as a squamous cell papilloma of skin. Benign tumours of glandular tissues are called adenomas and may be solid or papillary, e.g. solid or papillary adenoma of thyroid.

Malignant tumours. The generic name for malignant tumours of epithelium is carcinoma, e.g. carcinoma of skin. The common skin car-

Table 1.1 Nomenclature of common tumours

Tissue	Basic cell type	Benign tumour	Malignant tumour
Skin	Squamous epithelium Basal cell Pigment cell	Papilloma Melanoma (naevus)	Squamous carcinoma Basal cell carcinoma[1] Malignant melanoma
Alimentary tract Lips, mouth, tongue, oesophagus	Squamous epithelium	Papilloma	Squamous carcinoma
Stomach Small bowel (rare) Large bowel	Columnar epithelium	Papillary adenoma	Carcinoma
Nasopharynx, larynx, lungs[2]	Bronchial (respiratory) epithelium	Adenoma (rare)	Carcinoma
Urinary system Bladder	Urothelium (transitional epithelium)	Papilloma	Carcinoma
Solid epithelial organs Liver, kidney, prostate, thyroid, pancreas, pituitary, etc.	Specific epithelium	Adenoma	Carcinoma

Table 1.1 —*continued*

Tissue	Basic cell type	Benign tumour	Malignant tumour
Gonads			
Ovary	Surface epithelium	Serous cystadenoma Mucinous cystadenoma	Serous cystadenocarcinoma Mucinous cystadeno- carcinoma
	Germ cells	Teratoma	Teratocarcinoma Choriocarcinoma
Testis	Germ cells	Teratoma	Seminoma Embryonal carcinoma Choriocarcinoma Malignant teratoma (rare)
Mesenchyme			
Fibrous tissue	Fibrocytes	Fibroma	Fibrosarcoma
Fat	Adipocytes	Lipoma	Liposarcoma
Bone	Osteocytes	Osteoma	Osteosarcoma
Cartilage	Chrondrocytes	Chrondroma	Chrondrosarcoma
Smooth muscle[3]	Smooth muscle cells	Leiomyoma	Leiomyosarcoma
Striated muscle[4]	Muscle cells	Rhabdomyoma	Rhabdomyosarcoma
Blood vessels	Endothelium	Haemangioma	Haemangiosarcoma
Lymph vessels	Endothelium	Lymphangioma	Lymphangiosarcoma
Nervous system			
Nerve cells[5]			Neuroblastoma[5] Retinoblastoma
Supporting cells	Astrocytes Oligodendrocytes		Astrocytoma[6] Oligodendrocytoma[6]

Tissue of origin	Cell type	Benign tumour	Malignant tumour
Covering cells (Central nervous system)	Meningeal cells	Meningioma	
Covering cells (Peripheral nervous system)	Perineurium } Endoneurium }	Neurofibroma	Neurofibrosarcoma
Reticuloendothelial system White blood cells	Myeloid cells Monocytes Granulocytes		Myeloid leukaemia Monocytic leukaemia Granulocytic leukaemia
	Lymphocytes		Lymphatic leukaemia
Red blood cells	Erythrocytes		Erythroleukaemia
Lymph nodes	Lymphocytes	Lymphoma	Lymphosarcoma
	Fixed reticuloendothelial cells		Reticulum cell sarcoma Hodgkin's disease
Embryonic type tissues	Mixed tissues	Teratoma	Teratocarcinoma

[1] Invades locally; does not metastasize.
[2] Lung tumours usually arise from lining epithelium of bronchi.
[3] Muscle of intestine, bladder, blood vessels, etc.
[4] Muscles under voluntary control, e.g. limb muscles; tumours very rare.
[5] Nerve cell tumours in the very young only.
[6] No absolute distinction between benign and malignant tumours possible; do not metastasize.

cinomas may arise from the differentiated squamous cells or from the less differentiated basal cells, so that skin carcinomas may be described as squamous cell carcinomas, or basal cell carcinomas. They may grow as flat plaques (sessile) or as warty outgrowths (papillary). So that a tumour may for example be described as a papillary squamous cell carcinoma of skin. Its grade and the extent of invasion may also be given. The final pathologist's report may read 'moderately well differentiated (Grade II) squamous carcinoma of skin. The structure is mainly papillary but there is invasion of the underlying connective tissue; muscle is not involved'. This report tells the oncologist that the tumour is made up of squamous cells which are known to be sensitive to X-irradiation and that the extent of spread is limited, i.e. that it could easily be removed by local surgery. The final decision on treatment would then depend on the exact position of the tumour and whether surgery or irradiation would be easier or leave less scarring, etc.

Malignant tumours of glandular tissues are also carcinomas but are sometimes described as adenocarcinomas, e.g. adenocarcinoma of breast, implying that the tumour has a glandular structure. As with the skin tumours, the cell type can be described (e.g. columnar cell or cuboidal) and if the cell of origin is known, this too can be added (e.g. ductal cuboidal cell adenocarcinoma of breast). The gross pattern of growth (sessile or papillary), and extent of spread can also be defined. Adenocarcinomas have a wider range of cellular patterns than tumours of covering epithelium. The cells may be arranged as large or small tubules or solid cords (trabeculae) or masses and this pattern will also be described. In some cases the tumour grade can be assessed.

Most tumours still retain some of the structural features of the cells from which they have arisen and, as we have seen, this allows the pathologist to make a rough assessment of the degree of malignancy by the extent to which the tumours have departed from the normal (grading); it also may allow the source of a secondary tumour to be established. But there are still problems. Some tumours may be so dedifferentiated that they no longer retain any structure which indicates the tissue of origin. In others some cells may develop in an abnormal way. A common event is that tumour cells from a glandular organ such as the breast, which are normally columnar in structure, may develop into squamous cells resembling those in skin tumours. This process is known as metaplasia and, although confusing to the pathologist, does not as a rule influence the degree of malignancy. A final point is that in many tumours the structure is not homogeneous and more than one cell type, growth pattern, or grade of tumour may be present. All these features will be indicated in the pathologist's report.

1.10.2 *Tumours of mesenchyme*

Benign tumours. Benign tumours of mesenchyme are described by the cellular tissue from which they arise (see Table 1.1), although confusion may be induced if Latin or Greek roots are introduced. Benign tumours of fibrous tissue are fibromas, benign tumours of bone may be described as osteomas and benign tumours of blood vessels as angiomas, but as can be seen from the Table the principles are simple.

Malignant tumours. The generic name for malignant tumours of mesenchyme is sarcoma and, as with carcinomas, this is qualified by the cell of origin and growth patterns. Thus a malignant tumour of bone cells is called a bone sarcoma or osteosarcoma but this can be qualified to describe behaviour. A tumour made of cells forming bone could be described as an osteogenic sarcoma and one with bone destroying cells described as an osteolytic sarcoma. Tumours derived from blood vessels are angiosarcomas, and so on. The extent of spread of sarcomas can also be defined and in principle sarcomas may also be graded in the same way as carcinomas, depending on the degree of dedifferentiation, but in practice this is rarely done since most of the sarcomas are in fact very rapidly growing.

1.10.3 *Tumours of the reticuloendothelial system*

This is a very complicated field. Benign tumours of the reticulo-endothelial system do occur but, since tumours in this system vary considerably in their degree of malignancy and since the tumours may affect the whole system which is widely distributed throughout the body, it is difficult if not impossible to distinguish between a malignant tumour which has spread and a benign tumour which has originated in several different sites, i.e. has a multicentric origin.

The tumours are usually divided into two main groups: those arising from blood forming cells—leukaemias; and those arising from fixed cells of the reticuloendothelial system—lymphosarcomas or reticulum cell sarcomas. In the first group, the tumour cells develop from precursor cells in the bone marrow and pass into the blood stream in the same way as normal blood cells so that the blood is filled with abnormal cells. Any of the stem cells of the bone marrow may give rise to leukaemias which may show any degree of differentiation, so that there may be undifferentiated stem cell leukaemias, or leukaemias with cells which retain some differentiated characters of normal white blood cells—myeloid (granulocytic or monocytic), lymphoid, or very rarely from red blood cell (erythroid) precursors. Although the striking feature of the leukaemias is that most of the tumour cells are in the blood stream, the cells may also penetrate normal tissues and form metastatic deposits in almost any organ. The biology of the leukaemias is described in Chapter 3. The fixed cells of the reticuloendothelial system in lymph nodes, etc. may give rise to a whole range of tumours derived either from the lymphoid cells (lymphosarcomas), or from the fixed macrophage like cells (reticulum cell sarcomas). Hodgkin's disease and Burkitt's lymphoma fall into this ill-defined category.

1.10.4 *Tumours of the nervous system*

Benign and malignant tumours arise in the nervous system but, most remarkably, malignant tumours hardly ever spread outside the brain or spinal cord. Tumours of the nerve cells proper—neurons—only appear in the embryo or very shortly after birth. These are called neuroblastomas or, if they arise from the specialized nerve cell layer in the eye (the retina), retinoblastomas. Almost all other tumours in the brain and spinal cord arise from the supporting cells, e.g. astrocytes which give rise to astrocytomas, etc. or from the coverings of the brain (the meninges) which give rise to meningiomas. More details are given in Table 1.1. As with tumours of other sites, tumours of the nervous system can be graded by assessing the degree of differentiation.

1.10.5 *Tumours of mixed tissues*

Very rarely tumours which contain a whole range of different tissues may be found. These tumours, known as teratomas, are thought to arise from primitive cells of embryonic type and are usually found in the testis or ovary, but may occur elsewhere. They are sometimes benign but very often malignant change occurs in one component tissue.

1.11 Tumour staging and the spread of tumours—metastasis

Tumour metastasis is the major practical problem and the commonest cause of death in clinical cancer. Tumours invade the surrounding tissues and may grow out of the organ in which they arise and involve surrounding tissues (Fig. 1.2). During this local invasion, tumour cells may penetrate the lymphatics and be carried to the regional lymph nodes where they are arrested. Some are destroyed but others may grow and produce new tumours. If tumour cells get into blood vessels they may be carried to any organ in the body. Again many are destroyed but others grow into secondary tumours. There are many unexplained problems. Carcinomas often involve lymph nodes but sarcomas rarely do. Some tumours give rise to secondary deposits more frequently in particular organs than others. Metastasis in the lungs, liver and bone are common since these organs have many small blood vessels in which tumour cells in the blood become trapped, yet other organs like muscle and spleen, which also have many small blood vessels, are rarely the site of tumour deposits. Some of these problems are discussed in more detail in Chapter 2.

Tumour staging is used to give an assessment of the extent of spread of tumours. One of the more commonly used systems is that established by the International Union Against Cancer. This TNM system is based on an assessment of the primary tumour T, the regional lymph nodes N, and the presence or absence of metastases M. Each of these categories is qualified by a number which indicates the precise extent of involvement according to clearly defined criteria.

1.12 How tumours present—some effects of tumours on the body

Tumours can only be diagnosed if they produce some effects (see Chapter 16). Tumours of the skin or of organs which can be easily examined such as breast, often present as a lump. Many cells in tumours die and these dead cells release enzymes which damage the overlying tissues so that a non-healing ulcer may form. Blood vessels at the base of the ulcer are damaged so that bleeding occurs. In the bowel or the urinary system, blood may be present in the stools, or in the urine, so that bleeding is a common presenting symptom in these organs. Many of the effects produced by tumours are due to the position of the tumour which may press on or destroy surrounding tissues or affect nerves and cause pain. Tumours, in the bowel for example, may cause obstruction either because the tumour mass grows into the cavity of the bowel, or by growing into the wall and destroying the muscle which normally moves the contents down the intestine. Tumours of the brain may present with headache caused by increased pressure inside the skull; tumours involving the bile ducts leading from the liver may cause jaundice, and so on. The physical effects obviously depend on the exact site of the tumour. Some tumours, particularly those which arise from hormone producing organs, may cause hormonal effects either by continuing to produce an excess of the hormones which the normal organ produces or they may cause a hormone deficiency by damaging the remaining normal gland cells. Less commonly they may produce abnormal hormones or hormones may be produced in tumours of organs which do not normally produce these substances, e.g. some lung tumours may produce hormones normally produced by the pituitary gland. Anaemia due to bleeding from the tumour or due to some toxic effects on the bone marrow is a not uncommon presenting symptom. As well as these effects, many tumours may cause general wasting and loss of appetite (tumour cachexia) sometimes even though the primary tumour is still fairly small. The cause is unknown but it is thought to be due to some toxic product of the tumour.

But as well as these harmful effects, some tumours may stimulate the defence systems of the body so that they react against the tumours. Unfortunately we know very little about the way in which this occurs but it seems very likely that some of the unexplained differences in the growth and development of tumours in different individuals may be due in part to this host defence reaction. This is an important area in which research is still in its early stages, but promising results are beginning to appear. For many years it has been known that the body sometimes produces substances that destroy cancer cells. Two of the substances, tumour necrosis factor (TNF) derived from macrophages, and lympho-toxin (LT) derived from lymphocytes, have now been identified and their genes isolated. Using modern gene technology, it is possible to produce these substances in large enough quantities for clinical trials as a treatment.

1.13 How does cancer kill?

As we have seen, many cancers develop in older people and a substantial number of patients do not die as a consequence of the disease but of some unrelated condition such as heart disease, incidental infections or even as a result of an accident. Tumour related events may cause death directly or indirectly depending on the site of the tumour and the extent of spread. A common cause of death is due to involvement of vital organs, either by direct local invasion or from distant metastases, for example in the brain, lung, or liver. Rarely, death may be due to haemor-rhage but more often anaemia and unexplained wasting may lead to decreased resistance to infection so that terminal bronchopneumonia or infection of the urinary tract (pyelonephritis) is common. In many cases it is not possible to establish the immediate cause of death.

1.14 Experimental methods in cancer research

Much of our knowledge of the development and growth of tumours is derived from a close study of cancers in patients by clinicians and pathologists. This has allowed us to define many of the problems to which we should like to find answers and although the application of new techniques in cell and molecular biology to human tumours continues to provide us with valuable information, other methods have to be used to study changes which cannot be easily observed in man. These include, for example, observations on cell behaviour in the very early stages of carcinogenesis, the direct effects of carcinogens on the genome, the direct effects of drugs on tumours, and so on. Although cancer is a disorder of cells, it is influenced by changes in the environment in the host, so that for experimental analysis, we need methods which allow us to study the changes which occur in isolated cells as well as in the whole animal. We also need standardized methods for producing tumours and for some purposes we need to transplant tumours into a new host to study the effects of a different environment on growth and behaviour.

The induction of tumours by giving or applying carcinogenic agents to animals is an essential experimental tool not only for studying the process of carcinogenesis (see Chapters 7, 8, and 9) but also for screening drugs or chemicals before use in man or for industrial processes. For some purposes, one needs samples of the same tumour for testing. The usual way to do this is to transplant the tumour into another animal. In ordinary populations there are large differences between individuals so that transplanted tumours (or normal tissues) are recognized as foreign by the new host and destroyed by the immune system. To avoid this, scientists have developed many 'pure line' (inbred) strains of mice. To do this, mice have been selected and inbred for many generations so that each individual in the colony is genetically almost identical with any other (syngeneic). Tumours and normal tissues in these animals can be transplanted easily. A further refinement is that tumours can now be specially prepared and stored frozen in ampoules in liquid nitrogen at $-193°C$ until needed for retransplantation into mice. Inbred strains particularly prone to develop a particular type of cancer or with a particular sensitivity to carcinogens have also been developed, so that the genetic basis for some tumours can be studied.

For human tumours or tumours from species in which no inbred strains are available, transplants can be made into animals in which the immune system has been impaired by treatment or in which there is a congenital defect in the immune system. One group of mice which have a congenital defect of this type also shows loss of hair. These 'nude' mice are used to maintain transplants of human and other tumours. Tumour or normal tissue grafts between individuals of the same species are allografts, between genetically identical individuals (e.g. identical twins or inbred strains) are isografts, and between foreign species (e.g. human tumour in nude mice) are xenografts. Unfortunately, not all tumours can be transplanted for reasons so far unknown.

For direct observation of tumour and normal cells isolated from their normal environment, tissue culture techniques are used. These methods allow studies on the direct effects of agents on living cells and the separation of different cell types from a mixed cell population, as well as the characterization of cell products. The most commonly used technique is cell culture in which fragments of tissue, tumour or separated cells are put into sterile glass or plastic containers in a fluid nutrient medium and maintained at body temperature in an incubator, in an atmosphere of air and carbon dioxide (usually 5 per cent) similar to that *in vivo*. If the cultures are successful, cells grow out from the explants and fill the container. They can then be removed and transplanted to other containers or treated for storage in liquid nitrogen. These populations are mixed, but single cells can be isolated and large numbers of genetically identical daughter cells (a clone) can be grown up from it and used for a more detailed study. Many tumour cell lines have been established and stored although only a small population of tumours will give rise to cell lines which can be maintained indefinitely. So far normal cells can only be maintained for relatively short periods, but have been used to study the induction of neoplastic transformation under closely controlled conditions. Cell culture can also be used to study the effects of drugs and the effects of cells on each other (cell interactions). A modification of the technique allows pieces of tumour or normal tissue to be maintained in an organized form ('organ cultures'). This method is particularly useful for looking at the effects which involve more than one cell type, e.g. some hormone effects. Cell culture has proved to be an essential basic technique for the development of modern cell and molecular biology, as will be seen later.

Further reading

Cairns, J. (1975). The cancer problem. *Scientific American* **233**, 64–78.
—— (1978). *Cancer: science and society*. W H Freeman Co., San Francisco.
—— (1981). The origin of human cancers. *Nature* **289**, 353–7. (Highly individual but stimulating reviews.)
Foulds, L. (1969). *Neoplastic development 1*. Academic Press, London. (A classic discussion—but detailed.)
Pierce, G. B., Shikes, R., and Fink, L. (1978). *Cancer: A problem of developmental biology*. Prentice-Hall, Englewood Cliffs, New Jersey. (A review on cancer as a disorder of development.)

For detailed information on specific topics, consult the following specialized review series.

Cancer surveys. Oxford University Press. Published quarterly. Each issue deals with clinical, experimental and epidemiological aspects of a single topic.
Advances in cancer research. Academic Press. Published annually. A series of specialized reviews.

2

The spread of tumours

I. R. HART

2.1 Introduction

2.1.1 *Significance of tumour spread*

Metastasis is 'the transfer of disease from one organ or part to another not directly connected with it. It may be due to the transfer of pathogenic organisms or to the transfer of cells as in malignant tumours'. This transfer of cells is one of the fundamental problems of clinical oncology. Surgical removal, often combined with irradiation, frequently is successful in the treatment of primary tumours but widespread dissemination often defeats this mode of treatment. Cancer spread is responsible for a large proportion of cancer deaths and the relentless and seemingly intractable movement from primary site to distant organs is a major factor in people's fear of neoplastic disease.

2.1.2 *Pathogenesis of the process*

Tumour dissemination is a complex process where the eventual outcome depends on the result of a number of interactions between the tumour cells and host cells. There are five major steps involved in metastasis, though it should be realized that the process is a dynamic one which may pass from one step to another without interruption and a number of the steps will be operating concurrently. Following tumour development and growth there must be (i) invasion and infiltration of surrounding normal host tissue with penetration of small lymphatic or vascular channels; (ii) release of neoplastic cells, either as single cells or as small clumps, into the circulation; (iii) survival in the circulation; (iv) arrest in the capillary beds of distant organs; and (v) penetration of the lymphatic or blood vessel walls followed by growth of the disseminated tumour cells (Fig. 2.1). If all

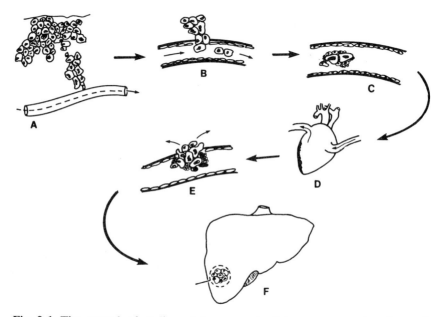

Fig. 2.1 The spread of malignant tumours. A. Primary tumour invades and spreads into adjacent normal tissue, eventually coming into contact with small blood vessels or lymphatics. B. These small vessels are penetrated by tumour cells which are released into the circulation. C. In the circulation a number of interactions occur between the released tumour cells and circulating host cells such as platelets, lymphocytes and monocytes. D. The passage of individual neoplastic cells or small emboli throughout the body is made possible by a number of junctions between the lymphatics and blood vessels; few tumour cells survive this passage. E. Those tumour cells that survive must arrest in distant organs, possibly in mixed clumps containing both neoplastic cells and platelets or lymphocytes, breach the integrity of the vessel wall and move out into the surrounding normal tissues. F. Growth of such extravasated tumour cells gives rise to secondary tumour deposits (here shown growing in the liver) and the process may be repeated.

these steps are completed, the result will be formation of a secondary tumour in a distant organ.

2.1.3 *Tumour progression/evolution*

As mentioned in Chapter 1, tumours do not come into being with all their characteristics already developed. This view of cancer as static populations of cells has been replaced by one in which they are seen as much more dynamic entities where there is gradual acquisition of new characters as the tumour develops. This process has been termed tumour progression and, while there are exceptions, the general trend is for tumours to go from bad to worse. Thus with tumour progression there is a movement towards a more aggressive behavioural pattern and the ability to invade and metastasize may not be manifested until relatively late in the course of neoplastic development. Some of the possible mechanisms involved in this process of evolution and progression will be discussed later in the Chapter but, for the present, it should be remembered that the fully malignant tumour cell, i.e. one that is able to invade and metastasize, may differ considerably in its character from a cell in the early stages of the transformation process.

2.2 Mechanisms of tumour invasion

Two of the five steps outlined in the pathogenesis of cancer spread depend on the ability of tumour cells to invade or infiltrate into areas of normal tissue. There is no evidence to show that the mechanisms used to gain access to the circulation are any different from the mechanisms used by the cells in moving out from the vessels in which they have become arrested so that both steps will be considered together here.

In general the mechanisms of tumour invasion are poorly understood though the three most likely possibilities are that it occurs as a result of: (i) mechanical pressure, (ii) release of lytic enzymes, and (iii) the increased motility of individual tumour cells. Obviously these mechanisms are not mutually exclusive and it is possible that in a given tumour any combination of the three may be involved and that the relative importance of each may vary depending both on the tumour type and its anatomical location.

The rapid proliferation of neoplastic cells may build up pressure which forces sheets, or fingers, of tumour cells along lines of least mechanical resistance in a manner somewhat analogous to the way that plants force their roots through the soil. Invasion, according to this hypothesis, is thus just a direct consequence of uncontrolled growth; pressure from the growing mass occludes (blocks) local blood vessels leading to local tissue death and a reduction in mechanical resistance which further aids the process.

While it is true that the gross appearance of many malignant tumours conforms with this picture with finger-like projections of tumour cells emanating from the main growth, it is also true that there are many observations that cannot be explained by this hypothesis. Some highly invasive tumours grow more slowly than their benign counterparts; histological examinations often reveal clumps of neoplastic cells which in serial sections reveal no connection with the main tumour, and cancer cells often invade and penetrate loose tissues where it would not seem to be possible to build up any pressure effect.

Areas of normal host tissue adjacent to areas of tumour invasion are often severely disrupted and show considerable amounts of lytic damage. Because many animal and human tumours have higher levels of proteases and collagenases than corresponding benign or normal tissue, the concept that malignant tumours produce and secrete lytic enzymes that degrade normal tissue has become firmly established in the literature. However, technical difficulties have made any correlation between malignant behaviour and increased proteolytic enzyme activity difficult to interpret. Direct sampling of tissue (biopsy) may damage tissue and this may give rise to elevated levels of enzyme activity. Furthermore, tumours are not composed solely of neoplastic cells but contain both stromal and infiltrating reticuloendothelial cells. Many of the infiltrating cells, such as polymorphonuclear leukocytes and monocytes, contain high levels of those enzymes most likely to be involved in tissue degradation; indeed their presence may well contribute to the eventual invasive behaviour of the tumour either by releasing their own lytic enzymes or by behaving as inadvertent 'guides' for infiltrating neoplastic cells. Since the number of these infiltrating cells varies from tumour to tumour, or even between different parts of the same tumour, their contribution to overall enzyme activity also varies considerably. Immunohistochemical staining for different collagenases and proteases has located many of these enzymes at the periphery of growing tumours, frequently at the sites of overt tissue damage and tumour cell invasion. However, the central portions of tumours often are necrotic and the peripheral staining observed may reflect the production of these enzymes by living cells rather than direct involvement in invasion. For these reasons, perhaps the most compelling evidence on the role of proteolytic enzymes in tumour invasion has come from experimental studies where it has proved possible to examine enzyme production by tumour cells grown in tissue culture and then to correlate this capacity with the subsequent invasive behaviour of the cells after transplantation into animals. Using this approach it was possible to establish positive correlations between invasion and high levels of the enzymes cathepsin B, type IV collagenase and plasminogen activator. These correlations are not universal in as much as different researchers have found conflicting results depending on the tumour types used. With data derived from naturally-occurring tumours in man, the circumstantial evidence linking proteolytic enzymes with a role in tumour invasion is strong but the exact nature of the enzymes involved is still not established.

Evidence for the role of tumour cell motility in invasion is also equivocal. The finding of individual tumour cells or small clumps of tumour cells separate from the main tumour mass is difficult to explain without invoking the concept of tumour cell motility. Cinematography has been used to show that tumour cells in the body, as in tissue culture, are capable of active movement and migration. To what extent this ability is used in tumour invasion is unknown but it seems highly likely that the neoplastic cells do move through normal tissues by active locomotion. If motility does play a role in invasion, the next step is to determine to what extent is such movement directional in nature. Tumour cells in tissue culture can move towards substances which attract them (chemotactic factors) and changes in the surfaces on which they move may also affect the direction of movement. It is tempting to speculate that such mechanisms operate *in vivo* but, because of the difficulties in assessing such responses in the whole animal, firm evidence is lacking.

It should be pointed out that tissues vary considerably in their ability to withstand tumour invasion. Tumours rarely penetrate the walls of arteries, arterioles or even the larger veins while they readily invade capillaries and lymphatics. Such resistance is in part due to greater mechanical strength of the larger vessels but there is also a suggestion that certain of the tissues resistant to invasion, such as cartilage or the elastic fibres surrounding the larger vessels, are resistant because they release anti-proteolytic factors that inhibit proteases. The presence of these factors in tissues with a natural resistance to invasion provides further support for the idea that proteolytic enzymes may play a role in mediating tumour spread.

2.3 Dissemination of tumour cells via lymphatics and/or blood vessels

Once tumour cells enter the lumen of lymphatic or blood vessels, they either remain at the site of penetration and grow there with a consequent occlusion of the vessel, or they release cells which are carried away in the lymph or blood. The release of individual cells or small emboli (clumps) has led to the suggestion that the cells of malignant tumours are less strongly attached to each other than are cells of benign tumours and are more readily detached from the primary mass.

It is a common clinical observation that carcinomas, which are epithelial in origin, generally spread in the lymphatic system as well as in the blood while the sarcomas of mesenchymal origin appear to spread via the haematogenous route. But this may be an arbitrary division. There are connections between the lymphatics and the blood vessels, and radio-labelled circulating tumour cells have been shown to be capable of moving between these two systems, either through direct veno-lymphatic communications (anastomoses) or from the lymphatics into the thoracic duct which empties into the jugular vein and the venous circulation. The preferential involvement of the lymph nodes with metastatic carcinoma may be a reflection of organ specific growth (see on) rather than a tendency to infiltrate specifically one system only. Alternatively it may be that there is a greater concentration of lymphatics in epithelial structures and a greater increase in the likelihood that these vessels rather than blood vessels will be penetrated.

In this chapter, the spread of tumours by either the lymphatic or the haematogenous route will be considered as a common process. From clinical observations and from experimental studies it is known that the mere presence of neoplastic cells in the circulation does not constitute metastasis. The process is inefficient and most of the cells released into the circulation die without forming a metastatic deposit. The death of many of the released cancer cells may be attributable to the controlling influence of the host's immune response (see on) but much may simply be the result of non-specific factors such as turbulence. The environment in the circulation is generally thought of as being hostile to disseminating tumour cells, but some of the interactions to which cells are exposed may aid their survival. Aggregation, either with other tumour cells or with host cells such as lymphocytes and platelets, may result in the formation of larger emboli which are more easily filtered out in distant capillary beds. Surrounding the tumour cells by aggregating blood cells may also provide a protective outer layer which prevents damage to the central tumour cells.

To leave the circulation, cells must be arrested and implant in the capillary bed of an organ. Generally tumour cells do not adhere to the walls of the large vessels where, presumably, blood flow is sufficiently vigorous to sweep away attaching cells. Even though tumour cells are deformable (not rigid) and can pass through capillaries of narrower bore than their resting diameter, it is in the capillary bed that the cells are generally arrested. This arrest may be due to passive filtering, as in the case of emboli rather than individual cells, or it may represent an active process. It can be shown that tumour cells, like platelets, do not adhere to intact endothelium but attach preferentially to exposed basement membrane. Tissue culture studies suggest that the tumour cells themselves might stimulate endothelial cell retraction and loss, though the shedding of endothelial cells from the wall is a normal physiological process and the basement membrane is frequently being exposed at various sites in the vascular system. Some proteins such as fibronectin and laminin are involved in the attachment of normal cells to each other and to basement membrane and may also play a part in determining both the specificity and the kinetics of tumour cell attachment. Such factors promote attachment of neoplastic cells *in vitro* and cell surface receptors for these proteins have been isolated from both tissue culture and spontaneously derived tumour cells. However, endothelial damage leads to platelet adherence, and tumour cell/platelet clumps may attach passively to the areas of endothelial retraction; arrest of the circulating neoplastic cell could then occur in the absence of any active ability or proclivity to attach to basement membrane.

2.4 Patterns of metastatic spread

Some tumours often metastasize to particular organs. Thus osteosarcomas normally give rise to pulmonary metastases whereas neuroblastomas most commonly spread to the liver; the reason for this organ selectivity is unknown but two hypotheses have been proposed. In the 'mechanistic theory' the eventual site of metastasis development is a consequence of the anatomical location of a primary tumour; the number of viable tumour cells delivered to the capillary bed in the first organ encountered is due to the pattern of blood flow. While this undoubtedly is true for some tumours it does not explain all patterns of tumour spread. Muscle is well vascularized and the kidney receives up to 25 per cent of cardiac blood output yet both these organs are infrequently involved in metastasis formation. Almost one hundred years ago Paget suggested the 'seed and soil' hypothesis, wherein the provision of a fertile environment (the soil) in which compatible tumour cells (the seed) could grow was the determining factor in deciding metastatic sites. Failure of an organ to develop metastases was not a consequence of the failure of disseminating cells to reach that site but was because of the inability of the organ to provide a favourable environment for growth. This hypothesis, perfectly suited to the Victorian era, with its biblical overtones of seeds falling on stony ground, has received strong support in recent years both from experimental results and clinical studies on the use of shunts to relieve extensive exudation of fluid in the peritoneal cavity (ascites) in terminally ill patients with abdominal cancers. Many of these patients produce considerable volumes of fluid in the abdomen leading to marked distress and discomfort; relief can be obtained by withdrawal of this fluid (paracentesis), but the procedure often needs to be repeated almost daily.

To provide such patients with relief from this unpleasant consequence of their tumours, it has proved possible to insert an artificial shunt from the abdomen into the jugular vein; fluid is thus continually returned to the venous circulation and the uncomfortable build up of ascites is avoided. Within the ascitic fluid are large numbers of viable tumour cells and returning them to the jugular veins means the first capillary bed encountered is that located in the lungs. In spite of this, many patients who survive with this treatment for a number of weeks or more show no evidence of pulmonary metastases, even though many millions of viable cells have been passed into their lungs where, according to the mechanistic theory of metastasis development, they should have been filtered out of the circulation. While these results are most compatible with the 'seed-soil' hypothesis, there is no information on the number of cells retained in the lung. It is also possible a third mechanism may be responsible for determining site specific metastasis. It has been suggested that there are specific interactions between cell surface proteins of tumour cells and organ specific proteins on the endothelial cells lining the capillaries or the exposed basement membrane in the capillary beds of different organs. Metastasis in this instance would not be the result of the increased delivery of tumour cells to the organ but the result of enhanced retention by selective adhesion.

2.5 The role of the immune system in modulating metastasis

The immune system reacts against foreign proteins either by direct attack by cells of the system or by the production of soluble antibodies against the proteins. The influence of the immune system on tumour growth is complicated and is discussed in detail in Chapter 15. As far as metastasis is concerned it must be noted that the process occurs in the presence of a mass of antigenic material, i.e. the primary tumour, so that this phenomenon might be thought to be highly susceptible to immune modulation. Results from experimental systems have confirmed this idea and shown that the immune system can exert a profound influence on the eventual outcome of the metastatic process. Interestingly, the immune system does not always exert an inhibitory effect on tumour spread but acts as a 'double-edged' sword. Thus lymphocyte aggregation with circulatory tumour cells can increase the size of emboli and assist in their arrest and lodgement. Furthermore, lymphocytes are capable of inducing angiogenesis (new growth of blood vessels to vascularize tissues) and may facilitate the provision of nutrients to a proliferating secondary tumour.

A subpopulation of lymphocytes, termed NK cells (see Chapter 15), has been implicated as being of great importance in regulating metastatic spread in experimental animals. Athymic nude mice have high levels of these cells and it has been suggested that the known infrequency of metastatic spread of allogeneic and xenogeneic tumours implanted into these mice might be attributable directly to the efficacy of the NK cell system. Suppression of NK cell activity by various techniques has led to enhanced metastasis of certain tumours though, to repeat a refrain that is becoming very familiar in this Chapter, there appear to be no simple generalizations that can be drawn from such experiments since in other experimental systems the effect of NK cell depletion on metastasis seems to be minimal.

Mononuclear phagocytes also appear to play a role in determining metastatic spread. Correlations have been established between the macrophage content of a series of tumours of similar histological origin and an inability to metastasize. Differences in absolute numbers of macrophages found in metastasizing or non-metastasizing tumours may be matched by differences in the functional capacity of such infiltrating cells. Thus there are reports that macrophages isolated from non-metastasizing or regressing tumours are cytotoxic whereas macrophages from progressing/metastasizing tumours are non-cytotoxic or may even stimulate tumour growth. Additionally circulating monocytes are cyto-toxic to various tumour cells *in vitro* and if these cells are capable of exerting such effects *in vivo* it is possible that these cells in conjunction with NK cells may make a significant contribution to the elimination of circulating tumour cells. Active research is going on in this area.

The exact role of humoral (antibody mediated) immunity in the modulation of metastasis is no more clear than that of the cell mediated arm. Once again it would seem evident that any tumour capable of evoking an humoral immune response would be more susceptible to such a response while circulating as individual cells or as small emboli. Antibodies directed against tumour antigens have been identified in many experimental tumour systems and against a few naturally-occurring human tumours. In cases of human melanoma there is a strong suggestion that the presence of circulating antibody correlates with the absence of metastasis. Antibody plus complement may lead to direct lysis of circulating cells or may facilitate removal of such cells by mononuclear phagocytes. Physical coating of the cells with antibody might interfere with certain of the steps in the metastatic sequence such as aggregation or adherence. Much more work remains to be done before any definite conclusions can be drawn.

2.6 Tumour cell heterogeneity

2.6.1 *Differences between primary and secondary tumours*

All cells in a single tumour are not identical but there is range of population of cells expressing many different characters (phenotypes). Cells in a tumour may show differences in structure, e.g. morphology, growth rate, karyotype (chromosome pattern) or behaviour, e.g. invasion and metastasis. This diversity is a consequence of tumour progression and some of the possible mechanisms involved in generating this diversity will be discussed below. The concept of heterogeneity is accepted by most pathologists, biologists and clinical oncologists. What is far more contentious is the idea, developed from experiments with transplantable rodent tumours, that metastases are derived from pre-existing subpopulations of cells in the primary tumour. Metastasis is an inefficient process and the majority of tumour cells released into the circulation do not give rise to secondary tumours. Do those few cells that survive do so fortuitously in a completely random manner, or is metastasis a selective process which allows the emergence of a pre-existent subpopulation of cells? Such cells presumably would possess certain characteristics that differ from those of the majority of cells. If only a few cells are capable of metastasizing then therapy should be targeted against those cells; the vast mass of cells in the tumour would not be life threatening. Again evidence for and against this concept comes from experimental studies because of the difficulties of analysing such characteristics in human tumours. Some workers have been able to show that cells derived from metastases are more metastatic than cells from the primary tumour whereas others, working with different tumour systems, have been unable to demonstrate this phenomenon. It seems highly likely that the process is a combination of both elements. Were metastasis entirely selective then it could be demonstrated in animal systems by the repeated selection of metastatic cells until 100 per cent efficiency was obtained; the injection of 100 metastatic cells should then lead to an eventual tumour burden of 100 metastatic nodules. This has never been achieved, even after selection; metastasis remains inefficient probably because metastasis is largely a random event where the destruction and elimination of circulating tumour cells is haphazard, regardless of whether cells are capable of forming metastatic tumours or not. There is, however, a selective aspect of the process, which is why metastatic variants can be isolated from heterogeneous populations of cells both by selection techniques and cloning procedures. This could help explain why there are many examples in the literature of differences between primary tumours and their metastases in terms of enzyme levels, karyotypes, drug sensitivity and cellular oncogenes. Alternatively, since tumours are known to be heterogeneous, it is possible that the selection for these differences is fortuitous and is not associated with the process of metastasis *per se.* Whether metastatic deposits in cancer patients are the result of the proliferation of selected subpopulations of cells would seem to be the most important question in the pathogenesis of cancer spread.

2.6.2 *Epigenetic and genetic mechanisms for generating phenotypic diversity*

Since tumours are so obviously heterogeneous for a wide variety of characteristics, what is the source of this diversity? Studies based on individual markers in leukaemias and lymphomas have shown that these cancers appear to be almost universally monoclonal in origin, i.e. descended from a single transformed cell; the situation in the solid tumours is less clear-cut and there is a certain amount of evidence to suggest that some carcinomas might be multicellular in origin. Even if such tumours are monoclonal in origin, by the time of presentation in the clinic there has been tumour progression and the generation of diversity. To explain this diversity Nowell suggested that the transition from normal to transformed cell carried with it the acquisition of inherent genetic instability. This genetic instability, he suggested, allowed trans-formed cells to mutate at a·higher rate than normal cells so that new variants were being produced continuously. Many of these variants would be eliminated by metabolic or immunological mechanisms but certain of these variants would possess selective growth advantages and these clones would grow to dominate the tumour populations. According to Nowell, sequential selection over time would lead to the emergence of sublines which would be increasingly abnormal both genetically and biologically. Genetic alterations occurring in progressing tumours could range from point mutations to gross aberrations such as loss or gain of complete chromosomes. These topics are discussed in more detail in Chapter 11. Certainly the malignant solid human cancers, which are able to metastasize, commonly show a degree of aneuploidy (variation in chromosome number) and mitotic variation. The hypothesis that neo-plastic cells have greater genetic instability and mutate at a faster rate than normal cells has been tested experimentally. The measurement of mutation rates at different sites (loci) in the cellular genetic material (genome) has shown that, in experimental tumours, transformed cells are more genetically unstable than their normal counterparts. A similar change appears to accompany the transition from low to high metastatic activity. This last observation may help explain how metastatic cells develop from the original tumour cell population but, as with many findings in cancer research, raises many new questions.

The mechanisms by which these alterations in gene activity may influence tumour growth and metastasis may include overexpression of normal gene products, gene amplification or mutation (aberration in gene structure and function). Alternatively epigenetic (non-genetic mechanisms altering gene expression) factors may be responsible for changes in metastatic behaviour. These mechanisms are discussed in detail elsewhere (Chapters 10 and 11) but active research in this field is opening up exciting possibilities not only in the general area of tumour growth but possibly in understanding the process of metastasis.

2.7 Experimental models/approaches to metastasis

It is apparent that relatively little is known about the exact mechanisms of tumour spread. In part this is a reflection of the complexity of the process and the fact that tumours of all types may not use identical mechanisms. In part it also reflects the difficulties involved in studying a dynamic process by essentially static observations. There is a wealth of data gathered on naturally-occurring tumours in man from histological, surgical and autopsy procedures. Many of the mechanisms likely to be involved have been inferred from these observations rather than by direct demonstration through experimental analysis. Biochemical studies on material from primary and secondary tumours obtained at the same time frequently is difficult because of problems in obtaining the material, so that considerable reliance has to be placed on the use of transplantable tumours in experimental animals to study the process of metastasis.

There are many advantages, and not a few disadvantages, associated with these animal models. The advantages arise from the ability to standardize procedures and the ease with which tumour cells growing as implants or as cell lines in tissue culture can be manipulated. The major disadvantage of the models is that the majority of the tumours represented are of mesenchymal origin, since these cells grow more readily in tissue culture whereas, as pointed out in Chapter 1, the vast majority of human solid cancers are epithelial in origin. Information derived from studies on mesenchymal cells may not be applicable directly to epithelial cells and there is a great need for the development of more realistic models of tumour spread (see Chapter 7). It may be that the use of epithelial lines of human tumour cells injected into athymic nude mice will provide such models. Notwithstanding these reservations about currently available transplantable tumour systems, it is true that a considerable amount of information has been derived from experimental studies and much of this has come because of the awareness of the cellular heterogeneity existing in tumours. While there has been some controversy over whether or not metastatic subpopulations of cells do pre-exist in the parental tumour, there is no doubt that general acceptance of this concept has led to the development of some powerful experimental tools. From a single parental tumour one can isolate sublines or variants which exhibit different metastatic capacities. When these differences are relatively stable, comparisons can be made between the variants to determine factors responsible for these phenotypic differences. Comparisons between metastatic and non-metastatic tumours of different origin, a situation somewhat akin to comparing apples and oranges, are thus avoided.

Many of the associations between malignant behaviour and the possession of specific properties described in this Chapter have been established using these analyses, and in the future it is certain that more associations will continue to be identified so that we may develop a more complete understanding of the pathogenesis of cancer spread. Until now modern molecular biology has played little part in unravelling this process but, given the availability of appropriate model systems, this is a situation that is likely to change dramatically over the next few years.

Further reading

Fidler, I. J., Gersten, D. M., and Hart, I. R. (1978). The biology of cancer invasion and metastasis. *Advances in Cancer Research* **28**, 149–205.

Liotta, L. A., and Hart, I. R. (eds.) (1982). *Tumour invasion and metastasis.* Martinus Nijhoff, The Hague.

Nowell, P. C. (1976). The clonal evolution of tumour cell populations. *Science* **194**, 23–8.

Prehn, R. T. (1976). Do tumors grow because of the immune response of the host? *Transplantation Reviews* **28**, 34–42.

Willis, R. A. (1972). *The spread of tumours in the human body.* Butterworth, London.

3

Biology of human leukaemia

MELVYN F. GREAVES

3.1 Cell lineages and differentiation of blood cells

3.1.1. *Cellular pedigrees*

Much of our current picture of the heterogeneity of leukaemias and lymphomas and the possible role played by particular molecular changes at the DNA level has been critically dependent upon our understanding of the normal cell lineage structure and differentiation programme of haemopoiesis. The different families of mature white and red cells are clearly demarcated by morphology and function but are descended by a succession of steps from the same population of multipotential stem cells in the bone marrow (and yolk sac or liver in embryogenesis) (Fig. 3.1).

It is important to appreciate that the blood forming tissues are arranged in lineage hierarchies with successive steps of amplification (in numbers) and genetic restriction (in differentiation options). The founder cells are considered to be stem cells by the criteria that they not only give

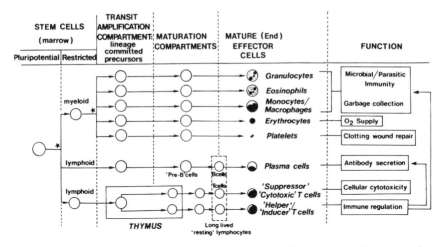

Fig. 3.1 Blood cell lineages and function. The asterisks indicate that our understanding of developmental potentialities and the sequence or pattern of commitment at these apparent 'junctions' in the lineage tree are still very incomplete.

rise to maturing progeny but can maintain their own numbers (i.e. 'self-renew') almost indefinitely. Stem cells are, however, heterogeneous in their capacity to self-renew and other, more mature cells, not normally considered as stem cells, may have very extensive self-renewal capabilities which can be revealed under certain circumstances. Mature, immunocompetent lymphocytes are particularly impressive in this respect since they may survive (as intermitotic cells) for 10 years or more and can be maintained for long periods *in vitro* provided the appropriate growth factor (Interleukin 2 or IL2) is present.

Our understanding of the control of haemopoiesis, though incomplete, is still considerably in advance of what we know of the developmental physiology of other tissues. As illustrated in Figure 3.2, interactions between stem cells, committed progenitors and stromal elements (fibroblasts, epithelial cells, macrophages, and perhaps extracellular matrices) appear crucial in blood cell maturation. Several polypeptide, hormone-like growth factors regulate the growth and differentiation of haemopoietic cells (e.g. Interleukin 1, 2, and 3, and granulocyte-macrophage colony stimulating factor or GM-CSF). These regulatory factors are frequently derived from activated T lymphocytes but may be released from a wide variety of tissues. A key, as yet unresolved, issue is whether these same proteins are mediating the control exercised by the stromal elements. It is widely anticipated that alterations in stromal interactions and/or in growth factor recognition and response will be critically

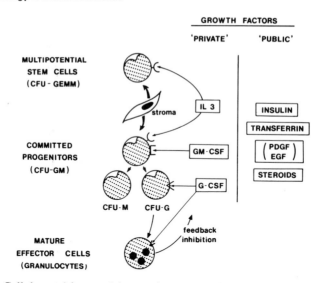

Fig. 3.2 Cellular and humoral interactions regulating growth and maturation in the haemopoietic system.

'Private' growth factors are those specific for, and acting directly upon, haemopoietic cells. 'Public' factors are circulating factors which regulate the growth of blood forming and other tissues. They may act directly upon blood forming cells or, as in the case of epidermal growth factor (EGF) and platelet derived growth factor (PDGF), influence haemopoiesis indirectly via effects on the stromal elements of blood forming tissue. CFU-GEMM, colony forming units of mixed cellularity (usually macrophage, erythroid, granulocyte and megakaryocyte); CFU-M, colony forming unit-monocyte/macrophage; CFU-G, colony forming unit composed of granulocytes only; IL 3, Interleukin 3; GM-CSF, granulocyte-macrophage colony stimulating factor; G-CSF, granulocyte colony stimulating factor.

involved in leukaemogenesis (see Chapter 12). Direct evidence for this is not available at present.

The precise role played by stromal cells and 'growth' factors in the differentiation process which restricts stem cell progeny to a single lineage is unknown although part of the process appears to involve random or stochastic events. This important question will only be answered when we have access to substantial numbers of essentially normal multipotential stem cells which can be maintained, cloned, and manipulated *in vitro*.

3.1.2 *Topographical compartmentalization of blood cell types*

A considerable amount of architectural organization exists in bone marrow, lymph nodes, thymus, and spleen and is probably important for cell differentiation, traffic, and function. Haemopoietic progenitor cells are found predominantly in the bone marrow with smaller numbers present in the blood and spleen, particularly during regeneration. A three-dimensional matrix and organizational heterogeneity also exists within the marrow consisting of bone, extracellular matrices, and blood cells.

A striking topographical compartmentalization exists for lymphoid cells. Thus T cells differentiate initially in the thymic cortex and are then released into the blood-lymphatic circulation with B lymphocytes derived from the bone marrow. Within lymph nodes and spleen fairly discrete areas consisting of predominantly T cells or B cells exist in association with other cells which are involved in immune responses, e.g. dendritic reticulum cells. Figure 3.3 shows a lymph node germinal centre which is a site for B cell proliferation, surrounded and infiltrated by T cells. As anticipated from this pattern of cell distribution, acute leukaemias originate from progenitor cells in the bone marrow whereas lymphomas originate predominantly from thymus or lymphoid tissue. The diversity of histopathology in lymphomas reflects in part the multiplicity of T and B cell subsets but also the topographical restriction, homing and traffic routes of particular cell types and the variable degree of architectural disruption in neoplasia.

3.1.3 *Markers of differentiation and proliferation*

Blood cell differentiation is characterized as in other tissues by morphological changes and functional activity. Biochemical markers of differentiation are required to identify earlier stages of maturation since immature cells are morphologically indistinguishable. Monoclonal antibodies, each of which recognizes only one specific antigen (see Chapter 15), have been especially useful in this respect. Lysosomal enzymes, enzymes involved in nucleotide metabolism (e.g. adenosine deaminase) and terminal deoxynucleotidyl transferase (TdT) have also been extensively used.

More recently, molecular markers have been developed which identify either unique, cell type specific products or genetic rearrangements at the immunoglobulin locus or the locus for T cell receptor characteristic of particular stages of differentiation in lymphocytes. The latter 'markers' are proving of special value in the analysis of lymphoid leukaemias and lymphomas (see on) since they not only identify lineage commitment prior to its *expression* at the protein and functional level but are *clonal* in nature and so can be operationally used as tumour specific markers. Figure 3.4 illustrates clonal rearrangements of immunoglobulin genes that can be identified in DNA from B cell leukaemias. Similar rearrangements occur in the α and β genes of the antigen receptor on T lymphocytes.

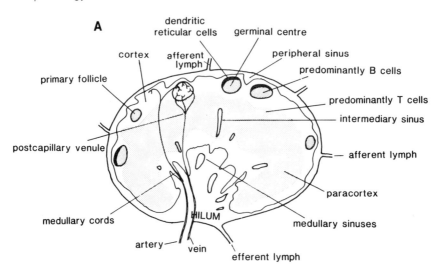

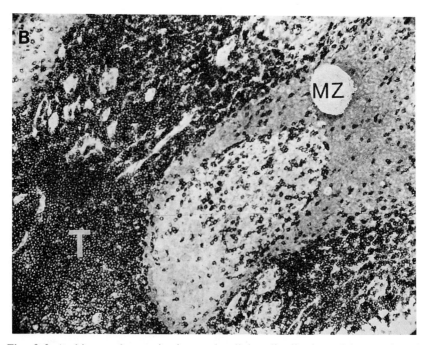

Fig. 3.3 Architectural organization and cellular distribution of human lymph nodes. (A) Topography of lymph node. (B) Immunoperoxidase staining of germinal centre area of lymph node with monoclonal anti-T cell antibody showing paracortical T cell area (T), pale germinal centre (B) and its mantle zone (MZ), both showing some degree of T cell infiltration.

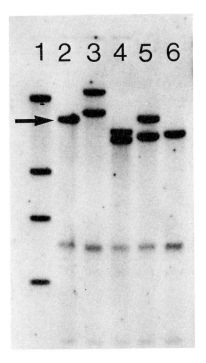

Fig. 3.4 Southern blot analysis of clonal Ig gene (μ) rearrangements. The restriction endonuclease BamHI has been used to digest DNA from human haemopoietic cells. The DNA was then electrophoresed, blotted onto nitrocellulose, and hybridized with a ^{32}P labelled Cμ probe. Track 1: Molecular weight markers. Track 2: Germline μ DNA (from a myeloid cell line). Tracks 3–6: DNA from different B lineage leukaemias showing various, *clonal* alterations, e.g. track 3, both alleles rearranged; track 4, both alleles rearranged; track 5, one allele rearranged, one allele remains germline; track 6, one allele deleted, one allele rearranged. Note that during normal B cell differentiation both heavy μ chain gene regions usually rearrange but only one produces a functional product (allelic exclusion).

These rearrangements occur within a limited region of individual chromosomes and constitute the normal mechanism of clonal diversification that accompanies lymphoid cell differentiation. Those same loci, and others, may be involved in rearrangements (especially translocations between different chromosomes—see Chapter 11) which are intimately linked to the *leukaemic transformation* process.

Multiple antigenic changes occur on the cell surface during haemopoiesis and lymphoid cell maturation. These have been extensively documented using monoclonal antibodies in conjunction with flow cytometry, tissue section staining and immunochemical procedures. As an example, Figure 3.5 represents an outline of the phenotypic changes associated with T cell maturation. Note that as maturation proceeds some 'markers' are lost and others gained. Some 'markers' are associated with discrete stages of differentiation, e.g. T6 and TdT in the thymic cortex, whereas others are associated with active proliferation, e.g. T9, the transferrin receptor in the subcapsular thymic cortex, and T4, the IL2 receptor on activated major T cells. An appreciation of the complexity and diversity of cellular phenotypes and their modulation by differentiation and proliferation provides an important framework for the analysis of leukaemic cells, and of course the same probes (antibodies, DNA, etc.) used to analyse normal differentiation and function can be readily applied to malignant cell populations.

Many of the cell surface antigens identified by monoclonal antibodies and used as cell type specific markers have now been analysed by biochemical and genetic techniques. Most are glycoproteins and in some

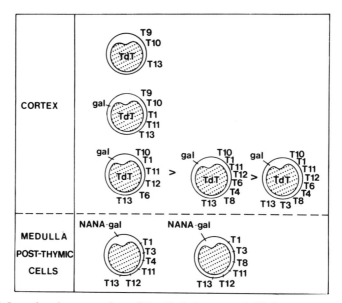

Fig. 3.5 Intrathymic maturation of T cells in humans. A likely sequence of early T cell differentiation stages which occur within the thymus as revealed by monoclonal antibody studies. The numbers (T1, 3 etc.) are an arbitrary code for T cell surface protein antigens. TdT, terminal deoxynucleotidyl transferase; Gal, terminal-D-galactosyl-1(1,3)N-acetyl-D galactosamine (recognized by peanut lectin, *Arachis hypogeae*); NANA-gal, terminal neuraminic acid galactose (therefore not recognized by peanut lectin); >, cell population more numerous than. Note: Thymic medulla cell types have a very similar antigenic phenotype to mature, circulating T cell subsets.

cases the antigenic component is carbohydrate associated with protein and/or lipid.

3.2 General features of haematological malignancy

Cancers of the blood-forming and lymphoreticular tissues can be broadly subdivided into the leukaemias, lymphomas, and myelomas. Within these major categories are subtypes identified by clinical, haematological, and histopathological features. Whilst there is broad agreement on the variety of leukaemic types, their classification and relationship to normal cells is obscure.

Leukaemias have been recognized for more than a century and are characterized, by definition, by an excess of white cells in the blood. Clinically, acute leukaemias will usually present with symptoms reflecting a disturbance of normal bone marrow function, e.g. anaemia, bruising, and infection. Myeloma will also present with manifestations of the side effects of the disease process, such as osteolytic lesions and impairment of kidney function by the immunoglobulins (myeloma proteins) secreted by the tumour cells.

Diagnosis is problematical in situations where the disease process is indolent or mild, e.g. persistent lymph node enlargement (lymphadenopathy), increase in number of blood lymphocytes (lymphocytosis), or myeloid dysplasia (bone marrow abnormalities). These conditions may be pre-leukaemic in nature, leading after months or years to overt malignancy. New karyotypic and molecular markers may provide a more precise means to evaluate the state of haemopoietic cells in such pre-malignant conditions (see on).

3.2.1 Incidence, geographic distribution, and aetiology

The blood cell malignancies represent around 5 per cent of all cancers in the Western World but are major cancers in certain age groups or geographic/ethnic settings. Thus acute leukaemia (mostly acute lymphoblastic leukaemia) is the major paediatric cancer in the West whilst Burkitt's lymphomas associated with Epstein Barr virus (EBV) are dominant tumours in tropical Africa. Intestinal lymphoma has been a common cancer in certain Mediterranean countries and in the Middle East but may now be declining, at least in certain areas (e.g. Israel). There are other marked differences in the incidence and geographic distribution of blood cell cancers (Table 3.1). Thus chronic lymphocytic leukaemia (CLL) and the follicular variety of lymphoma are relatively rare in orientals whilst an aggressive form of T cell lymphoma/leukaemia, adult T cell leukaemia or ATL, is common in individuals born in southern Japan, the Caribbean and West Africa. These latter

Table 3.1 Uneven geographic distributions of leukaemia/lymphoma

USA/Europe
Incidence rate *2–4*× that of Japan for chronic lymphocytic leukaemia (CLL),
non-Hodgkin lymphoma (NHL) (follicular), Hodgkin's disease, and myeloma
(except *extra-nodal* lymphoma and for ATL in Nagasaki/Kyushu region)
Japanese immigrants to USA
B-CLL remains low; NHL (follicular) increases
Southern Japan, Caribbean and West Africa
HTLV associated adult T cell leukaemia (ATL) high
Tropical Africa and southeast Asia
EBV associated Burkitt's lymphoma (malaria associated)
Mediterranean region
Intestinal immunoglobulin-producing (IgA$^+$) lymphomas common
Nigeria
Relatively high incidence of chronic lymphocytic leukaemia in young female
adults
Tropical Africa
Apparent low incidence of common ALL (cf. T-ALL and AML) in black
children[1]
Similar picture (until recently) in black children in the USA

[1] Could be due to preemptive death from infection obscuring true incidence rate.

leukaemias are associated with a C type retrovirus—HTLV (human T cell
lymphotropic virus type 1).

Burkitt's lymphoma and ATL are at present the only human
leukaemias or lymphomas whose aetiology is known to involve infectious

Table 3.2 Causes of human leukaemia?

Inherited, genetic defects e.g. Bloom's syndrome Fanconi's anaemia Congenital, genetic defects e.g. Down's syndrome[1]	rare
Environmental carcinogens irradiation chemicals (benzene?) viruses (EBV, HTLV) Spontaneous mutation[3]	+ host background influence[2]

[1] These children have a 20-fold increased rate of acute leukaemia.
[2] Genetic and immunological.
[3] Postulated for leukaemias such as childhood ALL that may have a constant low
incidence rate irrespective of environmental or genetic background.

viruses (see Chapter 9). Evidence for other environmental or genetic factors that may be 'candidate' aetiological agents or cofactors for these diseases is relatively sparse and the causative agents involved in most human leukaemias and lymphomas are unknown (Table 3.2). It is clear from the atomic bomb experience in Japan that irradiation can cause or initiate acute and chronic (granulocytic) leukaemia in humans (see also Chapter 8). From the study of both experimental and naturally occurring leukaemias and lymphomas in animals we might anticipate that chemical carcinogens, viruses, and irradiation may all have a role to play in the different varieties of human disease. Genetic factors appear to be of marginal significance but there are some instructive exceptions to this, e.g. the chromosome breakage disorders such as Bloom's syndrome and Fanconi's anaemia (see Chapter 5).

It is also possible that in certain leukaemias no environmental factor or inherited susceptibility may be involved. Some of our own recent work indicates that acute lymphoblastic leukaemia (ALL) in children may have a remarkably constant, low incidence rate (approx 3.0 per 10^5/year) irrespective of country or ethnic group; we suggested that *spontaneous mutation, in utero*, might therefore be responsible for initiating this type of leukaemia.

In studying the aetiology and biology of leukaemia it is important to bear in mind that, in common with most other cancers, these diseases are multifactorial and a succession of events, possibly involving different agents and cofactors, may well be necessary for the evolution of the malignant clone. Indeed, as discussed below, the multi-step nature of cancer is well illustrated by (i) Burkitt's lymphoma, (ii) the transition of myeloid dysplasia to frank acute myeloblastic leukaemia (AML), and (iii) the blast crisis (acute leukaemic phase) of chronic granulocytic leukaemia (CGL).

Finally, in the context of aetiology, it is important to emphasize the link between immunodeficiency, immunoregulatory disorders and lymphoma. This association has attracted increasing attention as a major problem in heart or kidney transplant recipients and in other individuals who may be immunologically compromised, e.g. patients with the acquired immunodeficiency disease syndrome (AIDS). Many of these patients develop lymphomas that are EBV associated. In these conditions, and possibly in lymphoma in general, as will be discussed in detail later, it is considered that defective immune regulation by T cells may allow B cells to proliferate extensively and acquire, by random genetic errors, molecular changes which precipitate rapid selection of malignant clones. Some of the likely genetic events underlying such patterns of cellular evolution can now be identified.

Table 3.3 Major features of leukaemic cell populations

Non-random chromosome changes
Uncoupling of maturation and proliferation (maturation 'arrest')
Conservation of normal differentiation linked phenotypes
Clonal dominance: Markers
    X chromosome linked glucose-6-phosphodehydrogenase polymorphism
      (G6PD.A, B alleles)
    Chromosome changes
    Gene rearrangements
      Immunoglobulin light and heavy chains (B lymphocytes)
      T cell receptor chains (T lymphocytes)
Clonal evolution

3.3 Common biological features of leukaemic cells

Table 3.3 lists the major features of leukaemic cells that have been well documented. These characteristics can be linked by a model of leukaemogenesis (Fig. 3.6). The key cell is the *clonogenic* leukaemic cell which emerges and assumes dominance by virtue of very rare (clonal) genetic events in the 'target cell' population (e.g. bone marrow progenitor cells). More than one genetic event may be involved and in some cases the genes involved may be already identified protooncogenes (e.g. c-*myc* in Burkitt's lymphoma, c-*abl* in CGL) (see Chapter 10). In most leukaemias and lymphomas these genetic alterations are brought about by translocations between different chromosomes (see Chapter 11). Significantly, *different* subtypes of leukaemia and lymphoma have distinct chromosomal rearrangements and therefore, we presume, different genes are involved.

In acute leukaemia, and probably in lymphoma also, the dominant cell population deviates only minimally from the normal and retains a relatively normal phenotype in relation to its developmental and proliferative status. This fidelity of phenotype provides the basis for new classification schemes and differential diagnosis. The crucial alteration in leukaemia appears to be one which alters the probability of maturation (and thus death) versus self-renewal in favour of the latter, such that immature cells which are normally transitory accumulate in apparent maturation arrest. This partial uncoupling of maturation and proliferation can be illustrated by maturation 'windows' (Fig. 3.6) whose width reflects the extent of residual maturation competence or the stringency of arrest (W^1; Fig. 3.6), and the compartments within which cells will accumulate (W^2; Fig. 3.6) and thus represent the dominant leukaemic cell population. The clonogenic cells may represent a small proportion of the total leukaemic

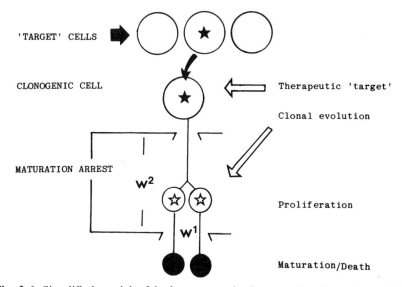

Fig. 3.6 Simplified model of leukaemogenesis. See test for discussion of this model.

population (usually 0.1–10 per cent), but are crucial since they are responsible for the maintenance of the disease and further clonal evolution associated with malignant progression. These cells therefore represent the major therapeutic targets. Note also that since differentiation arrest is seldom absolute the clonogenic leukaemic cell can have a *different* phenotype from the bulk of leukaemic tissue as clearly illustrated by chronic granulocytic leukaemia (see on).

In the light of these concepts, leukaemic cell heterogeneity observed between patients with dissimilar or similar leukaemias and in an individual patient at diagnosis or during relapse can be ascribed to (i) the target cell population initially involved, (ii) the stringency of maturation

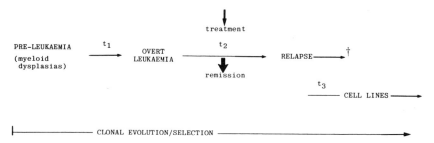

Fig. 3.7 Progression of leukaemia. t_1, t_2, t_3 variable time intervals. †=death.

Table 3.4 Major phenotypic characteristics of blast cells in acute leukaemia

	ALL		AML
	Type 1 pre-B (common ALL null ALL)	Type 2 pre-T (T-ALL)	
Cell surface antigens			
HLA, DR/SB	+	−	+ or −
T lineage (WT1/3A1)	−	+	−[1]
CALLA[2]	+ or −[3]	+ or −[4]	−
B lineage (B-4, PI153)	+	−	−
Myeloid lineage (MY9)	−	−	+
Enzymes[5]			
TdT	+	+	−[6]
Peroxidase	−	−	+
Focal acid phosphatase	−	+	−
Lysosomal hydrolase isoenzymes	+	−	−
Purine degradation enzymes			
5′NT	H	L	L
ADA	I	H	L
PNP	I	L	(V)
Gene rearrangement[7]			
Ig	+	−	−
T cell receptor β chain	−	+	−

[1] Some AML may express the WT1/gp40 antigen.
[2] See Chapter 15.
[3] Proportion positive is related to age of patients.
[4] Approximately 15 per cent positive.
[5] 5′NT = 5′ nucleotidase; ADA = adenosine deaminase; PNP = purine nucleoside phosphorylase. H = High levels; L = low levels; I = intermediate levels; V = variable levels.
[6] Approximately 5 per cent positive.
[7] Partial or aberrant rearrangements of immunoglobulin as T cell receptor B chain genes may also be found in the inappropriate lineage, e.g. immunoglobulin in T leukaemic cells.

arrest, and (iii) the expression of abnormal cellular features associated with progression. This diversity is not only clinically important but is a crucial feature to take into account when attempting to identify underlying molecular events. Over a period of several years a sequence of different genetic events may occur progressively to uncouple the leukaemic clone (Fig. 3.7). The developmental level of target cells is, however, of overriding importance as it probably governs and restricts both the range of potential aetiological agents and the phenotypic and clinical features of any emerging leukaemia.

3.4 Phenotypic analysis of leukaemic cells and implications for mechanisms of leukaemogenesis

3.4.1 *Phenotypic diversity*

Leukaemia and lymphoma cells can be characterized and classified in relation to normal cell types using enzymatic, immunological, and molecular markers. Simple morphological correlates are also still very useful, particularly for those countries or hospitals with minimal laboratory facilities, since they usually distinguish quite readily between most lymphoid leukaemias and the various subtypes of myeloid leukaemias, and may even identify subtypes of lymphoid leukaemias. The light microscopic appearance of stained smears of EBV associated Burkitt's lymphoma/leukaemia and HTLV-1 associated adult T cell leukaemia, for example, are quite distinct.

Table 3.4 illustrates in a simplified diagrammatic form the major phenotypic differences between acute myeloblastic leukaemia and acute lymphoblastic leukaemia in humans. The latter consists of two major subtypes corresponding to progenitors of the T and B lymphocyte lineages. Within a single cell lineage, diverse cellular phenotypes can dominate and be associated with quite distinct clinical entities as illustrated by the four types of T cell leukaemia/lymphoma analysed with monoclonal antibodies and flow cytometry in Figure 3.8.

No unequivocally leukaemia specific antigens have been identified to date despite frequent claims to the contrary and concerted attempts to find them. The most logical, though perhaps unpalatable, interpretation is that they do not exist. There may be two important exceptions to this. Immunoglobulin producing B cell tumours produce only a single cell surface immunoglobulin type which, though a normal gene product, is operationally leukaemia/lymphoma specific. The other potentially leukaemia specific determinant may be an antigen associated with a consistently mutated region of a protooncogene such as p21^{ras} (see Chapter 10). As yet, however, it is unclear how frequently this family of genes is involved in human leukaemia.

Another clinically relevant phenotypic variable is the proliferative activity of the leukaemic clone. This can be assessed by investigation of receptors associated with proliferation, such as the transferrin receptors or, in the case of mature T cells, receptors for IL2; an alternative and more usual procedure is to measure DNA synthesis or DNA content. The latter can be conveniently carried out at a single cell level by flow cytometry using fluorescent dyes, such as propidium iodide, which inter-

T-ALL

T-NHL

T-Sezary

T-CLL

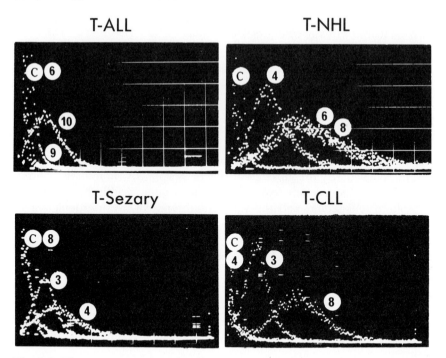

Fig. 3.8 Fluorescence activated cell sorter analysis of cell surface antigens in various subtypes of human T cell leukaemia. Vertical axis: relative cell number. Horizontal axis: relative fluorescence intensity. T-ALL, T (or thymic) acute lymphoblastic leukaemia; T-NHL, T non-Hodgkin lymphoma (in a child and therefore of thymic subtype); T-Sezary, a cutaneous neoplasm of adults; T-CLL, T-chronic lymphocytic leukaemia, a rare neoplasm of adults; C, control antibody. 3, 4, 6, 8, 9, 10 = various monoclonal antibodies (T-series) reactive against T cell surface determinants (compare with Fig. 3.5).

calate with DNA. From such analyses the proportion of cells in cycle can be estimated giving values which often differ between subtypes of a leukaemia and between leukaemic subpopulations from different sites of the same individual. In ALL and non-Hodgkin lymphoma those subtypes with the larger growth fraction, or more rapid proliferation, generally respond well initially to chemotherapy (since dividing cells are more sensitive), but also more readily relapse and so have a worse prognosis. The most likely explanation of this response pattern is that rapidly proliferating cancers spawn drug resistant mutants at a relatively fast rate.

On the basis of these phenotypic studies it is possible now to align different types of leukaemia with their nearest normal counterparts in haemopoietic differentiation. Such a scheme, simplified (especially with respect to the B cell lymphomas), is illustrated for those leukaemias and lymphomas involving lymphoid cells in Figure 3.9. A similar scheme

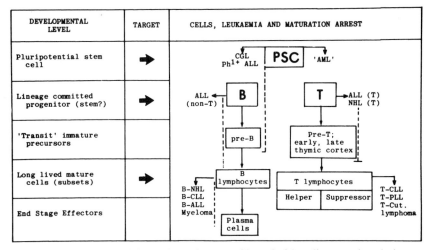

DEVELOPMENTAL LEVEL	TARGET	CELLS, LEUKAEMIA AND MATURATION ARREST
Pluripotential stem cell	➡	CGL, Ph^{1+} ALL **PSC** 'AML'
Lineage committed progenitor (stem?)	➡	ALL (non-T) **B** **T** ALL (T) NHL (T)
'Transit' immature precursors		pre-B Pre-T; early, late thymic cortex
Long lived mature cells (subsets)	➡	B-NHL, B lymphocytes, T lymphocytes, T-CLL
End Stage Effectors		B-CLL, B-ALL, Myeloma, Plasma cells, Helper, Suppressor, T-PLL, T-Cut. lymphoma

Fig. 3.9 Phenotypes of the major subtypes of lymphoid malignancy in relation to normal cells. ➡ Possible, initial 'target' cell (see text). - - - - variable extent of maturation competence (*in vivo*). T-cut. lymphoma = T cutaneous lymphoma. For other abbreviations see text.

could be drawn up for the myeloid lineages. Considerably more hetero-geneity in both normal and leukaemic cell populations exists than can be easily accommodated in such a figure. With respect to T-ALL, for example, cellular phenotypes corresponding to the different stages of intrathymic differentiation illustrated in Figure 3.5 can be readily identified.

Most subtypes of leukaemia and lymphoma are, as already mentioned, associated with specific or 'non-random' chromosome changes which are usually reciprocal translocations (see Chapter 11). The genes involved in most of these changes have not yet been identified, but we can assume that for each leukaemia with a consistent, reciprocal translocation at least two genetic regions are necessary and one or both of these must have an activity which is selectively associated with the growth, differentiation or function of the particular types predominantly involved in the disease. The clearest example of this possibility comes from Burkitt's lymphoma and other B cell malignancies in which a commonly expressed proto-oncogene, c-*myc*, becomes associated with a rearranged immuno-globulin gene locus and, by a process still incompletely understood, is altered in its transcriptional control (see Chapters 10 and 11).

3.4.2 *Identification of target cell populations for initial selection and subsequent progression in leukaemia: the lessons from CGL*

Phenotypic 'maps' as illustrated in Figure 3.9 provide reasonably accurate guides to the approximate levels of maturation arrest in leukaemia in relation to the normal blood cell lineages and maturation compartments. The developmental level of a particular leukaemia may suggest, but does not necessarily identify, the precise target cell population involved in the genetic events responsible for initiating the disease. This point is well illustrated by a consideration of chronic granulocytic leukaemia (CGL).

CGL occurs in association with a special chromosome marker—the Philadelphia (Ph¹) chromosome (see Chapter 11) and is an almost universally fatal disease. Its rate and pattern of malignant progression is extremely variable although a clear two-stage process is usually evident. A chronic phase, characterized by excessive numbers of immature granulocytes, gives rise to a second or acute phase called 'blast crisis', in which immature blast cells predominate. The latter have a diversity of phenotypes but approximately two thirds are myeloblastic and one third is lymphoblastic; rare blast crises involve erythroid cells or megakaryoblasts. Also, blast crises can be a mixture of different cell types or can switch from predominantly lymphoid to myeloid (or vice versa).

In 'lymphoblastic' blast crises, the blast cells are indistinguishable (except by karyotype) from common ALL cells and may synthesize immunoglobulin chains and have rearranged genes.

Chromosome studies indicate that the changes seen in blast crisis development reflect intra-clonal evolution. The explanation for these remarkable phenotypic shifts, which accompany malignant progression, lies in the original 'target cells', the selection of different clonogenic cells, and the altered stringency of maturation arrest (see Fig. 3.10 and Table 3.5). Chromosome and isoenzyme studies have demonstrated that CGL

Table 3.5 Multistep pathogenesis of CGL

Step	Event/marker	Cell	Consequence	Clinical outcome
1	?	Pluripotential stem cell	Clonal advantage and normal differentiation	Preleukaemia, myeloid dysplasia
2	Ph¹ $9q^{c-abl} \rightarrow 22q$	Multipotential stem cell	Clonal dominance+ (a) Normal differentiation (b) Excessive granulocyte production	CGL
3	Additional chromosome markers	Multipotential stem cell or lineage restricted progeny	Clonal dominance with minimal differentiation	CGL blast crisis

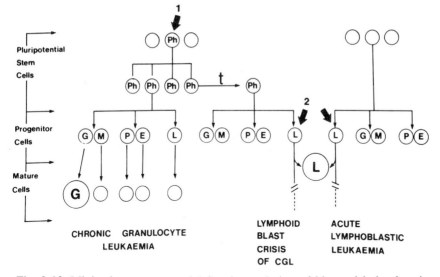

Fig. 3.10 Minimal, two step model for the evolution of blast crisis in chronic granulocytic leukaemia (compared with possible origin of acute lymphoblastic leukaemia). Ph, Philadelphia chromosome; G, M, P, E and L, precursors for granulocytes, monocytes, platelets, erythrocytes, and lymphocytes respectively; t, variable time.

originates in pluripotential stem cells. In the relatively benign, chronic stage of the disease the Ph[1] positive clone is dominant in the marrow and most, if not all, dividing progenitors of different lineages are Ph[1] positive. However, only in the granulocytic lineage is the total number of maturing progeny elevated. Differentiation itself is relatively normal although the majority of granulocytes may not be fully mature. Blast crisis can be interpreted as a second or sequential genetic alteration involving the selection of a single clonogenic cell in which proliferation is now effectively uncoupled from maturation. If this clonogenic cell is committed to the B cell lineage then blast crisis mimicking common or pre-B ALL results. Alternatively, if it is a granulocytic progenitor then myeloblastic blast crisis resembling AML results. Interestingly, some patients present clinically with Ph[1] positive acute leukaemia with no evident prior chronic phase, indicating either that the first selective event was bypassed or, more likely, that the two events occurred in relatively quick succession in a preclinical phase.

The subsequent clinical course of CGL blast crisis compared with ALL or AML is very revealing. 'Lymphoid' blast crises respond initially to therapeutic protocols appropriate for ALL, i.e. those incorporating prednisolone and vincristine; this probably reflects the steroid sensitivity of normal lymphoid progenitor cells in marrow. Remission, however, in contrast to that seen in ALL, is always short lived and relapse occurs soon thereafter with selection of new clonogenic cells from within the Ph[1] positive stem cell pool which are not steroid sensitive. Myeloid blast crises seldom remit and, with increasing chemotherapy, severe bone marrow damage, concurrent infection and death are likely. For these reasons, high dose chemotherapy (and irradiation) combined with stem cell replacement by marrow transplantation (see Chapters 17 and 18) is now generally considered the best therapeutic option for patients with CGL.

The dramatically different clinical course of Ph[1] negative ALL versus Ph[1] positive 'ALL'/CGL blast crisis provides a vivid example of the clinical importance of 'target' cell and clonogenic cell identity as well as illustrating the impact that maturation competence has on the biological phenotypes of leukaemic cells which dominate during different stages of a cancer.

Stem cell origins, patterns of shifting phenotypes, and imposition of maturation arrest analogous to those observed in CGL are probably common in solid tumours also. In the brain, the progression of relatively well differentiated astrocytoma to a more anaplastic glioblastoma mimics, in cellular phenotype or cytopathology, primary glioblastoma (i.e. highly malignant glioblastoma multiforme), but this progression has often been traditionally misinterpreted as reflecting dedifferentiation. The more likely interpretation is that, by analogy with CGL, some astrocytomas originate in normal glioblasts and that only after an additional (rare) genetic event(s) occurs which uncouples maturation from proliferation do glioblast phenotypes dominate.

There are some interesting lessons to be learnt from CGL. Apart from its clinical relevance, the biology of these leukaemias illustrates a diversity and varied evolutionary pattern which nevertheless strikingly parallels components of normal differentiation (Table 3.6).

The sequential involvement of different genes which can confer selective (clonal) advantage is likely to be a common feature not only of CGL but of most leukaemias and lymphomas. Thus in Burkitt's lymphoma, which represents the best studied 'model' at the molecular level, three distinct genetic events and other important associated factors can be identified. (i) Transformation (or immortalization) of B cells by EBV with defective T cell surveillance against EBV infected cells (as a consequence of immunodeficiency associated with malaria and malnutrition). (ii) Continuous, rapid proliferation of EBV 'transformed' B cells *in vivo* predisposing to other independent genetic events including chromosome breaks and reciprocal translocations. These may occur essentially at random and are independent of the EBV genome but

Table 3.6 Lessons from CGL

Cause of possible event 1 is unknown

Oncogenic events 1, 2, 3 are
  Spaced *variably* in time
  Can occur in different cell types (but within a single clone)
  Probably involve different protooncogenes

Step 1/2: Ph[1] involves c-*abl* plus a key gene (*bcR*) on chromosome 22q[1]

Phenotypic 'switches' reflect
  Stem cell origin
  Normal differentiation linked phenotypes
  Maturation arrest (not dedifferentiation or aberrant differentiation)

Stem cell origin makes cure by conventional eradication therapy unlikely, although
  bone marrow transplantation is a possible alternative

[1] See Chapters 10 and 11.

alterations which juxtapose c-*myc* with immunoglobulin heavy or light chain loci have a strong selective advantage for the growth of the transformed B cells in which they occur. (iii) Continued growth of the malignant clone *in vivo* (if the patient has not yet died) or *in vitro* (as established cell lines) may select for additional, genetic changes associated with further growth advantage and/or independence from exogenous growth factors. We have seen that, in a stem cell leukaemia such as CGL, successive independent genetic events can occur in distinct cell types (though intraclonally derived); in Burkitt's lymphoma and other mature lymphoid neoplasms it is more likely that the clonal progeny at approximately the same developmental level sustain the succession of molecular alterations.

3.4.3 *Age associated vulnerability of 'target' cells*

The association between malignancies of lymphoid progenitors (i.e. ALL) with childhood reciprocates with the predominant association of mature lymphoid malignancy (e.g. CLL, myeloma, most B-non-Hodgkin lymphoma) with adult life. This remarkable correlation of cancer type with age is relevant to the possible aetiology and/or pathogenic mechanisms involved. One plausible explanation for this age association invokes the concept of available 'target' cells 'at risk' of leukaemogenic events. Thus during early development, when there is considerable proliferative demand on lymphoid progenitors, these cells are relatively at risk compared with adult life where the turnover in pre-B and pre-T cells is likely to be extremely slow. Evidence for an age associated vulnerability of lymphoid progenitors to leukaemogenesis comes from observations on atomic bomb survivors. Acute lymphoblastic leukaemia was predominantly seen in individuals who were less than 15 years old at the time of exposure.

In contrast, throughout adult life, mature immunocompetent lymphoid cells are at risk due to their inherent proliferative potential and their long life span which increases opportunities for exposure to one or a succession of leukaemogenic events. In this context, breakdown of immunoregulation (primarily by T cells) could predispose towards lymphoproliferative disorders and eventual rare 'spontaneous' genetic events could endow additional clonal growth advantage, expressed clinically as lymphoma or leukaemia. Patients with inherited or acquired immunodeficiency diseases or individuals immunosuppressed for transplantation are especially at risk of such events and it is striking that mature B cell lymphomas are the usual neoplasms in both paediatric and adult patients that have malignancy associated with immunodeficiency. Burkitt's lymphomas in children are an apparent exception to the otherwise striking association between lymphoid progenitor malignancy and childhood, but can be readily explained on the basis of the presence of special co-factors (especially malaria) which are immunosuppressive for the childhood population at risk.

In these respects lymphoid neoplasms are in principle similar to other tumours which have marked age associations. Thus the typical tumours of childhood, e.g. neuroblastoma, connective tissue sarcoma, Ewing's sarcoma, Wilms' nephroblastoma, and rhabdomyosarcoma, originate in cells which proliferate in early development but rarely if at all in adult life, whereas the more common but exclusively adult epithelial carcinomas probably originate in tissue stem cells continually proliferating and exposed over decades to potential carcinogens. In contrast to lymphoid malignancies, CGL and AML do not appear to conform to this pattern. This difference could reflect the proliferative demand on multipotential and myeloid restricted progenitors both in early development and throughout adult life.

3.4.4 *Reversibility of 'maturation arrest'*

Considerable interest has focused on the possible reversibility of maturation arrest in leukaemia. If the central defect(s) is (are), as postulated, basically regulatory in nature then it might be possible to induce terminal maturation and thus exhaust the leukaemic clone as a non-toxic alternative to chemotherapy. This idea has been championed by Sachs in particular, who has provided ample evidence for differentiation induction of rodent myeloid leukaemic cells *in vitro* and *in vivo*.

Human leukaemic cells and leukaemic cell lines can be induced by agents such as retinoic acid, vitamin D3, phorbol esters, and dimethyl-sulphoxide to undergo some further maturation. However, sensitivity to these inducers is extremely variable and the real clinical potential of this approach remains uncertain. This general strategy may well become more effective when we know more about the biochemical basis of the maturation–proliferation uncoupling process and the biological activity of protooncogene coded proteins.

3.5 Practical implications of leukaemic cell biology

Our understanding of the biology of both normal haemopoiesis and leukaemia in humans, though still incomplete, is in several respects considerably more advanced than our knowledge of normal epithelia and carcinomas which constitute the major human cancers. Although the relevance of leukaemia and lymphoma to the major clinical problem of metastasis (see Chapter 2) can be debated, it is important to consider to what extent a better grasp of cancer cell biology as exemplified by the leukaemias can be translated into real practical benefits for patient management.

Although still an issue of considerable debate, the benefits already derived from leukaemic cell biology are, in this author's view, consider-able (Table 3.7) especially in terms of standardized, differential diagnosis and the introduction of new forms of therapy (see Chapters 15 and 18).

Table 3.7 Clinical utility of monoclonal antibodies in leukaemia/lymphoma

Differential diagnosis
    Equivocal diagnoses improved
    Incorrect diagnoses reversed (AML/ALL)
    'Undifferentiated' leukaemias typed
    'Cryptic' erythroleukaemias revealed
    Diagnostic subgroups identified (ALL, CGL, blast crisis)
    Non-haemopoietic neoplasms distinguished (neuroblastoma, carcinomas)

Monitoring
    Extra-medullary relapse (central nervous system, testis)
    Thymic cells (T^+/TdT^+) in marrow

Therapy
    T cell removal from allogeneic marrow (*ex vivo*)
    Removal of leukaemic cells from autologous marrow (*ex vivo*)
    In vivo treatment?

Further reading

Catovsky, D. (ed.) (1981). The leukemic cell. In *Methods in hematology* Vol. 2. Churchill Livingstone, Edinburgh and New York.

Ciba Foundation Symposium 84. *Microenvironments in haemopoietic and lymphoid differentiation.* (1981). Pitman, London.

Farber, E. (1984). The multistep nature of cancer development. *Cancer Research* **44**, 4217–23.

Fialkow, P. J., Jacobson, R. J., and Panayannopoulou, T. (1977). Chronic myelocytic leukaemia: Clonal origin in a stem cell common to the granulocyte, erythrocyte, platelet and monocyte/macrophage. *American Journal of Medicine* **63**, 125–30.

Ford, A. M., Molgaard, H. V., Greaves, M. F., and Gould, H. J. (1983). Immuno-globulin gene organization and expression in haemopoietic stem cell leukaemia. *EMBO Journal* **2**, 997–1001.

Greaves, M. F. (1982). 'Target' cells, cellular phenotypes and lineage infidelity in human leukaemia. *Journal of Cellular Physiology* Suppl. 1, 113–26.

—— (1982). 'Target' cells, differentiation and clonal evolution in chronic granulocytic leukaemia: A 'model' for understanding the biology of malignancy. In *Chronic granulocytic leukaemia* (ed. M. T. Shaw) pp. 15–47. Praeger, New York.

——, Delia, D., Newman, R. A., and Vodinelich, L. (1982). Analysis of leukaemic cells with monoclonal antibodies. In *Monoclonal antibodies in clinical medicine* (eds. A. J. McMichael and J. W. Fabre) pp. 129–165. Academic Press, London.

—— and Janossy, G. (1978). Patterns of gene expression and the cellular origins of human leukaemias. *Biochimica et Biophysica Acta* **516**, 193–230.

Klein, G. (1982). The role of specific chromosomal translocations and trisomies in the origin of some murine and human tumours of lymphoid origin. *Cancer Surveys* **1**, 299–308.

Knapp, W. (ed.) (1981). *Leukemia markers.* Academic Press, London.

Louie, S. and Schwartz, R. S. (1978). Immunodeficiency and the pathogenesis of lymphoma and leukaemia. *Seminars in Hematology* **15**, 117–38.

Pierce, G. B., Shikes, R., and Fink, L. M. (1978). *Cancer. A problem in developmental biology.* Prentice Hall, New Jersey, USA.

Rowley, J. D. (1984). Consistent chromosome abnormalities in cancer. *Cancer Surveys* **3**, 360–570.

Yunis, J. J. (1983). The chromosomal basis of human neoplasia. *Science* **221**, 227–36.

4

Epidemiology of cancer

M. C. PIKE

4.1 Introduction

Cancer epidemiology is the study of the pattern of cancer in populations and is essentially statistical, i.e. its methods and conclusions are expressed in terms of probabilities, e.g. 'Japanese women have less than a quarter the breast cancer risk of US women', 'women who have a baby before age 20 have only half the chance of getting breast cancer of women without children', or 'men exposed to benzene have an increased risk of leukaemia'. Its fundamental aim is, of course, to identify preventable (i.e. avoidable) causes of cancer, but it also has a critical role to play in many other areas of cancer research, particularly in the evaluation of screening tests to detect cancer at an early (more curable) stage.

The most basic task of cancer epidemiology is simply to describe the occurrence of human cancer, noting differences, for example, between males and females, between persons of different ages, between different socio-economic classes, between persons in different occupations, between different time periods, between different areas of a country and between different countries. This descriptive epidemiology has been a most fruitful source of ideas as to the possible causes of various cancers. For example, the enormous rise of lung cancer in men, but not in women, between 1920 and 1945 in certain countries, including the UK, suggested that some recently introduced habit of men, but not women, must be responsible, and cigarette smoking was the prime candidate. More recently the finding of large differences in the occurrence of colon cancer between different countries has led to intense investigation of the possible role of various aspects of the normal diet (not contaminants, but fat or fibre content) as factors in the aetiology of this cancer.

4.2 Descriptive epidemiology

4.2.1 *Incidence rates*

To describe the differences in occurrence of a particular cancer between different groups in a meaningful way the most useful concept is that of an incidence rate—this is (for all practical purposes) the probability of an individual in the particular group (the reference group) being newly diagnosed as having the particular cancer within a year. In epidemiological studies these probabilities are usually expressed not as fractions or decimals but as 'per 100 000', so that, for example, an incidence rate expressed as '200 per 100 000' is the same as an incidence rate of 0.2 per cent or 0.002. The incidence rate, for example, of breast cancer in females in England and Wales (E and W) in 1978 was 85.2 per 100 000 (estimated by noting that there were 25 204 900 females in E and W on 1 July 1978 and that 21 486 new breast cancer cases were diagnosed in females in E and W in that year: 21 486/25 204 900=0.000852 or 85.2 per 100 000). We would estimate the equivalent figure for 1976–8 as 84.7 per 100 000 calculated by dividing the 64 085 new breast cancer cases in the three years by the appropriate population of females. Incidence rates are commonly affected by the sex distribution of the people in the reference group, and in this Chapter I shall always be referring to single sex reference groups, e.g. the incidence rate of lung cancer in UK females in 1972.

4.2.2 *Age specific incidence rates*

Incidence rates are almost invariably strongly affected by the age of the people in the reference group. For aetiologically meaningful comparisons, incidence rates must be worked out separately for groups of persons all of a similar age. The collection of such incidence rates over a span of age groups is referred to as an age specific incidence curve.

Table 4.1 and Figure 4.1 show the age specific incidence figures for cancer of the colon in females in E and W in the period 1976–8. These particular age specific incidence rates display the age incidence pattern

Table 4.1 Age specific incidence of cancer of the colon in females in England and Wales (1976–8)

Age	Rate per 100 000
0–4	0.00
5–9	0.02
10–14	0.12
15–19	0.47
20–24	0.66
25–29	0.96
30–34	1.76
35–39	4.54
40–44	8.38
45–49	13.41
50–54	23.61
55–59	39.21
60–64	54.89
65–69	81.08
70–74	113.04

of most of the important cancers, that is, a rapid increase in incidence with age: there is an enormous rise in incidence from early childhood to old age (a more than 100-fold increase between age 25 and age 70). It has been found most useful to plot both the incidence rate and age on logarithmic scales because the 'log-log' plot so obtained is often very close to a straight line (see Fig. 4.2).

This straight line pattern of the logarithm of incidence against the logarithm of age holds, as we have stated, for many cancers at different sites, and deviations from it have often provided important insights into the aetiology of particular cancers. Two of these are breast cancer and testicular cancer.

The age specific incidence curve for breast cancer in females in E and W in 1976–8 is shown in Figure 4.3: there is a roughly linear relationship of the logarithm of incidence with the logarithm of age until about age 50, but then the rate of increase of incidence with increasing age clearly slows down. This incidence curve therefore strongly suggests that something occurs around age 50 in women that acts as a brake on breast cancer occurrence—the obvious candidate is menopause or ceasing menstruation. This protective effect of menopause has now been definitely established (see on), and this observation continues to play a central role in research into the causes of breast cancer.

The age specific incidence curve for cancer of the testis in males in E and W in 1976–8 is shown in Figure 4.4: there is a peak in incidence

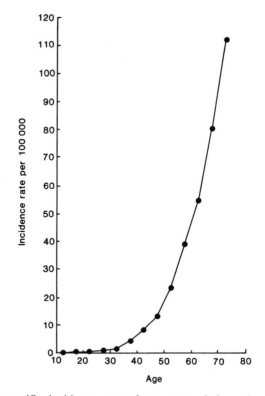

Fig. 4.1 Age specific incidence rates for cancer of the colon in females in England and Wales, 1976–8.

around age 30 and then a steady fall in incidence (in national statistics there is a second peak in incidence in old age but these old age tumours are mostly lymphomas not the germ cell tumours which comprise the overwhelming majority of the tumours in younger men). Such a pattern suggests that there is a limited group of susceptible men in the population and that they have almost all got the cancer by middle age. For this and other reasons it is reasonable to postulate that the 'susceptible men' are those that have been exposed to some 'carcinogenic agent' either during development in the uterus or in the first few years of life. Research into this hypothesis has only just begun.

If the incidence rates for a particular cancer are changing rapidly, then the log–log plot of incidence against age for a particular calendar period will not show the true relationship between incidence and age. If the incidence rates are increasing as they did for lung cancer when cigarette smoking became common then the incidence at old age will be low

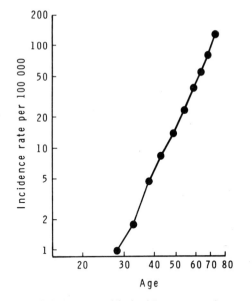

Fig. 4.2 Log-log plot of the age specific incidence rates for cancer of the colon in females in England and Wales, 1976–8.

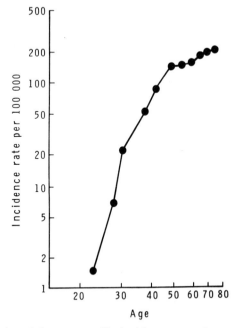

Fig. 4.3 Log-log plot of the age specific incidence rates for cancer of the breast in females in England and Wales, 1976–8.

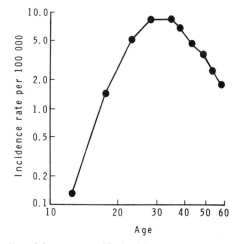

Fig. 4.4 Log-log plot of the age specific incidence rates for cancer of the testis in males in England and Wales, 1976–8.

relative to the incidence that the population now providing the incidence at young ages will display when they reach old age. The log-log plot will thus have too shallow a slope and may even reach a peak before old age and then decline. The opposite phenomenon will be observed if the incidence rates are decreasing. The correct interpretation of age specific incidence curves, therefore, also requires an understanding of their changes over calendar time.

4.2.3 *Age standardized incidence rates*

Comparisons of age specific incidence curves between different groups usually show that the pattern of change with age is very similar in the different groups, and only the level of incidence varies (Cook *et al.* 1969). For example, Figure 4.5 shows the age specific incidence of stomach cancer in men in Japan (Miyagi Prefecture) in 1973–7 and in the USA in 1969–71. For these situations, comparisons between the different groups can be made simply by giving a single number representing the level of incidence for each group. The single number chosen is usually taken either as the sum of the incidence rates at each single year of age between, for example, 0 and 64 (the cumulative incidence method) or some weighted average of the age specific incidence rates (the age standardized incidence method). The cumulative incidence method gives a number that is approximately the probability that a person gets the specific cancer between the summed over ages (if he does not die from any other cause), while the age standardized method gives the incidence in a standard group whose age structure is represented by the weights

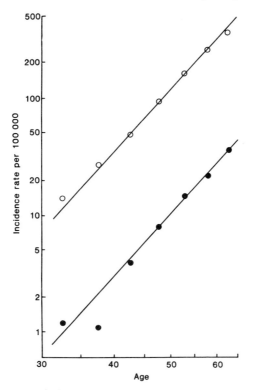

Fig. 4.5 Log-log plot of the age specific incidence rates for cancer of the stomach in males in Miyagi Prefecture, Japan, 1973–7, (○), and in the USA (Third National Cancer Survey), 1969–71, (●).

used in calculating the weighted average: the methods give essentially the same comparative information.

If the pattern of change of incidence with age is not similar in the groups being compared then single numbers cannot, of course, adequately represent the differences between the groups. Cumulative incidence rates or age standardized rates will still provide valuable information on the occurrence of cancer in the different groups; they will, however, need to be supplemented with a description of the age specific patterns in the different groups.

Comparisons of cumulative or age standardized incidence rates between different groups is one of the most commonly used and one of the most useful epidemiological methods. Inter-country comparisons of age standardized rates suggest that some 80–90 per cent of the current total cancer rate in the UK is caused by environmental and/or behavioural factors and is thus potentially preventable.

4.2.4 *Comparisons between populations*

Table 4.2 shows the cumulative incidence rates (ages 0–74) of breast cancer in different populations: the rates vary over a more than seven-fold range. Japan, China and black Africa have the lowest rates, while the highest rates are observed in North American whites.

Japanese and Chinese immigrants to the USA have breast cancer rates intermediate between those of Asia and the USA, and at young ages their rates more closely resemble those of the USA; their cumulative incidence of breast cancer is now little different from that of women in the UK (in this Chapter, figures for the South Thames Cancer Registry, which covers south London and south-east England, will be used to represent the UK). Breast cancer rates of African blacks are also greatly affected by migration to the USA. Blacks in Africa have rates less than one-fifth that of US whites, whereas US blacks have almost three-quarters that rate.

Table 4.2 Cumulative incidence rates (ages 0–74) of breast cancer in different populations [1]

Population	Cumulative incidence rate (%)
USA, San Francisco, white	8.9
Canada, British Columbia	8.8
Switzerland, Geneva [2]	8.3
Israel, Jews, Israel/Europe/USA born	6.5
USA, San Francisco, black	6.4
New Zealand, white	5.8
Sweden	5.8
New Zealand, Maori	5.7
USA, Hawaii, Japanese	5.3
UK, South Thames [3]	5.2
Brazil, São Paulo	5.1
Norway	4.9
USA, San Francisco, Chinese	4.8
Finland	3.7
Colombia, Cali	2.9
Israel, Jews, Africa/Asia born	2.9
China, Shanghai [2]	2.2
Singapore, Chinese	2.2
Nigeria, Ibadan	1.7
Japan, Osaka	1.3
Senegal, Dakar [2]	1.3
Israel, non-Jews	1.2

[1] From IARC Sci. Publ. No. 15: *Cancer incidence in five continents,* Vol. 3 (Waterhouse *et al.* 1976), unless otherwise noted.
[2] From IARC Sci. Publ. No. 42: *Cancer incidence in five continents,* Vol. 4 (Waterhouse *et al.* 1982).
[3] South London and south-east England.

These dramatic effects of migration on breast cancer rates show that environmental (probably dietary) and/or behavioural factors are the major determinants of breast cancer risk. If these environmental and/or behavioural factors could be identified and UK women (and their families) were prepared to adopt those of the low risk populations of Asia and black Africa, then the UK breast cancer rate could be reduced to 23 per cent (1.2/5.2) of its current rate, i.e. we would have prevented (or avoided) some three-quarters of current UK breast cancer.

Breast cancer is not unusual in showing large differences between incidence rates in different populations; for most cancer sites the pattern of disease in migrants comes to resemble that of their host country in a few generations as they adopt the local life style. Table 4.3 shows the cumulative incidence rates at the common cancer sites in the UK and the percentage reduction in these rates if the lowest observed rate could be achieved in the UK: the reductions are over 70 per cent for most of the major sites, and there is thus tremendous potential for preventing cancer

Table 4.3 Comparison of South Thames, UK, cumulative incidence rates (ages 0–74) for common cancer sites with the lowest incidence population[1]

Primary site of cancer	Cumulative incidence rate (%)		
	South Thames	Lowest incidence area	Potential reduction
Males:			
Lung and Bronchus	9.54	0.08	99%
Bladder	2.24	0.40	82%
Stomach	2.14	0.75	35%
Prostate	1.64	0.34	79%
Colon	1.53	0.16	90%
Rectum	1.26	0.12	90%
Pancreas	1.07	0.18	83%
Females:			
Breast	5.23	1.22	77%
Lung and Bronchus	1.79	0.08	95%
Colon	1.51	0.15	90%
Cervix	1.39	0.39	72%
Ovary	1.27	0.28	78%
Endometrium	0.96	0.13	86%
Stomach	0.87	0.43	51%
Rectum	0.80	0.26	68%

[1] IARC Sci. Publ. No. 15: *Cancer incidence in five continents*, Vol. 3 (Waterhouse *et al.* 1976).

if the causes of the extreme variations in site specific cancer rates can be identified.

4.3 Identifying the causes

A comprehensive overview of our current understanding of the causes of the whole range of international variations has recently been made by Doll and Peto (1981) and their conclusions are summarized in Table 4.4. The figures were calculated for the USA, and these are given in the Table, but very similar figures apply to the UK.

The evidence that tobacco (more particularly cigarette smoking) is the major identified avoidable cause of an enormous cancer burden is overwhelming, and tobacco is unique in this respect. Certain occupational factors (e.g. asbestos exposure) are equally well established but, as Table 4.4 shows, their contribution to the general cancer burden is much less. Protective 'reproductive' factors, particularly early age at first birth and high parity, are well established and could theoretically make a substantial contribution to the reduction of the present large burden of cancers

Table 4.4 Proportions of cancer deaths in the USA attributable to various factors [1]

Factor or class of factors	Per cent of all cancer deaths	
	Best estimate	Range of acceptable estimates
Diet	35	10–70
Tobacco	30	25–40
Reproductive and sexual behaviour	7	1–13
Occupation	4	2–8
Alcohol	3	2–4
Geophysical factors	3 [2]	2–4
Pollution	2	<1–5
Medicines and medical procedures	1	0.5–3
Food additives	<1	−5 [3]–2
Industrial products	<1	<1–2
Infection	10?	1–?

[1] From Doll and Peto (1981).

[2] 'Only about 1 per cent, not 3 per cent, could reasonably be described as avoidable. Geophysical factors also cause a much greater proportion of non-fatal cancers (up to 30 per cent of all cancers, depending on ethnic mix and latitude) because of the importance of UV light in causing the relatively non-fatal basal cell and squamous cell carcinomas of sunlight exposed skin' (Doll and Peto 1981).

[3] 'Allowing for a possible protective effect of antioxidants and other preservatives' (Doll and Peto 1981).

of the breast, ovary and endometrium, but this is not a practical policy for prevention; practical use of the information we have gained on these reproductive causes will have to come from a fundamental understanding of the biology of how they operate. Although diet is allocated the highest percentage in Table 4.4, it has also been given the widest range of 'acceptable values': this is because although there is strong indirect evidence that diet plays a major role in determining the incidence of most common cancers, there is little reliable evidence as to which precise changes in diet would produce the desired effects.

In this Chapter I shall illustrate the nature of the research findings underlying these conclusions by considering three cancer sites, lung, breast and testis, in some detail, and then give a brief description of the known (and strongly suspected) risk factors for the complete range of cancer sites.

4.3.1 *Lung cancer*

Table 4.3 shows that lung cancer is by far the most important cancer of UK men and it is also, after breast cancer, the most important cancer of UK women. This cancer occupies a unique position among the important cancers in that we have known for at least 35 years the cause of some 90 per cent of it, namely cigarette smoking. This is clearly avoidable. Epidemiological research into lung cancer causation may rightly be claimed as a triumph of cancer research. Present epidemiological research interest in lung cancer is mainly focused on how best to reduce the lung cancer risk among persons apparently unable to stop smoking, by altering the constituents of cigarettes (tar and nicotine content, etc.), by identifying subgroups of persons at especially high risk of lung cancer if they smoke, and by measuring the risk from passive smoking, i.e. from being exposed to other persons' cigarette smoke. The latter may be particularly important: if passive smoking does cause a significant amount of disease then more stringent control of smoking in public places would clearly be called for.

Figure 4.6 shows the trends in male and female lung cancer mortality in E and W from 1916 to 1970. Some of the increase in the earlier period is due to improvements in diagnostic accuracy, but the size of the male risk and its continuing increase persuaded scientists and public health officials in the years immediately after World War II that the reason for the increase warranted urgent study. That cigarette smoking could be the cause of the increase was suggested by a number of people and, unbeknown to scientists in the UK and USA, two studies conducted in Germany in the late 1930s and early 1940s had, in fact, found a strong association of lung cancer and cigarette smoking. By the end of 1950 a further six case control studies had been published; these studies all

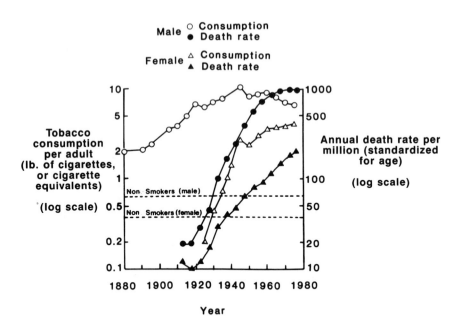

Male ○ Consumption
● Death rate

Female △ Consumption
▲ Death rate

Fig. 4.6 Trends in male and female lung cancer age standardized mortality rates in England and Wales, 1911–80, and cigarette sales per adult expressed as cigarette equivalents (0.3 lb. of pipe tobacco equals 1 lb. of cigarettes. See Doll and Peto, 1976). The dashed lines are lung cancer rates found in lifelong non-smokers in cohort studies conducted in the 1950s and 1960s. Note that the observed national rates early this century were lower than these rates and these differences in all likelihood are a reasonable measure of the improvements in diagnostic accuracy that have been achieved over the years. (Figure kindly supplied by Professor Sir Richard Doll.)

compared the cigarette smoking history of lung cancer cases to that of similar men without the disease (controls) and all showed a clear relationship between increasing risk and increasing exposure. Figure 4.6 also shows how, with women taking up smoking, their lung cancer rates have also increased and how well knowledge of the smoking habits of a population predicts its lung cancer rates some two to three decades later.

There was naturally a great deal of reluctance to accept the findings of the early case control studies—cigarette smoking was, after all, an almost universally accepted habit—and a great number of further epidemiological studies were therefore soon initiated, partly in order to answer criticisms that had been made of the case control studies, but also to find whether smoking was associated with cancers of other sites. A number of these further epidemiological studies were cohort studies, i.e. studies in which large numbers of people with different smoking habits were identified (in the UK the smoking habits of a large number of doctors were recorded) and their subsequent mortality experience monitored. These cohort studies not only confirmed the lung cancer/cigarette smoking association but soon established that smoking was also causally associated with cancers of the tongue, mouth, pharynx, larynx, and bladder, and probably with cancers at a number of other sites.

Studies of the relationship of cigarette smoking to lung cancer have also led to a deeper understanding of a number of aspects of carcinogenesis. Possibly the most important of these is the enormous importance of the duration of cigarette smoking in contrast to the cumulative numbers of cigarettes smoked. The incidence of lung cancer caused by smoking 'c' cigarettes per day for 't' years is not proportional to the cumulative dose, i.e. 'ct', of cigarette smoke, but to 'ct$^{4.5}$', i.e. to 'c' times duration of smoking raised to the fourth or fifth power. For example, at age 60 a man who has smoked 10 cigarettes per day from age 20 (400 cigarette years total dose) has 11 times the lung cancer risk of a man who has smoked 20 cigarettes per day but only from age 40 (also 400 cigarette years total dose).

An important facet of this enormous effect of duration of smoking is the large effect of age at starting to smoke on lung cancer incidence: each one year delay in starting to smoke at a fixed daily cigarette consumption decreases one's lung cancer risk by some 10 per cent.

These epidemiological studies have also shown that stopping smoking has an almost immediate effect on lung cancer risk. The absolute difference between the ex-smoker's lung cancer rate and the lung cancer rate of a non-smoker stays effectively constant with length of time after stopping, rather than continuing to increase as it does for the continuing smoker. These effects of age at starting to smoke and lung cancer incidence after stopping smoking imply that the incidence of lung cancer in a population in late middle age or old age (the ages effectively shown by age standardized incidence rates) depends not only on current cigarette consumption in the population but on the cigarette consumption of young adults 40 or more years before, and changes in population cigarette consumption may take a long time to show up in the lung cancer death rates of older people.

The tobacco industry responded to the ever mounting evidence of the carcinogenic effects of cigarette smoke by reducing the tar and nicotine content of cigarettes, first by introducing filters and later by modifying the tobacco. The tar content of the cigarette is probably the relevant constituent as regards lung cancer and the average tar yield per cigarette declined from approximately 30 mg/cigarette in 1960 to 25 mg/cigarette in 1970 and then to 15 mg/cigarette in 1980.

The average number of cigarettes smoked by men in Britain was approximately 10.5/day from 1950–70 but then declined steadily to reach 8/day in 1980. The average number of cigarettes smoked by women in Britain was only 4/day in 1960, rose to a maximum of 7/day in the early 1970s and subsequently declined to 6/day in 1980.

The combined effect of the changed constituents of cigarettes and the average number of cigarettes smoked is shown in Table 4.5. There has been a dramatic reduction in male lung cancer incidence at young ages, and male lung cancer rates are, in fact, now declining at all ages; we can now look forward in this country to an overall reduction of more than 75 per cent in the male lung cancer rate even if no further reduction in tar content or cigarette smoking takes place, and an even greater reduction if further 'pressure' is exerted on the tobacco industry and the smoker. Female lung cancer rates are also showing a sharp decline at young ages, and although lung cancer rates of older women are still rising (due in large part to the early adoption of smoking by the present cohort of older women), we can also confidently look forward to a substantial reduction in female lung cancer in the not too distant future.

Two aspects of the relationship between cigarette smoking and cancer—identifying the genetic constitution of the smoker who is most at risk of lung cancer, and the carcinogenic effects of exposure to other people's cigarette smoke (so-called 'passive' or 'involuntary' smoking)—are presently the focus of much interest.

Although all smokers would probably get lung cancer if they lived long enough, there is clearly a large difference between the age at onset of the

Table 4.5 Changes in lung[1] cancer mortality rates in England and Wales, 1946–83

| Age | Death rate per 100 000 | | | | | Reduction from peak rate to 1983 |
	1946–50	1956–60	1966–70	1976–80	1983	
Males:						
30–34	3.6	3.5	2.5	1.6	1.0	72%
40–44	23.6	25.1	21.6	13.8	11.8	53%
50–54	95.4	124.8	116.0	99.6	76.3	39%
60–64	171.7	331.5	369.5	332.0	304.3	18%
70–74	140.0	387.8	621.0	662.5	656.0	1%
Females:						
30–34	1.2	1.4	1.1	0.8	0.8	43%
40–44	4.8	6.0	8.1	6.2	5.3	35%
50–54	11.7	16.9	28.4	35.9	29.9	17%
60–64	22.1	32.8	51.5	84.6	92.4	—
70–74	31.6	44.5	73.1	110.5	140.8	—

[1] Bronchus and pleura. The highest rate for each age group is underlined.

disease in different persons with the same smoking habits. These differences in age at onset of lung cancer do not prove that different people have different susceptibilities to cigarette smoke induced lung cancer, it may all be simply a matter of chance; they do, however, strongly suggest that there may be different genetic susceptibilities involved. The host factor that has excited most interest are the genes coding for the enzymes that control the metabolic oxidative activation of various chemical carcinogens. The different levels of such enzymes, which are known to be genetically controlled in many animal species, would give rise to wide inter-person variation in the generation of carcinogenic derivatives of the chemicals in cigarette smoke.

A number of polycyclic aromatic hydrocarbons (PAHs) that occur in cigarette smoke are potent carcinogens, and the activity of one of the above enzyme systems—aryl hydrocarbon hydroxylase (AHH)—is known to vary in animals and is closely linked to their susceptibility to some PAH induced cancers. At least 16 studies have compared the AHH activities of lung cancer cases with controls; although the first few studies showed a clear difference between the cases and the controls, the results of subsequent studies have been most confusing and in many cases contradictory. The reasons for the contradictory results are probably methodological, such as the use of different cell types to measure AHH activity, and different assay conditions. The use of cryopreserved tissue may enable one to circumvent some of these problems, and Kouri et al. (1982) have found much higher AHH activities in lung cancer cases than in controls using this technique. The higher AHH activities were not directly related to cigarette smoking history or tumour type, but, of course, whether the high AHH activity was the cause or the result of lung cancer could not be answered by such a study. Although work on the relation between AHH and human lung cancer is difficult, establishing such a genetic link is clearly of the greatest interest and further work on this system is to be encouraged.

Recently the oxidative metabolism of the chemical compound debrisoquine has been shown to be genetically determined in man, and the first study comparing its metabolism in lung cancer patients and controls has been reported (Ayesh et al. 1984). Very large differences were found between the cases and the controls. The authors concluded that although this oxidation process may not be involved in chemical carcinogenesis, and in particular cigarette smoke carcinogenesis, the gene may be closely linked with genes which are. Whatever the underlying basis of these results is, they are, as with the AHH results, clearly of the greatest interest, and further results are eagerly awaited.

There is good evidence that parental, particularly maternal, smoking increases respiratory disease rates in young children, and evidence is slowly accumulating that pulmonary function of non-smokers is adversely affected by exposure to the smoking of their spouses. Since cigarette smoke is clearly carcinogenic, it is reasonable to assume that involuntary smoking will also cause a certain amount of lung cancer; the epidemiological question of interest is not really whether or not involuntary smoking causes lung cancer, but how much. Although sidestream smoke contains higher levels of certain highly carcinogenic chemicals (*N*-nitrosamines) and has a smaller particle size than mainstream smoke, one may be able to get a rough idea of the lung cancer risk of involuntary smoking by measuring the passive smokers' blood (or urine) levels of some constituent of tobacco smoke. Studies of urinary cotinine (Wald *et al.* 1984) suggest that the lung cancer rate of the average non-smoking spouse of a smoker should be increased some 10 per cent, i.e. the equivalent of smoking about one tenth of a cigarette per day. This small but not negligible effect adds considerably to the other reasons, e.g. nuisance, eye and respiratory irritation effects, for no longer permitting smoking in enclosed public places. A number of recent direct studies of the lung cancer effects of passive smoking have shown moreover that the carcinogenic effects of such exposure may be much greater (see Loeb *et al.* 1984 for references): risks of two-fold or more have been found in studies in Japan, Greece and the USA. These large risks have, however, not been found in all studies and the matter is being very actively pursued.

Although cigarette smoking is by far the major cause of lung cancer, exposure to a number of other substances has created a substantial added risk of lung cancer for workers in certain industrial occupations. The most important of these exposures has been to asbestos. A substantial number of men were previously exposed to high levels of asbestos, particularly in the shipbuilding and insulation industries, and these men have experienced very high lung cancer rates. This risk is now universally recognized and the asbestos levels permitted in industry have been very substantially reduced over the last decade. Occupational exposure to polycyclic aromatic hydrocarbons from the combustion of fossil fuels has also been an important source of added lung cancer risk. High level PAH exposure has occurred particularly to men working in the fumes from coke ovens and in coal gas manufacturing. Other substantial risks to small groups of workers have resulted from exposure to radiation from radon in the air of certain mines, and from exposure to some aspect of the manufacture or refining of chromates, nickel and copper.

The general population has been exposed in the past to significant amounts of PAHs in urban air, mainly from the uncontrolled burning of coal. Such general air pollution may have contributed to as much as 10 per cent of all lung cancer in heavily polluted cities, but, with the passing of various clean air acts over the years, general air pollution has been reduced dramatically and current levels are unlikely to be making more than a small contribution to lung cancer risk.

4.3.2 Breast cancer

There has been slow but steady progress over the last two decades in our understanding of the aetiology of breast cancer. The large variation in international rates have provided the stimulus to much valuable work. Hormones appear to hold the key in humans just as they do in certain animal species (see Chapter 13).

Epidemiological research has established that early menarche, late age at first birth and late menopause are three major risk factors for breast cancer (Table 4.6). A delay of two to three years in age at menarche has been found to reduce breast cancer risk by up to a half. The earlier a woman gives birth to her first child, the greater the reduction in breast cancer risk; women with a first birth under age 20 have about one half the risk of nulliparous women, but nulliparous women do not have as high a risk as women whose first birth is after age 35. Similarly the earlier a woman has her menopause the greater the reduction in her breast cancer risk; women with natural menopause before age 45 have only one half the risk of women whose menopause occurs after age 55. Post–menopausal weight also appears to be important. Studies have found an

Table 4.6 Effects of age at menarche, age at first birth, age at meno-pause, and post-menopausal weight on breast cancer risk[1]

Risk factor		Relative risk
Menarche (yrs.)	≦ 11	1.00
	12	0.90
	≧ 13	0.50
First birth (yrs.)	≦ 19	0.83
	20–24	1.00
	25–29	1.30
	30–34	1.57
	≧ 35	2.03
	Nulliparous	1.67
Menopause (yrs.)	40–44	1.00
	45–49	1.27
	50–54	1.47
	55–59	2.03
Post-menopausal weight (kg.)	≦ 59	1.00
	60–69	1.61
	≧ 70	1.81

[1] From Pike and Ross (1984).

approximately 40 per cent increase in breast cancer risk for a 20 kg increase in post-menopausal weight.

Before one can undertake serious discussion of the possible effect of any other factor as an explanation, or partial explanation, of a particular aspect of the pattern of breast cancer occurrence in different populations, one needs to consider whether these four risk factors (menarche, first birth, menopause, and post–menopausal weight) by themselves are an adequate explanation. The distribution of age at menopause appears to vary very little between populations, but there are large differences in the distributions of the other risk factors. Detailed study of the extent to which such differences between Japanese and American women could explain the large differences between their breast cancer rates has been undertaken. Age at first birth has not differed greatly between the two populations, but Japanese females born around 1900 had an average age at menarche two and one half years later and they weighed some 22 kg less at age 70 than the 1900 cohort of US white women. Although these differences steadily decreased over the years with the improved nutrition of the Japanese, they could account for as much as two thirds of the difference in the observed breast cancer rates in the two countries. They could not, however, acccount for all the difference—US white women still have 2.5 times the breast cancer rate of Japanese women even after allowing for these factors—and dietary differences have been the focus of much attention as the additional factor needed to explain both the international pattern of breast cancer occurrence and the changes in rates with migration.

International breast cancer incidence and mortality rates are particularly highly correlated with per capita consumption of fat (Fig. 4.7). The

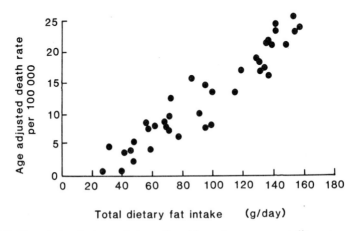

Fig. 4.7 Correlation between international breast cancer mortality rates and per capita consumption of fat.

international correlations between per capita consumption of fat and animal protein (and certain other dietary constituents such as meat) are so high, however, that it has not been possible to disentangle their separate effects. Epidemiological study of individual breast cancer cases and controls have provided some support for a role for fat consumption, but the studies have found only small differences between cases and controls, generally no larger than the differences in total calorie consumption; moreover, a large prospective study has found no relationship between serum cholesterol levels and breast cancer incidence. Further progress in evaluating dietary factors is most likely to come from a deeper understanding of how they might influence breast cancer risk at a cellular level.

The association of breast cancer with age at menarche and age at menopause almost certainly implies that ovarian activity is an important determinant of breast cancer risk, and detailed study of ovarian hormones and how they may be affected by diet offers a most exciting challenge with the hope of discovering facts that may be truly useful in preventing breast cancer. Ovarian oestrogen activity appears to be of particular importance. There is abundant evidence that oestradiol, the most important of the circulating oestrogens, is involved in breast cancer risk, and recent studies have found that the 'packaging' (binding) of oestradiol is markedly different in breast cancer cases (oestradiol not so tightly bound to sex hormone binding globulin, so more is 'available' to breast tissue), and that the oestradiol in British women is much less tightly bound than that of low breast cancer risk Japanese women. The increasing breast cancer risk associated with increasing weight may also, at least in part, be a binding effect; sex hormone binding globulin levels decrease with increasing weight so that 'available' oestradiol increases— the mechanism of this decrease in sex hormone binding globulin is not yet understood. The finding that circulating oestradiol in Japanese women is tightly bound is obviously potentially of great preventive value if the reason is, as one suspects, some aspect of everyday diet (e.g. a direct effect of a low consumption of fat). The effects of particular aspects of diet (total calories, proportion of calories from saturated fat, etc.) on various aspects of hormone metabolism is the focus of much current research, and further significant progress can confidently be expected.

During the first half of the menstrual cycle, before ovulation takes place, the ovary mainly produces oestrogens, but after ovulation it also produces a second hormone, progesterone, in significant amounts. Combination type oral contraceptives (COCs), the commonly prescribed type, contain both a synthetic oestrogen (usually ethinyl oestradiol) and one or other of a variety of synthetic progestogens (drugs which mimic the action of progesterone). COCs effectively stop the ovaries functioning and, if this were the only effect of the pill, COC use should reduce a woman's risk of breast cancer, since this state mimics the menopause (a state known to be associated with a reduced risk of breast cancer). Epidemiological studies have, however, found little evidence of such a protective effect of COC use. The reason for this would appear to be that the synthetic hormones in COCs act directly on the breast, effectively replacing the action of the ovarian hormones. For mature women the action on breast tissue, that is relevant to breast cancer causation, of COCs available up to the mid-1970s appears to be very similar to such action of her own ovarian hormones, so that her breast cancer risk is neither decreased nor increased. If this reasoning is correct, and the hormone dose in even the lowest dose pills does not provide maximal action on breast tissue, then one may reasonably suspect that the newer low dose COCs may actually reduce breast cancer risk when taken by mature women. For very young women, however, whose cycle lengths tend to be longer and who frequently fail to ovulate, there is some evidence, although very controversial, that COC action on her breast tissue may be greater than the breast tissue action of her ovarian hormones, i.e. that COC use increases her risk of breast cancer. The question we face here is whether the hormone dose in COCs can be reduced sufficiently to pose no risk to these young women while still providing effective contraception. This is an area of very active research and debate, in particular as to what role, if any, the different progestogens have to play in the actions of COCs on breast tissue.

Following the above reasoning, one would expect that oestrogens taken around the time of the menopause or in the post-menopausal period would increase the risk of breast cancer. A number of studies have now found just such an effect, i.e. a small, but not insignificant, increase in breast cancer risk after using oestrogens for a number of years. Such hormone replacement therapy also has, however, many important beneficial effects, such as reducing heart disease and bone loss, and the optimum manner of prescribing this very important therapy is the subject of much current research.

At present, the only advice for preventive action against breast cancer that can be confidently given without fearing that it may involve losses in some other area of health is to avoid obesity. There are recent research results, however, so far unconfirmed, that suggest that increased strenuous activity both in childhood and through the teenage and later years will lead to a significant decrease in breast cancer risk, not only through delaying menarche but also by changing the menstrual cycle pattern in a protective way. Further results of research in this area are awaited with great interest.

4.3.3 *Cancer of the testis*

Table 4.7 shows that there is a very marked international variation in the

Table 4.7 Cumulative incidence rates (ages 15–49) of cancer of the testis in different populations [1]

Population	Cumulative incidence rate (%)
Switzerland, Geneva [2]	0.30
USA, San Francisco, white	0.28
Norway	0.28
New Zealand, white	0.24
New Zealand, Maori	0.22
UK, South Thames [3]	0.19
Canada, British Columbia	0.19
USA, San Francisco, Chinese	0.18
Sweden	0.15
Israel, Jews, Israel/Europe/USA born	0.11
Finland	0.06
USA, San Francisco, black	0.06
Brazil, São Paulo	0.06
Colombia, Cali	0.05
Singapore, Chinese	0.05
China, Shanghai [2]	0.04
Israel, Jews, Africa/Asia born	0.04
Japan, Osaka	0.03
Nigeria, Ibadan	0.01
Senegal, Dakar [2]	0.01
USA, Hawaii, Japanese	0.01
Israel, non-Jews	0.01

[1] From IARC Sci. Publ. No. 15: *Cancer incidence in five continents*, Vol. 3 (Waterhouse *et al.* 1976), unless otherwise noted.
[2] From IARC Sci. Publ. No. 42: *Cancer incidence in five continents*, Vol. 4 (Waterhouse *et al.* 1982).
[3] South London and south-east England.

incidence of testicular cancer. There has also been a large increase in the incidence rate of the tumour over time in many countries; in E and W the incidence rate has increased steadily since the turn of the century and the current rate is at least six times the rate in 1900. These differences have not, unfortunately, been the source of clues to the underlying aetiology of the tumour. However, the well known increased risk of testicular cancer in cryptorchid (i.e. undescended) testes and the distinctive age specific incidence pattern of germ cell cancers of the testis (Fig. 4.4) both strongly suggest that *in utero* events may be important in the genesis of the tumour.

Three case control studies have begun to explore the gestational events of the relevant pregnancies (Table 4.8 gives the results from the most recent of these). All three studies found an increased risk in the male offspring of women exposed early in pregnancy to either diethylstilbo-estrol (DES), oestrogens or the oestrogen/progestogen combinations

Table 4.8 Risk factors for (germ-cell) cancer of the testis [1]

Risk factor	Relative risk
Cryptorchidism	9.0
In utero, first trimester exogenous hormone exposure	8.0
Maternal weight (QI [2]) < 19	1.0
19–21	1.6
$\geqq 22$	2.9
Birth weight, < 2.7 kg	3.2

[1] From Depue *et al.* (1983).
[2] Quetelet's index (QI) = (weight in kg)/(square of height in metres).

used in hormone pregnancy tests (now no longer used). In the study of Depue *et al.* (1983) there were nine hormone exposed mothers of cases and five had had only a single exposure as a result of a pregnancy test.

Increased maternal weight immediately before the pregnancy has also been found to be associated with an increased risk of cancer of the testis. The clearest gradient of risk was obtained when weight was expressed in terms of Quetelet's index (QI=weight in kg divided by the square of height in metres), an increase in QI from 18.5 to 22.5 increased the risk of testicular cancer approximately 2.5-fold: for a 1.68 metre (5ft.6in.) woman, this is an increase of only 12 kg from approximately 52 to 64 kg. This is a particularly exciting finding. As we noted above in our discussion of breast cancer, increasing weight has a strong inverse relationship with sex hormone binding globulin levels, so that increased bioavailability of oestrogens during the first trimester of pregnancy may be the mode of action of this risk factor.

'Excessive' nausea of pregnancy, as indicated by treatment with drugs, was also found to be a risk factor for testicular cancer in first-born pregnancies (Depue *et al.* 1983). It is difficult to separate the effect of severe nausea from the effect of the drugs used to treat it, but the fact that the risk appeared to be confined to first births argued strongly that the severe nausea itself was the risk factor. The cause of nausea of pregnancy is not known, but it almost invariably starts in the first two months of gestation when oestrogen levels rise rapidly in the mother.

The risk factors discussed above all appear to relate to events in the first trimester of pregnancy when the testis is being formed. The other main risk factor identified for cancer of the testis is prematurity, as measured by a low birth weight: this suggests that events in the last few weeks of pregnancy are also important in the aetiology of the disease.

Investigating maternal factors for cancer of the testis is clearly very difficult and subject to a great deal of errors of recall since mothers of testicular cancer cases cannot easily recall events 20 to 40 years in the past. Fortunately the maternal risk factors (exogenous hormone exposure, increased maternal weight and prematurity) bear a close relationship to the maternal risk factors for cryptorchidism (Depue 1984), and these factors are much easier to investigate since true cryptorchidism can be reliably diagnosed three months after birth. One current study in Oxford is investigating not only events in the actual pregnancy but also the precise menstrual, contraceptive and reproductive history in the period immediately before conception. This study should also cast some light on the doubling in the apparent frequency of cryptorchidism in E and W between 1962 and 1981 (Chilvers *et al.* 1984); since true cryptorchidism is associated with a large increase in risk of testicular cancer, this increase in cryptorchidism clearly also needs investigating for its potential impact on future testicular cancer rates.

Testicular cancer is uniformly rare in black populations, including blacks in the USA whose cancer of the testis rates are only a fifth of the rates in US whites. This suggests that genetic factors may play a particularly important role in these germ cell tumours; however, no such factor has as yet been identified.

4.4 Risk factors

Table 4.9 summarizes the known and suspected risk factors for each cancer site in order of the percentage of all cancer deaths caused by the tumour in E and W in 1979. The incidence and mortality figures give a rough guide to the relative importance of the site as a source of cancer; the relation between the incidence and mortality figures indicates the fatality rate associated with the particular cancer; and the male to female ratio for sites common to both sexes suggests the importance of exposure to sex specific risk factors. The publication of Doll and Peto (1983) should be referred to for a fuller description of these results. Certain aspects of Table 4.9 are particularly noteworthy.

4.4.1 *Bladder cancer risk factors*

This cancer is particularly intriguing. Although epidemiological studies suggest that cigarette smoking accounts for about half the cases in Britain, the mortality rate from the disease did not increase as lung cancer did, with the enormous increase in smoking this century, but if anything decreased (incidence figures are suspect due to the possibility of an increased tendency to classify benign papillomas as carcinomas).

Bladder cancer has also been shown to be caused by occupational

Table 4.9 Risk factors and certain basic information for England and Wales by specific cancer site [1]

Site	Incidence (%)	Mortality (%)	M:F	Risk factors
Lung	18.6	27.0	2:1 to 5:1	Smoking Asbestos Polycyclic aromatic hydrocarbons Arsenic Nickel refining Chromates Bis chloromethyl ether
Large bowel	12.1	12.9	1.3:1	Diet: meat (?), fat (?), lack of fibre (?) Genetic: polyposis coli
Breast	10.8	9.5	0.01:1	Early menarche Late menopause Late first birth Obesity Diet: fat (?)
Stomach	7.4	8.8	2.2:1	Blood group A Diet: inadequate preservation of food (?) Low socio-economic class
Pancreas	2.8	4.7	1.7:1	Smoking
Prostate	4.6	3.8	M	Diet: meat (?), fat (?)
Bladder	4.7	3.3	4.2:1	Smoking Aromatic amines Schistosomiasis Certain anti-cancer drugs (rare)
Ovary	2.3	2.9	F	Low parity Early menarche Late menopause Obesity Diet (?) Decreased by oral contraceptive use
Oesophagus	1.8	2.8	1.9:1	Smoking Alcohol Nutritional deficiencies (?)

Table 4.9 —*continued*

Site	Incidence (%)	Mortality (%)	M:F	Risk factors
Leukaemia	2.0	2.6	1.5:1	Ionizing radiation Benzene Phenylbutazone (?) Genetic: Down's syndrome, ataxia telangiectasia, Bloom's syndrome, Fanconi's anaemia Viruses: HTLV I
Brain and nervous system	1.8	2.3	1.5:1	Certain occupational exposures (?)
Kidney	1.4	1.8	2.2:1	Smoking Aromatic amine exposure Analgesic nephropathy from phenacetin
Non-Hodgkin's lymphoma	1.4	1.7	1.6:1	Burkitt's lymphoma (rare)—Epstein-Barr virus (?) Immunosuppressive drugs (rare) Genetic: immunological impairment
Cervix	2.6	1.6	F	Multiple sexual contacts by self or partners Cleanliness (?) Herpes simplex virus (?) Papillomavirus (?)
Myelomatosis	0.7	1.2	1.3:1	Genetic factors (?)
Tongue, mouth and pharynx (excluding nasopharynx)	1.2	1.0	2.2:1	Smoking Alcohol
Endometrium	1.9	0.9	F	Low parity Early menarche Late menopause 'Unopposed' oestrogens Obesity Decreased by oral contraceptives
Gall-bladder and extra-hepatic bile ducts	0.7	0.8	0.9:1	Obesity, high parity (gall-bladder)

Table 4.9 —*continued*

Site	Incidence (%)	Mortality (%)	M:F	Risk factors
Liver	0.3	0.7	2.1:1	Cirrhosis Hepatitis B virus Anabolic steroids (rare) Oral contraceptives (rare) Angiosarcoma (rare): thorotrast, vinyl chloride
Larynx	1.0	0.6	6.9:1	Smoking Alcohol
Skin (melanoma)	0.8	0.6	0.6:1	Ultraviolet light (particularly high intermittent exposure (?)) Decreases with increased skin pigment Genetic: xeroderma pigmentosum
Hodgkin's disease	0.9	0.5	1.8:1	Epstein Barr virus (?)
Thyroid	0.4	0.3	0.5:1	Ionizing radiation
Bone	0.3	0.3	1.7:1	Ionizing radiation Paget's disease
Skin (non-melanoma)	> 11	0.3	1.7:1	Ultraviolet light Polycyclic aromatic hydrocarbons Immunosuppression
Pleura and peritoneum	—	0.2	3.4:1	Asbestos (particularly crocidolite)
Testis	0.4	0.2	M	Undescended testis Maternal weight Exogenous maternal oestrogens and progestogens (?)
Nose and nasal sinuses	0.3	0.2	2.0:1	Some aspects of nickel refining, and manufacture of isopropyl alcohol, hardwood furniture, and leather goods
Connective tissue	0.4	0.2	1.3:1	Immunosuppression

Table 4.9 —*continued*

Site	Incidence (%)	Mortality (%)	M:F	Risk factors
Nasopharynx	0.1	0.1	1.9:1	Epstein Barr virus (?) Salted fish (in China) (?)
Salivary gland	0.4	0.1	1.0:1	Genetic (rare): associated with breast cancer
Penis	0.2	0.1	M	Early circumcision decreases risk
Lip	0.4	0.04	13.6:1	Pipe smoking Smoking Ultraviolet light
Choriocarcinoma	0.01	0.005	F	—

[1] From Hirayama *et al.* (1980) and Doll and Peto (1983). The incidence figure is for UK cancer registries around 1970; the mortality for E and W, 1979: both expressed as proportion of all cancers.

exposure to a number of chemicals used in the dye and rubber industries; these chemicals (2-naphthylamine, benzidine, 3,3′-dichlorobenzidine, and 4-amino-biphenyl) belong to a class of chemicals, the aromatic amines, which are now known to be animal carcinogens. 2-naphthylamine is particularly carcinogenic; all 19 distillers in one factory developed bladder cancer, and it is no longer used in industry here. Certain other aromatic amines are suspected of causing bladder cancer, and it has been estimated that between 5 and 10 per cent of current bladder tumours are due to such occupational exposures.

The bladder cancer risk factors that have declined to compensate for the increased risk from cigarettes await discovery: decreased occupational exposure to aromatic amines will not account for the difference. Genetic differences in susceptibility to bladder cancer are suggested by some recent work, and further studies to establish this and to understand its biological basis may help us to identify these clearly very important, although declining, risk factors.

4.4.2 Smoking and alcohol

Smoking is a very important cause of cancer at all sites in the upper respiratory and digestive tracts, but for cancers of the oesophagus and larynx its effect is markedly dependent on alcohol consumption. For these two sites the harmful effects of cigarettes and alcohol act synergistically, i.e. their effects are more than additive and are, in fact, close to multiplicative. The results of one particularly large study of oesophageal cancer found that a non-drinking smoker of 20 cigarettes per day had a 1.7-fold increased risk, while a non-smoking drinker of 100 g of alcohol per day had a 7.2-fold increased risk, but a 20 cigarettes per day drinker of 100 g of alcohol per day had a 12.1-fold increased risk. Such synergism is found quite commonly with cancer risk factors, and shows that control of one risk factor may have a larger effect than one might predict from studies in which people, or experimental animals, were only exposed to the single agent.

4.4.3 Oral contraceptives

I noted above, in my discussion of breast cancer, that the effects of oral contraceptives (OCs) on the disease were the subject of much current research and heated debate, and we are very far from being able to write the last word on the subject.

The situation as regards the effects of OCs on the risk of cancer at other sites is much clearer. OC use causes a very small number of benign liver tumours (adenomas of the liver), and appear to cause an even smaller number of liver cancers after prolonged use. Much more importantly, OC use sharply reduces the risk of ovarian cancer, and use of combination type OCs (with each pill containing both a synthetic oestrogen and a synthetic progestogen) sharply reduces the risk of cancer of the endometrium (the lining of the uterus). Ovarian cancer has a particularly high death rate as it is so seldom diagnosed at an early (treatable) stage, and the protective effect of OC use is thus particularly important for this cancer. Although we cannot yet be sure if the protective effect of OC use will be lifelong, there are good theoretical reasons to suggest that it will be, and in this case some five years of OC use may reduce the lifelong risk of ovarian cancer by as much as 50 per cent. A similar level of protection may be achieved against the much less fatal cancer of the endometrium.

4.4.4 Diet

Diet could influence the risk of cancer in many ways. Obesity itself contributes directly to certain cancers, in particular to cancer of the endometrium, so that calories are important. The consumption of known animal carcinogens has some role to play. Aflatoxin, a fungal contaminant of peanuts, appears to be a major cause of liver cancer in certain tropical countries, and bracken fern consumption in Japan has been linked to cancer of the oesophagus. It has, however, not been possible to show that consumption of any other known carcinogens, such as polycyclic aromatic hydrocarbons in grilled meat, play a causative role in any human cancer.

Certain aspects of diet may influence the formation of carcinogens in the body; for example, the consumption of nitrites and nitrates may increase, and the consumption of vitamin C may decrease, the formation of the very potent animal carcinogens, nitrosamines, in the stomach. No such effects on human cancer risk have, however, been established, despite considerable and continuing efforts.

There is some, not as yet compelling, evidence that dietary 'fibre' may protect against cancer of the colon. There are a number of different varieties of fibre and the types that appear most likely to exert the greatest protective effect—the pentose sugar polymers—are abundant in unrefined cereals and most vegetables, although not potatoes.

Fat consumption is the most commonly considered dietary cause of human cancer, in particular cancer of the large bowel. There are strong international correlations between per capita fat consumption and cancer of the large bowel, and studies of Japanese migrants to Hawaii have found an increased fat intake and a much increased risk of bowel cancer. These correlational studies are, however, the crudest form of epidemiological evidence, and case control and cohort studies of fat consumption of individuals have provided little or no support for such a relationship. Moreover, prospective studies of serum cholesterol levels, which have provided the most compelling evidence of a link between fat consumption and heart disease, have found no evidence whatsoever of a relationship with large bowel cancer. It appears, therefore, that if a high fat diet does increase the risk of large bowel cancer it will have to be some element of such a diet that does not raise serum cholesterol levels; finding out what this element is, if it does exist, is not going to be easy.

Appropriate modifications of diet could probably alter the cancer risk at many sites. At present we have insufficient knowledge to confidently recommend any protective measures other than avoidance of obesity. However, increased consumption of vegetables, and a decreased consumption of fat are extremely unlikely to do any harm and will probably be beneficial, at least in terms of general health. This is a difficult field to study, mainly because of the great inaccuracies inevitably associated with recording individual dietary intakes over long periods (usually obtained through diet histories). Progress is, however, being made. Relating diet to biological factors found to influence cancer risk holds great promise for significant progress in this field.

Further reading

Ayesh, R., Idle, J. R., Ritchie, J. C., Crothers, M. J., and Hetzel, R. (1984). Metabolic oxidation phenotypes as markers for susceptibility to lung cancer. *Nature* **312**, 169–70.

Chilvers, C., Pike, M. C., Forman, D., Fogelman, K., and Wadsworth, M. E. J. (1984). Apparent doubling of frequency of undescended testis in England and Wales in 1962–81. *Lancet* **ii**, 330–2.

Cook, P. J., Doll, R., and Fellingham, S. A. (1969). A mathematical model for the age distribution of cancer in man. *International Journal of Cancer* **4**, 93–112.

Depue, R. H. (1984). Maternal and gestational factors affecting the risk of cryptorchidism and inguinal hernia. *International Journal of Epidemiology* **13**, 311–18.

——, Pike, M. C. and Henderson, B. E. (1983). Estrogen exposure during gestation and risk of testicular cancer. *Journal of the National Cancer Institute* **71**, 1151–5.

Doll, R., and Hill, A. B. (1950). Smoking and carcinoma of the lung. *British Medical Journal* **2**, 739–48.

——, and Peto, R. (1976). Mortality in relation to smoking: 20 years' observations on male British doctors. *British Medical Journal* **2**, 1525–36.

——, and Peto, R. (1981). *The causes of cancer: quantitative estimates of avoidable risks of cancer in the United States today.* Oxford Medical Publications, Oxford.

——, and Peto, R. (1983). Epidemiology of cancer. In: *Oxford textbook of medicine* (eds. D. J. Weatherall, J. G. G. Ledingham, and D. A. Warrell). Oxford University Press, Oxford.

Hirayama, T., Waterhouse, J. A. H., and Fraumeni, J. F. (1980). Cancer risk by site. UICC Technical Report Series (Geneva) 41.

Kouri, R. E., McKinney, C. E., Slomiany, D. J., Snodgrass, D. R., Wray, N. P., and McLemore, T. L. (1982). Positive correlation between high aryl hydrocarbon hydroxylase activity and primary lung cancer—analysis of cryopreserved lymphocytes. *Cancer Research* **42**, 5030–7.

Loeb, L. A., Ernster, V. L., Warner, K. E., Abbotts, J., and Laszlo, J. (1984). Smoking and lung cancer: an overview. *Cancer Research* **44**, 5940–58.

Pike, M. C., and Ross, R. K. (1984). Breast cancer. *British Medical Bulletin* **40**, 351–4.

Wald, N. J., Boreham, J., Bailey, A., Ritchie, C., Haddow, J. E., and Knight, G. (1984). Urinary cotinine as marker of breathing other people's tobacco smoke. *Lancet* **i**, 230–1.

5

Inherited susceptibility to cancer

W. F. BODMER

5.1 Introduction: cellular genetic basis for cancer

Epidemiological studies, especially of variations in cancer incidence in different populations and their migrants, as discussed in Chapter 4, strongly suggest that at least 80 per cent of cancer incidence is attributable in the broadest sense to environmental factors. Studies on the incidence of cancer in the relatives of patients with the disease support the view that, overall, the contribution of inheritance to cancer susceptibility is not as large as it is in some of the other major chronic diseases, such as heart disease and autoimmune diseases. At the cellular level, in the individual in whom cancer develops, genetic changes in the cells destined to form a malignant tumour clearly play a major role. In this Chapter I shall briefly review the evidence for the importance of genetic changes at the cellular level in the development of a cancer, and then discuss more extensively those situations where there is an inherited basis for cancer susceptibility and their potential inter-relationships with the changes at the cellular level.

Most of the fundamental ideas on the causation of cancer were suggested in the early years of this century, or earlier, while the idea that exposure to substances in the environment could be a cause of cancer goes back at least to Percival Pott in 1775. He pointed out that chimney sweeps tended to get cancer of the scrotum because they were continuously exposed to soot. Thus he was the first to identify clearly not only an environmental carcinogen, but also an occupational cancer.

The major fundamental ideas about the causes of cancer are

1. That genetic changes, or mutations, in somatic cells of the body are the main initiating events, and are responsible for tumour progression.
2. The related idea that changes in the chromosomes, either in their number or organization, are key events.
3. That the immune system plays a role in combating cancer through recognition of surface changes in cells.
4. That some cancers are caused by viruses.
5. That cancers represent a form of dedifferentiation or, more generally, perturbation of the differentiated state, that is associated with a loss of growth control.

Modern developments in genetics, cell biology and virology, especially in recent years at the molecular level, now make it possible to understand these fundamental notions. These ideas can all be interrelated through the basic assumption that a cancer develops through a series of genetic changes progressing from the initiated cell, whose progeny eventually give rise to the cancer, to the ultimate malignant cell.

5.2 Evidence for a genetic basis

There are at least five major lines of evidence to support this viewpoint of the genetic origin of cancers at the somatic level.

Cancers, as populations of cells, tend to breed true as far as their cell types are concerned. This is the fundamental basis for the histopathological diagnosis of a cancer as, for example, a particular sort of lymphoma or carcinoma. Staying true to type, however, says little more than that the cells of a cancer reflect, on the whole, the properties of the tissue from which they originated. Since the process of cellular differentiation, by which tissues acquire and maintain their particular characteristics, is not, in general, due to genetic changes in the sense of mutations, the evidence that a cancer tends to retain the characteristics of the tissue from which it is derived does little more than relate carcinogenesis to the process of differentiation. Differences between types of cells are based on differential gene expression. This emphasizes the possibility that some of the steps in tumour progression may not necessarily be mutations, but may involve aberrant control of gene expression by mechanisms analogous to those which control cellular differentiation. The term 'epigenetic' is often used to describe this situation, and to contrast it with genetic changes in the sense of mutations, namely alterations in the DNA sequence itself.

Genetic markers can be used to show that the vast majority of cancers are clonal in origin, that is are derived at some point by cell division from a single cell. The evidence for this depends on the fact that in female cells, which contain two X chromosomes, only one of them is active or fully functional thus ensuring that male (XY) and female (XX) cells have the same level of X chromosome activity. The female receives one of her X chromosomes from her mother and the other from her father, and the random process by which inactivation in somatic cells of one of the X chromosomes occurs means that in roughly half the cells it is the maternal X chromosome that is active and in the other half the paternal X chromosome. Thus, a female who is heterozygous for two forms, or alleles, of a gene on the X chromosome is a mosaic of cells, half of which on average express one allele and the other half the other allele. Glucose–6–phosphate dehydrogenase (G6PD) occurs in some populations, especially those of African origin, in two different forms, A and B, which can be distinguished by the technique of electrophoresis. A female who is heterozygous G6PDA/B is thus a mosaic of cells approximately half of which express G6PDA while the other half express G6PDB. A tumour in such an heterozygous female, if it is clonal, should not be a mosaic. All the cells of the tumour will either be G6PDA or G6PDB depending on which allele was active in the initiated cell from which the tumour was ultimately derived (see Fig. 5.1). Studies on tumours in G6PDA/B heterozygotes, pioneered by Gartler, Fialkow, and others, have shown that at least the vast majority of leukaemias are clonal in origin by this criterion. There are similar data in the mouse, using another X chromosome enzyme marker, to show that the vast majority of experimentally induced liver tumours are clonal in origin. This evidence, of course, only shows that at some point in the development of a tumour it becomes clonal. It does not rule out the possibility that epigenetic influences, such as for example persistent immune reaction or tissue repair, may create a cellular environment involving many cells which favours the initiation of a tumour. In such a situation the tumour could potentially be derived from any one of a number of cells in this altered cellular environment.

Chromosomal changes have been seen in tumours since the studies by Boveri and others in the early years of this century. However, as discussed in Chapter 11, it is only comparatively recently that highly specific chromosome changes have been identified that are, in some cases, quite characteristic of a particular tumour. The initial and classical example is the Philadelphia chromosome found in chronic granulocytic leukaemia (CGL). This is now known to be a translocation, namely an exchange of parts between two chromosomes (in this case 9 and 22), a specific genetic event. It is almost always seen in all CGL cells, and so clearly itself is evidence for at least one genetic step in the development

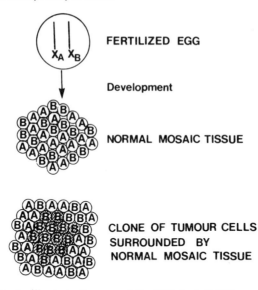

FERTILIZED EGG

Development

NORMAL MOSAIC TISSUE

CLONE OF TUMOUR CELLS
SURROUNDED BY
NORMAL MOSAIC TISSUE

Fig. 5.1 Scheme to illustrate the use of the X-linked G6PD marker to show the clonal origin of tumours. The female heterozygote carries the allele A for G6PDA on one X-chromosome, and B for G6PDB on the other X chromosome. The two forms of the enzyme can be distinguished by their different electrophoretic mobilities on a gel. During development the fertilized egg divides to give rise to the somatic tissues. Each somatic cell has only one active X and since the mechanism of inactivation appears to be random, normal tissues will usually be a mosaic of two different sorts of cells with respect to G6PD activity, one expressing the A variant and the other expressing the B variant. If tumours arise from a single progenitor cell, then all the cells of the tumour will be derived by division from this progenitor and express the same G6PD type as the cell which initiated the tumour. Thus, tissue from a tumour will express only one of the two alleles (G6PDB in the Fig.), whereas samples of normal tissue will express a mixture of the two.

of this particular tumour. Added to this is the observation that this specific change has never been seen in a normal cell, and so the frequency with which it is produced must be exceedingly low. The fact that the Philadelphia chromosome is found in all CGL cells is further evidence of the clonality of this tumour, since the probability of that chromosomal mutation occurring independently two or more times in the same tissue must be negligible.

The majority of cancer causing agents, or carcinogens, are also mutagens, namely cause genetic mutations (see Chapter 7). One of the most widely used simple carcinogen screening tests is a test for mutagenicity using bacterial strains, the so called Ames test. Many agents act directly on DNA to cause genetic mutations and, in this case, there is often a good parallel between their mutagenic and their carcinogenic activity. There are, however, at least three important limitations to this approach for the detection of carcinogens. The first is that many carcinogens are turned into an active form in the body by various enzymes, in particular the P450 mixed-function oxidases of the liver. In these cases, unless these enzymes are provided, usually as a liver extract, the test will be negative. The second limitation is that some agents can cause genetic changes, for example by interfering with chromosome organization, in a way that cannot be detected by bacterial mutagenesis assays. The third limitation is that the tumour promoters, which are chemicals that on their own cannot initiate a cancer, but which enormously increase the probability of a cancer developing once a cell is initiated, work by different mechanisms that cannot be detected by bacterial or other mutagenesis assays (see Chapter 7).

There are a number of rare inherited diseases that involve an inability to repair damaged DNA and so increase the mutation or chromosomal damage rates. These inherited syndromes are associated with marked increases in susceptibility to cancer (see later on).

A final piece of evidence for genetic changes in tumour cells comes from the exciting studies on oncogenes, mainly those identified in the oncogenic viruses. Using recombinant DNA techniques, specific genetic changes in the normal versions of the oncogenes have been demonstrated in a number of human and animal tumours, as discussed in several of the chapters in this book, especially Chapters 10 and 11.

The general notion that changes in gene expression in somatic cells, mostly due to mutation (which in the broadest sense includes, for example, chromosome translocation), underlie the origin of cancer, unites the major fundamental ideas about its causes. Mutation, chromosome changes, the effects of viruses, novel determinants on the surface of tumour cells and changes in the pattern of expression of differentiated gene products are all subsumed, in one way or another, under this general hypothesis, for which there is increasing direct experimental evidence.

Many lines of evidence suggest that tumour progression is a multistep process, presumably involving several successive genetic changes (see Chapter 7). Analysis of the increase in incidence of cancer as a function of age has been used by Doll, Armitage, Peto, and others to provide approximate estimates for the number of steps involved, which come to about four or five, at least for the carcinomas. This can, however, be no more than a very rough guess at the number of steps, and such estimates cannot clearly distinguish between genetic and epigenetic changes. One problem is that a single genetic change, for example in the control of a series of genes involved in a differentiation pathway, may lead to multiple changes in gene expression in one step. A possible example of this is intestinal metaplasia in the gastric epithelium. Intestinal metaplasia describes a focal region of the gastric epithelium which takes on, often almost completely, the phenotype of the intestine rather than the stomach. It is as if a switch has been thrown which changes the pattern of epithelial differentiation from that of the stomach to that of the intestine. This can be identified by a whole series of differences in gene expression associated with the intestinal phenotype. The significance of these lesions is that they appear to be the precursors to the vast majority of gastric carcinomas. Each change in gene expression during the progression from the initial cell to the final malignant tumour must give rise to a selective advantage, in terms of enhanced growth rate or independence of growth from the effects of the immediate environment of the tumour. Otherwise the change would not be seen in all, or at least a substantial fraction, of the cells of the tumour. In this sense, tumour progression is an evolutionary process at the somatic level within the individual. Heterogeneity within a tumour can clearly arise both from different evolutionary sublines within any given tumour, and also from variations in expression associated with environmentally determined differences in the stage of residual differentiation of the cells within a tumour.

5.3 General nature of inherited susceptibility

Mechanisms underlying inherited susceptibilities to cancer must be consistent with the general views described above as to its nature at the cellular level. There are, in principle, two basic types of mechanisms which can underlie an inherited susceptibility. The first could be through an influence on the particular cells from which a certain type of tumour is derived, and this can be thought of as essentially a tissue specific influence. The second may be through systemic effects, for example on the frequency with which mutations arise due to environmental effects, or on the efficiency with which potential carcinogens are metabolized. While the former mechanism should influence susceptibility to a particular form of cancer, the latter in principle may give rise to inherited susceptibility to a wide range of cancers.

In 1971 Knudson pointed out that there should be some relationship between the genetic changes in a somatic cell that give rise to a cancer and changes in these same genes in the germ line, which will be passed on in the usual way from parent to offspring following Mendelian laws of inheritance. This follows from the fact that, when one of the particular genetic changes involved in initiation or progression of a tumour occurs in the germ line, all the somatic cells of an individual who has inherited this particular change will already carry one of the steps required for malignant change. This should increase the chance that a tumour will develop in such an individual, and so lead to an inherited susceptibility to that particular cancer. Clearly, there could be such inherited changes which would involve, e.g., growth factors or their receptors, in a way that influenced the development of a variety of different tumours. In this sense, such a mechanism need not necessarily be tissue specific. Knudson emphasized that a corollary of these ideas was that identification of the gene involved in such an inherited susceptibility would also pinpoint a gene that might be involved in somatic changes in the same sort of tumour even when there was not an inherited susceptibility.

Retinoblastoma, a tumour of the eye in children, is a good example of the application of these ideas. About 40 per cent of cases of retino-blastoma occur as a clear-cut, dominantly inherited Mendelian condition. The remainder are sporadic, in the sense that their first degree relatives (parents, siblings, or grandchildren) have a very low increased risk of getting retinoblastoma. The inherited, or familial, cases are most often bilateral, while the sporadic cases are often unilateral and in this sense less severe. Knudson argued that the familial cases of retinoblastoma were those in which one of the genetic changes essential for the development of the tumour was already inherited through the germ line. He also argued that the change in the tumour was recessive, so that the relevant gene on both homologous chromosomes had to be mutated. In the inherited form, one of the genes was already mutated and so only one further mutation, in the normal gene on the homologous chromosome, was needed for the development of the tumour. In the sporadic cases, on the other hand, independent mutational events in both homologous genes were required, and this had a very low chance of occurring. Hence the difference between the inherited and sporadic forms. Recently, as described in Chapter 11, these ideas have received dramatic support from chromosomal, genetic and molecular studies. Thus, from the obser-vation that a proportion of the familial cases were associated with a specific abnormality on chromosome 13, it was eventually shown that all familial cases were probably due to a mutation at the relevant position on chromosome 13, while the tumours themselves, whether from a familial or a sporadic case, were recessive for a genetic change at this same position on chromosome 13. This clearly shows how the exceptional and rare familial cases with the chromosome 13 abnormality have provided the clue to identifying the position of a genetic change that takes place in all retinoblastomas, whether familial or sporadic.

Colonic tumours, in contrast, are amongst the most common of the carcinomas. However, in a rare dominantly inherited disease called poly-posis coli (Fig. 5.2), affected individuals have very large numbers of polyps, on average about a thousand, in the large intestine. These polyps

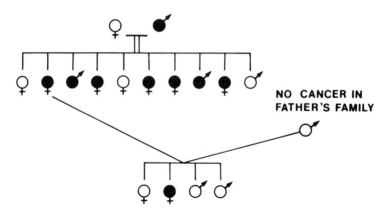

Fig. 5.2 Pedigree of the first clear-cut reported case of polyposis coli (Lockhart-Mummery, 1925, *Lancet* **i**, 427).
Filled in circles—affected.
Open circles   —unaffected.
The disease is passed down through three generations from one affected parent.
The pattern of inheritance is characteristic for a dominantly inherited trait.

progress to carcinomas with a high probability, so that almost invariably an untreated individual with polyposis coli develops one or more colon carcinomas. Fortunately, early screening of individuals from affected families can identify the polyps at a stage when they can be removed prophylactically and so development of a carcinoma can nearly always be prevented. So far, there are few clues to possible chromosome abnormalities associated with these tumours, but extensive family studies are now being carried out to identify the gene involved, using molecular techniques, as will be described later. Following Knudson's ideas and the lead from retinoblastoma, it may be hoped that the gene for polyposis coli, once identified, will also be a gene which is mutated in many non-familial colon carcinomas.

There are many examples of individually rare instances of clear-cut inherited susceptibilities to particular cancers. Each of these cases may be of fundamental interest in providing a clue to the genetic changes in non-familial cancers, even though the overall contribution to the incidence of cancer from these inherited susceptibilities is very small.

The best example of a systemic effect leading to an inherited susceptibility to cancer is the recessively inherited xeroderma pigmentosum, which is due to a deficiency in the ability to repair DNA. Xeroderma pigmentosum (XP) is characterized by a susceptibility to sunlight induced abnormalities of the skin, frequently followed by malignant skin cancer. Cells from individuals with the disease are unusually sensitive to the lethal effects of ultraviolet light and certain types of carcinogens, because they have defects in their ability to repair damaged DNA. It is now known that there are several different forms of the disease, probably due to different genetic mutations having similar effects. It seems likely that the reason why XP individuals predominantly get malignant skin cancers is that this tissue is most exposed to a mutagen, the ultraviolet light in sunlight. This exposure probably far exceeds that of internal organs from ingested mutagens, to which XP individuals would also be sensitive. There are, in fact, reports of patients with internal tumours. Several other diseases are also thought to be associated with DNA repair defects, or other related defects, giving rise to sensitivity to ultraviolet light or other carcinogens, and all of these appear to be associated with a very significantly increased susceptibility to cancer. Notable amongst these disorders are ataxia telangiectasia, which is now also known to be a collection of diseases associated with different mutations, Fanconi's anaemia and Bloom's syndrome (a multiple abnormality associated with sensitivity to sunlight and immune deficiency). These are all recessively inherited syndromes, probably involving some aspect of DNA repair leading to increased chromosome breakage and multiple abnormalities.

Inherited variations in the activity of enzymes that metabolize potential carcinogens are another source of inherited systemic suscepti-bilities to cancer. Amongst the best known such enzymes are the mono-oxygenases, or cytochrome P450 enzymes. These enzymes are known to metabolize many substances from inert into reactive, or carcinogenic, compounds. Thus, in the mouse there are differences between inbred strains in the level of the enzyme aryl hydrocarbon hydroxylase, which acts on certain hydrocarbons turning them into potent mutagens and carcinogens. These differences have been shown to be associated with differential effects of these hydrocarbons on the rate of tumour induc-tion. Similar studies in man were initially promising and suggested a single gene difference in susceptibility to induction of lung tumours by cigarette smoking, but these observations have not been confirmed. More recently data involving another analogous system have been published which looks very convincing (see Chapter 4).

Inherited variations in various P450 enzyme activities are associated in man with differential responses to a wide variety of drugs. This is due to the fact that the activity of the drugs is modified by these enzymes. One example studied by Smith and his collaborators involves differences in the ability to metabolize the drug debrisoquine. About 10 per cent of the population metabolize this drug slowly and so have severe side effects when given the drug at therapeutic doses. This reaction appears to be associated with a recessively inherited difference in the relevant hydroxyl-ating enzyme, the susceptible individuals being homozygous for a less active form of the enzyme. A controlled study of cigarette smokers with and without lung cancer has shown a striking six-fold lower frequency of the slow metabolizers of debrisoquine amongst lung cancer cases. If confirmed, this would be a most important example of an inherited systemic susceptibility to the carcinogenic effects of an environmental agent, cigarette smoke, due to differences in rates of carcinogen metabolism.

A third major example of inherited systemic effects concerns immune response differences. The major human histocompatibility (HLA) system controls two main sets of cell surface determinants which are involved in interactions between lymphocytes and other cells in the control of the immune response. The system is highly polymorphic, that is there are many differences between individuals with respect to the cell surface determinants; these differences make it necessary to match individuals for organ transplantation. HLA differences have also been shown to be associated with a variety of autoimmune or immune related disease, such as juvenile onset, insulin dependent diabetes mellitus, rheumatoid arthritis and ankylosing spondylitis, most probably through inherited differences in specific immune responses. A number of associations between HLA and different cancers have been suggested, most notably with nasopharyngeal carcinoma (NPC) and Kaposi's sarcoma, although in no case is the association as striking as that with the clear-cut autoimmune or immune related diseases. In the case of both NPC, associated with the Epstein Barr virus, and Kaposi's sarcoma, associated with a human T cell leukaemia virus, an inherited immune response difference to the virus or virally induced cellular determinants is a plausible mechanism for an inherited difference in susceptibility to the cancer. The association between HLA and Hodgkin's disease is described later.

5.4 Types of family data and their interpretation

The simplest inherited susceptibilities are those, such as retinoblastoma, polyposis coli, the DNA repair deficiencies and other inherited systemic susceptibilities, that follow a clear-cut Mendelian pattern of inheritance. In such cases, the nature of the genetic control is not in question, and the challenge is to identify the specific genes involved and interpret their functions at the molecular level. There are, however, many examples of inherited susceptibilities which are not so easy to interpret. For example, the associations of debrisoquine slow metabolizers or HLA variants and particular cancers were not identified through family studies, but by looking at the distribution of a particular genetic difference in patients with a given sort of cancer as compared to controls.

The classical approach to assessing a potential inherited contribution to a disease, in the absence of clear-cut Mendelian segregation, is to establish to what extent there is an increased incidence of the disease amongst the relatives of affected individuals. Often this involves specifically the study of twins, contrasting identical with non identical twins. If there is a major inherited component, then the disease incidence amongst coidentical twins of affected twins, the concordance, should be greater than that amongst conon identical twins. This is because the former share all their genes, while the latter on average share only half their genes, just as do any brothers or sisters. Studying twins brought up in the same household tends to average out the effects of environment. Twin studies tend to show a slightly increased concordance of cancer amongst identical as compared to non identical twins, but the effect is marginal and the data very hard to obtain. More generally, studies on the incidence of particular forms of cancer amongst relatives of patients as compared to that in the general population have often indicated an approximately two- to four-fold increase in incidence amongst relatives especially for breast and childhood cancers. It is, however, very difficult to interpret these relatively modest increases as necessarily due to genetic factors, since relatives also tend to share a common environment and this clearly could have a similar effect on incidence amongst relatives as do genetic factors. Thus, while such studies may suggest a limited genetic contribution to overall inherited susceptibility to certain cancers, they do not provide clear-cut answers and offer little or no prospect for further investigation.

Another approach to the problem of sorting out inherited susceptibilities, especially for the comparatively common cancers such as breast and colon cancer for which it is clear that the majority of cases do not show an obvious inherited component, is to ask whether there is, nevertheless, a subset of cases that tend to cluster in families. This would indicate a minority of cases associated with a clearly inherited susceptibility. Occasional very striking examples of clusters of cancers within a single family have often been described, and an example is shown in Figure 5.3. The difficulty with this approach is in assessing whether the familial clustering is really significant. Obviously for a relatively common cancer, some cases will cluster in families simply by chance, and appropriate statistical methods must be used to distinguish these from familial clustering due to Mendelian segregation of a gene associated with an increased susceptibility. Statistical models for the expected distribution of different genetic types can be fitted to such families, but such models rarely provide a clear-cut answer to the interpretation of familial clusters.

The study of familial clustering as a basis for identifying inherited susceptibilities is also subject to another major difficulty. This is the fact,

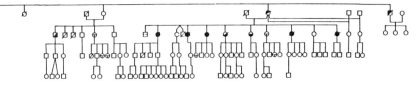

Fig. 5.3 Pedigree of a family with multiple cases of cancer (personal communication from Drs. S. Cartwright and J. G. Bodmer).
Circles=females; ◕ carcinoma cervix; ◔ carcinoma liver; ● carcinoma breast; ◕ carcinoma stomach; ⊕ cervical dysplasia; ⊕ ovarian cysts.
Squares=males; ■ carcinoma bronchus; ◢ skin basal cell carcinoma; ⊟ papilloma bladder.
A diagonal slash through the symbol symbolizes death of the individual.

easily demonstrated, that even if a disease does not show any obvious familial clustering, it may nevertheless have a major genetic component. Suppose, for example, there exists a dominant gene which increases the chance of getting a particular form of cancer by a factor of 10, say from one in a thousand to one in a hundred. If the gene is rare, then in most families where it occurs it will only occur once in one of the parents. Then, for example, only in $(1/100)^2 = 1/10\ 000$ of such families with two offspring will both of them have the cancer, and the chance that a sib of an affected sib will be affected is only $1/200$. Even if the gene gives rise to a 10 per cent chance of getting the cancer, only 1 per cent of families with two children with the gene present once in either parent will have pairs of affected sibs. Nevertheless, even when the gene frequency is as low as 0.05 per cent, it could still be contributing as much as 50 per cent to the total incidence of the particular form of cancer with which it is associated. Here, one would have a situation where a particular gene was responsible for 50 per cent of the incidence of one form of cancer, and yet because only 10 per cent of the people with the gene get the cancer, there would be very few examples of familial clustering. However, in those families where pairs of sibs are affected, most pairs will both carry the relevant susceptibility gene. And it is this that provides the clue to the objective study of such inherited susceptibilities. Because, if an inherited Mendelian marker difference can be found for a gene that is reasonably close to the one actually causing the inherited cancer susceptibility, then this marker will also tend to be associated with pairs of affected sibs. In other words, if one finds a genetic marker whose distribution amongst affected pairs of sibs is distorted as compared to Mendelian segregation, then this marker must be linked to a gene causing an inherited susceptibility.

This principle can be illustrated using the example of HLA and Hodgkin's disease. A weak association between certain HLA markers and Hodgkin's disease was first observed in 1967 by Amiel. This was subsequently confirmed by many other studies, but its significance is only due to the fact that the association was studied so extensively. The maximum relative risk, a simple measure of the relative increase in the frequency of a particular HLA determinant amongst people with Hodgkin's disease as compared to controls, was only about 1.3–1.6 as compared, for example, to relative risks of close to 100 or more for the association of HLA type B27 with ankylosing spondylitis. Now, although the vast majority of cases of Hodgkin's disease are sporadic, a small proportion, perhaps up to 3 per cent of cases, occur in families with two or more affected individuals. Within such families, HLA typing can establish whether the affected pairs of sibs with Hodgkin's disease are HLA identical (namely have inherited the same HLA chromosome complement from each parent), share only one HLA chromosome but not the other, or have neither chromosome in common. The expected frequency of these three situations on the assumption of Mendelian segregation, and in the absence of any association within the families between HLA and Hodgkin's disease, is 1:2:1. Overall, amongst 32 sib pairs studied in this way, 16 were found to be HLA identical, 11 shared one HLA chromosome and 5 none, a highly significant departure from the expected Mendelian 1:2:1 or 8:16:8. The data thus clearly show an association between the HLA segregation in the families and Hodgkin's disease. This is exactly as expected if there is a gene in, or close to, the HLA region which confers susceptibility to Hodgkin's disease. Thus, in the case of Hodgkin's disease, the family data provide the most convincing evidence for an association with the HLA system. This approach can clearly be generalized to any situation where there is more than one member of a family with Hodgkin's disease. The question asked is whether the HLA distribution is distorted amongst the individuals with Hodgkin's disease, as compared to what could be expected from the normal pattern of Mendelian segregation.

The HLA system was originally chosen for study in the case of Hodgkin's disease because of the association between the mouse H2 system (the equivalent to HLA) and certain types of virally induced leukaemias. For most examples of familial clustering of cancer, there is no such clue as to which genetic marker should be studied. In this case all that one can advocate is a systematic search for a genetic marker which is distorted in its segregation amongst individuals with cancer in the family. While this may seem a haphazard approach the range of genetic markers available for such studies is now vastly increased using recombinant DNA techniques (see Chapter 11), and so such systematic surveys are becoming a realistic possibility. Through them it should be possible to identify, for any significant familial clustering of an inherited cancer susceptibility, one or more genetic markers sufficiently close to the gene actually causing the susceptibility. Such a gene would be detected by a distortion in its expected Mendelian segregation amongst the individuals in the family who have cancer. In my view, this is now the only satisfactory way of establishing an inherited susceptibility, other than finding the gene which itself gives rise to that inherited susceptibility.

5.5 Genetic markers, DNA polymorphisms and genetic linkage

The human genes are distributed amongst the 23 pairs of human chromosomes. Genes on different chromosomes are combined and passed on at random from parent to offspring. Thus if an individual is heterozygous A1/A2 at one locus, and B1/B2 at a second locus on a different chromosome, then the combinations A1B1, A1B2, A2B1, and A2B2 are each passed on with a frequency of, on average, a quarter to each offspring. Suppose, on the other hand, that the A and B loci are on the same chromosome, so that, e.g., one of the pairs of homologous chromosomes in an individual carries A1B1 while the other carries A2B2. Then, if the genes are sufficiently close together, the combinations A1B1 and A2B2 will be passed on to the offspring more frequently than the 'recombinant' combinations A1B2 and A2B1. The frequency with which these recombinant, non–parental types are passed on is called the recombination fraction (r), and is an empirical measure of the distance between the A and B genes on the chromosome. The recombination fraction is thus less than half when genes are sufficiently close together on the same chromosome, and the genes are then said to be linked (see Table 5.1). Suppose for example the A1,A2 difference is the one that determines an inherited susceptibility to cancer, while the B1,B2 difference can be directly observed, as can for example the inherited HLA types. Then the latter difference B1,B2 is said to be a marker difference, and it will be distorted in its distribution amongst individuals in a family with cancer due to the linkage between the A and the B genes. Thus the closer together the two genes are the smaller is the recombination fraction r, and the greater will be the distortion in the distribution of the marker difference B1,B2 amongst individuals with cancer. For example, suppose A1 is a dominant susceptibility gene. Then, when linkage is close and the recombination fraction, r, very small, almost all the affected offspring of an A1B1/A2B2 individual will carry the B1 marker, whereas in the absence of linkage only one half would be expected to.

This is the general principle which underlies the analysis of the association between HLA and Hodgkin's disease discussed above. Clearly, the ability to detect a distortion in the marker distribution amongst individuals with cancer in families will be a function of how close the marker happens to be to the susceptibility gene. In practice, even a recombination fraction of 10 per cent would readily allow the detection of a segregation distortion. It can be calculated that approximately 250 markers regularly spaced at a 10 per cent recombination fraction interval are needed to cover the complete human chromosome set. This, therefore, in principle would be the maximum number of markers needed to be tested on a set of families in order to find one or more sufficiently close to the gene actually causing an inherited susceptibility for it to be identified.

Table 5.1 Linkage and recombination

	Parent	Gametic (egg or sperm) combinations			
No linkage	A1 B1 A2 B2	A1B1, A2B2, A2B1, A1B2 passed on to offspring with equal frequencies of $\frac{1}{4}$			
		Parental		Recombinant	
Linkage	A1B1* A2B2	A1B1	A2B2	A1B2	A2B1
	frequencies	$\frac{1}{2}(1-r)$	$\frac{1}{2}(1-r)$	$\frac{1}{2}r$	$\frac{1}{2}r$

A1, A2, and B1, B2 are alleles at loci A and B respectively.

*The line separating A1B1 from A2B2 indicates that A1B1 are together on one chromosome and A2B2 on the other.

r is the 'recombination fraction'; the smaller is r the fewer recombinants are produced, and the closer together are the genes A and B. When, on the other hand, r is $\frac{1}{2}$, the result is as if there were no linkage.

In the past such studies have been done using blood groups and enzyme differences, but the number of such differences is limited. Now, however, using recombinant DNA techniques a potentially unlimited source of genetic markers can be produced. Using a cloned DNA probe, differences in the sequence with which it is associated can be identified using restriction enzymes that cut the DNA at particular short sequences, together with the technique known as Southern blotting (Chapter 10). The incidence of differences between individuals at the DNA level is such that there should be no difficulty in finding a set of genetic differences (restriction enzyme fragment polymorphisms, see Chapter 11) that covers all the chromosomes at a reasonable recombination interval. These differences can now be used systematically in cancer families to look for markers that are associated with, or closely linked to, genes giving rise to inherited susceptibility to cancer.

5.6 Future prospects

Although inherited susceptibility to cancer may contribute no more than 20 per cent of overall cancer incidence, nevertheless this is both an important contribution in its own right and can help to provide major clues to the fundamental underlying causes of cancer, and to approaches for its prevention and treatment. Tissue specific inherited changes can provide clues to genetic changes taking place during tumour progression in non–inherited cancers. Inherited susceptibilities connected with systemic effects, such as deficiencies in DNA repair, carcinogen metabolism and immune response, provide major clues to potentially controllable environmental factors which cause cancer. In all cases, the ultimate challenge is to identify the particular genetic differences and their functional basis.

The use of DNA polymorphisms to find markers linked to cancer susceptibility genes in principle provides an avenue to the eventual identification of the susceptibility gene itself. The more closely the marker is associated within families with the cancer, the more likely it is to be near to the responsible gene and the greater the chance that eventually this gene may itself be identified. The technical problems are still formidable, but the rate of progress in recombinant DNA technology is such that one must surely expect the problem to be solved within the forseeable future. In some cases, an intelligent guess may provide a clue once the chromosomal region within which a susceptibility gene lies has been identified. This proved, quite dramatically, to be the case for the identification of the involvement of the c-*myc* oncogene in Burkitt's lymphoma cells and c-*abl* in chronic granulocytic leukaemia (see Chapters 3 and 11). Clearly, another set of genes worth investigating in great detail for their potential contribution to inherited cancer susceptibility are those for all the various P450 like mono-oxygenases (see Chapter 17). Sooner or later the genes for the DNA repair deficiency syndromes will also be identifed, and then the question of whether there is an increased risk of cancer associated with an individual who carries just one copy of a defective gene will become amenable to analysis using linked DNA polymorphisms. Hopefully, in the case of polyposis coli, a combination of cellular and molecular experiments looking for oncogenes in colorectal carcinoma cells together with marker linkage studies in the polyposis coli syndrome, might provide clues to the particular genetic changes involved in colon carcinomas.

A genetic marker that is reasonably closely linked to an inherited susceptibility may have considerable practical value even if it does not immediately lead to the identification of the specific genetic function involved in the susceptibility. First of all, such a marker may help to recognize heterogeneity in the predisposition, since different subsets of susceptibles may show different patterns of linkage to different genetic markers. Second, within families, the linked marker defines a high risk group, the identification of which may be very valuable. For example, individuals identified as being at high risk may be treated prophylactically, as is now the case for polyposis coli. Such individuals may also be useful for studies of the physiology of the difference between high and low risk groups, which should help to identify the underlying functional basis for a particular inherited susceptibility. It may also be possible to do case control studies comparing high and low risk groups within families, in order to identify factors that may interact with a genetic predisposition.

Sooner or later we shall have essentially the whole DNA sequence of the human genes and some definition of all the basic functional units. When this situation is reached, having found a linked marker for a particular inherited susceptibility, it may be possible simply to look up the genes with relevant functions that are in its neighbourhood, and through that, focus onto the actual genetic difference responsible for the inherited susceptibility. There can be no doubt that the application of recombinant DNA techniques, coupled with epidemiological and genetic studies, will in due course unravel the genetic contribution to the initiation and progression of cancers both at the germ line and somatic cell levels.

Further reading

Ayesh, R., Idle, J. R., Ritchie, J. C., Crothers, M. J., and Hetzel, M. R. (1984). Metabolic oxidation phenotypes as markers for susceptibility to lung cancer. *Nature* **312**, 169–70.
The paper on the association between debrisoquine metabolism and lung cancer due to cigarette smoking.

Bodmer, W. F. (ed.) (1982). Inheritance of susceptibility to cancer in man. *Cancer Surveys* **1**, 1–186.
Contains a range of articles covering most of the topics surveyed in this chapter.

Harnden, D., Morten, J., and Featherstone, T. (1984). Dominant susceptibility to cancer in man. *Advances in Cancer Research* **141**, 185–245.
A recent review of certain aspects of inherited susceptibility to cancer.

McKusick, V. (1983). *Mendelian genetics in man* (6th Edition). Johns Hopkins University Press, Baltimore.
The standard reference catalogue for inherited human diseases, including cancer.

Mulvihill, J. J., Miller, R. W., and Fraumeni, J. F. Jr. (eds.) (1977). *The genetics of human cancer.* Raven Press, New York.

An earlier collection of papers on cancer genetics which is still a very useful survey.

Omenn, G. S., and Gelboin, H. V. (eds.) (1984). *Genetic variability in response to chemical exposures,* The Banbury Report **16**. Cold Spring Harbor Laboratory, Cold Spring Harbor, New York.

A useful collection of papers on a whole variety of aspects of inherited differences in drug metabolism and their relationship to cancer incidence.

6

Structure of DNA and its relationship to carcinogenesis

BEVERLY E. GRIFFIN

6.1 Introduction

Cells and the intracellular substances secreted by them make up the structural elements of the body. Within the nucleus of the cell resides its genetic information in the form of the polymeric material, deoxyribonucleic acid, or DNA. The integrity of this DNA is essential for the proper functioning of cells, their interactions and, following naturally from this, the health of the whole organism. (There are a few well-documented exceptions to DNA as the repository of genetic information. Some viruses carry their genetic information in ribonucleic acids, or RNA (see Chapter 9). Among these are viruses, designated *retroviruses*, that warrant serious consideration in any discussion about the genesis of cancer in avian and mammalian species. They code for an enzyme that converts their genomic RNA into DNA, which provides the origin of the term 'retro' or backward flow of information.)

Simplistically, the history of the study of DNA might be divided into 'seven ages'. First was the age of the medical investigator, with the discovery by Miescher and colleagues in Germany over a century ago of a material in pus cells designated by them 'nuclein'. Their finding alerted the scientific world to the existence of a hitherto unknown, and possibly important, cellular component. The second age, that of the chemist, was necessary to provide the definition of the component parts of DNA (and RNA), their chemical nature, and how they are linked to make up the polymeric species. Following this comes the age of the geneticist and the discovery that DNAs, and not the previously suspected proteins, contain the genetic information essential for the continuity of any particular organism. In the fourth age the molecular biologist defined the mechanisms by which DNA could pass on its genetic information. From this group of scientists came the concept of the linear relationship whereby DNA specifies the structure of RNA which in turn specifies proteins (the so called 'central dogma' of molecular biology) and the concept of a triplet genetic code (see on). The virologist provided many of the material and experimental designs for testing hypotheses proposed by molecular biologists and for identifying regulatory mechanisms that control gene expression, both quantitatively and qualitatively. The sixth age of DNA, that of the present, belongs to the biotechnologists and genetic engineers who are rapidly turning academic exercises into practical reality, manipulating genes and their expression at will in the cause of medical or commercial progress, and in turn providing tools for probing the details of the biology of normal and abnormal cells. This 'history of DNA' should not end like the famous Shakespearean diatribe on the 'seven ages of man', terminating in 'second childishness and mere oblivion, sans teeth, sans eyes, sans taste, sans everything'. Rather, one would predict optimistically that the 'seventh age of DNA' will complete the circle, returning to the cell and the cell biologist, who can now draw on all the knowledge acquired over the last 100 or so years (as outlined briefly in the discussion that follows) to unravel the intricate interactions, balances and counterbalances in the normal cell, and contrast them with lesions that give rise to the malignant cell.

We now know that each specific character in an organism is coded by a gene, a unit of genetic information, which produces its effect by specifying the production of its particular protein. The genes consist of long strands of DNA (see on) arranged in a very specific order. The DNA exists in close association with a group of proteins also arranged in an ordered manner with the protein molecules acting as wedges which have the correct shape to form the strands into coils. The structural unit is a nucleosome (Fig. 6.1) which is made up of a short length of DNA (about 200 nucleotide pairs—see on) associated with a protein core of histones. The nucleosomes are attached to each other by a short piece of linker DNA (about 60 base pairs) like strings of beads which are themselves organized into coils or supercoils by associated non-histone proteins. Individual nucleosomes in themselves are too small to be genes (the average gene is thought to be about 1000 nucleotide pairs) and act as packing devices. When the genes are inactive, the DNA and protein molecules are closely packed. When the genes are active, that is, being transcribed (see on), the protein DNA complex opens up to allow the

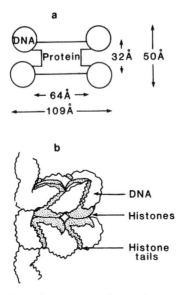

Fig. 6.1 Diagram showing substructure of a nucleosome. DNA strands in the nucleosome surround a core of histones, and are continuous with linker strands of DNA above and below; (a) cross section along axis, (b) from the side (from Richards *et al.* 1977, *Cell Biol. Inter. Rep.* **1**, 107–15).

process of gene expression to take place. Alterations in cell behaviour may be brought about by changes in the structure of the DNA—mutation—or by perturbations in the mechanisms which control gene expression. Although we now have a great deal of information on changes in DNA structure and their relationships to neoplastic development (to be discussed in this Chapter), our knowledge of gene expression control is much more limited. Research in this area and into the relationship between mutation and gene expression should ultimately lead to a better understanding of cancer and of its control.

6.2 Components of DNA

DNA is made up of three relatively simple chemical species, namely, four heterocyclic (nitrogenous) bases, a five carbon atom sugar (deoxyribose), and phosphoric acid. The bases themselves are of two types, one a six membered ring species designated a 'pyrimidine', and the other a fused five and six membered ring species designated a 'purine'. By convention, pyrimidines as classes are abbreviated as Y, purines as R, and the rings are numbered as shown in Figure 6.2. In spite of their apparent simplicity, purines and pyrimidines have the capacity for determining many of

	FORMULA	NAME

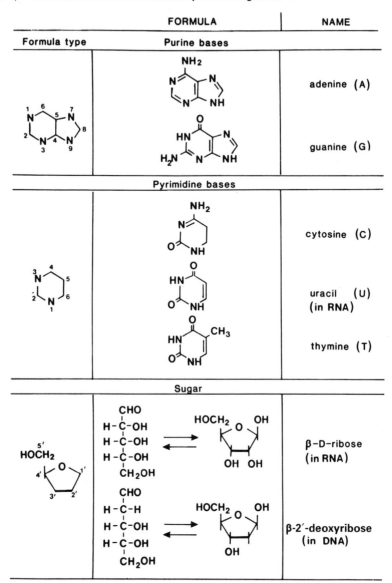

Fig. 6.2 Structures, numbering systems and abbreviations of the heterocyclic (nitrogenous) bases, and five carbon sugar moieties that are found in DNA and RNA. The numbering system currently in use for the six membered pyrimidine ring is to be regretted, since the original system wherein the corresponding rings in both purines and pyrimidines were numbered alike is a simpler system. Further, it was that used in the classical hydrolytic studies of Chargaff where he showed that, regardless of the system used for isolation of DNA, or its overall base content, there was a conserved correspondence between the ratios of A:T

the physical and biological properties of individual DNAs. Thus, it is important to understand their chemistry. The structures of the two pyrimidine residues, cytosine (C) and thymine (T), that exist in DNA are shown in Figure 6.2. Theoretically, both these species can exist in a number of tautomeric forms (see on), although the isomer shown in the figure is that normally found in DNA. Nonetheless, it is relevant to consider the other forms, as illustrated for cytosine (Fig. 6.3), since pyrimidines

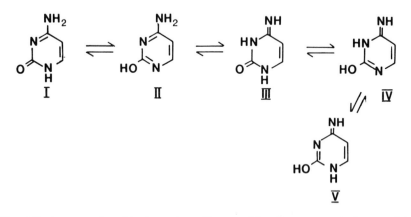

Fig. 6.3 An example of tautomerism, illustrated by the tautomeric forms of the pyrimidine base, cytosine. Form I is that commonly found in DNA, but forms III and V are also theoretically capable of existing under suitable conditions. Similar tautomeric forms can exist for the other bases that make up DNA (or RNA) and can often be 'trapped' as such by mutagenic and carcinogenic reagents.

trapped in one of these alternatives (as for examples by alkylation) can lead to mutations in DNA. The various species result from a simple form of keto–enol (or imino–amino) tautomerism, that is, the interconversion between a double bonded oxygen atom (=O) and its singly bonded hydroxyl (−OH) counterpart which occurs by shift of a pair of electrons and hydrogen moiety or, alternatively, by comparable mechanism, between an =NH and −NH$_2$ moiety.

Similarly, in the case of the two purines that make up DNA, guanine (G) and adenine (A), various tautomeric forms exist, but for native DNA,

and G:C. That is, the 'oxy' function in the 6 position of one purine was matched by a 6 amino function in the pyrimidine, and vice versa. This provided the basis for the well-known Watson Crick hypothesis of complementary structures in double-stranded DNA and ultimately to the 'double helix' of DNA.

The pentose sugar numbers carry a 'prime' designation when this moiety is linked to the bases, to distinguish them from numbers given to the latter.

those shown in Figure 6.2 persist. That is, for both pyrimidines and purines in DNA under normal circumstances the exocyclic oxygen atoms exist in the keto ($=O$) form, whereas the exocyclic nitrogens exist in an amino ($-NH_2$) form. This tautomeric preference in DNA can be altered, for example, by radical changes in pH or chemical modification, events frequently accompanied by important changes both in the physical and biological properties of the DNA.

Three of these heterocyclic bases, C, G, and A, also make up the building blocks of RNA. In the latter, however, the fourth residue, thymine (T), is replaced by a similar molecule designated uracil (U) that lacks a methyl group at position 5, for reasons that are not wholly understood. Similarly, in the DNA of many plants, 5 methylcytosine (5-MeC) is frequently found in place of cytosine (C), again for reasons that are yet to be defined, but may be related to the maintenance of fidelity of DNA. This base also occurs infrequently in mammalian DNA.

The role of modified or altered bases in DNA and RNA is clearly of great functional significance and may be important in control of gene expression in a cell. This is an area that is just beginning to be explored. In small RNA species called transfer (t) RNAs that are important in protein synthesis, many unusual modified bases are found as shown for one such tRNA in Figure 6.4. The relative absence of 'unusual' bases in DNA may reflect the fact that error free replication is vital to the maintenance of any specifics, and modifications could increase the likelihood of error.

In DNA (and RNA), the heterocyclic bases are covalently bound to the pentose sugar moiety, deoxyribose, via an N-glycosidic bond. This link traps the carbohydrate in one of its tautomeric forms, that of a β-D-deoxyribose, see Figure 6.2. (In RNA, the corresponding sugar moiety is β-D-ribose.) The combination of a heterocyclic base linked to the sugar is called a *nucleoside* (or deoxynucleoside), as shown (Fig. 6.5, see also Table 6.1).

The third component of DNA, phosphoric acid, is covalently linked to the pentose sugars by a phosphate ester bond to produce, initially, a *nucleotide*. Nucleotides *per se,* especially in the cases where the sugar component is ribose, have many functions in cells. For example, they further combine with other molecules of phosphoric acid to produce compounds (such as adenosine triphosphate) that act as energy sources in many biochemical reactions. They also combine with other organic molecules to produce coenzymes, or they cyclize to produce signalling molecules important in regulating cellular funtions.

A nucleotide, linked to another nucleoside via a phosphodiester bond, produces in an initial reaction a dinucleoside phosphate, which on phosphorylation gives a *dinucleotide*, part of the backbone of either DNA or RNA (see Fig. 6.5). The determination of the nature of the links

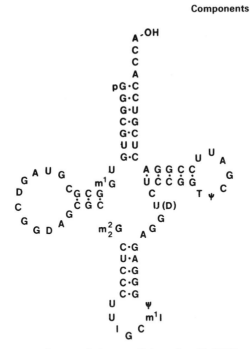

Fig. 6.4 The structure of one of the small transfer (t) RNAs, alanine tRNA, important in protein synthesis, showing some of the so-called 'minor bases' common to this kind of RNA, but not known to be ubiquitous in DNA or other RNA. Transfer RNAs carry amino acids to sites of protein synthesis on ribosomes. It can be seen that more than 10 per cent of this particular molecule is composed of bases such as methylated guanines (m^1G, M_2^2G) or inosine (I) which are not normal components of DNA. Similar types of modifications are found in other tRNAs. ψ is pseudouracil.

involved in generating these species was one of the important contributions of chemists of this field, since it provided the basis for our present understanding of the structure of DNA. It was found that the 5′ position of the deoxyribose in one nucleotide was covalently bound to the 3′ position of another by diester bonds with phosphoric acid (for number-

Table 6.1 Standard nomenclature

Base	Nucleoside	Abbreviation	Nucleotide
cytosine	(deoxy)cytidine	C	(deoxy)cytidylic acid
thymine	thymidine	T	thymidylic acid
(uracil)	(uridine)	(U)	(uridylic acid)
guanine	(deoxy)guanosine	G	(deoxy)guanylic acid
adenine	(deoxy)adenosine	A	(deoxy)adenylic acid

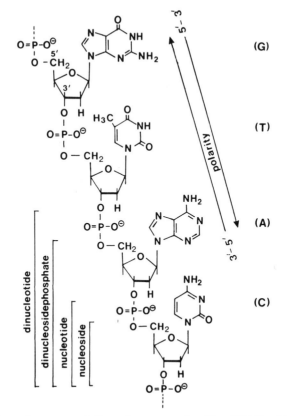

Fig. 6.5 Schematic representation of a tetranucleotide, GTAC, which illustrates the chemical linkages found in DNA, the terminology used to describe individual chemical entities and the concept of polarity, important in any consideration of the double-stranded nature of DNA. The polarity must also be known before the structure of a polypeptide (or protein) can be predicted from DNA sequence.

ing of the sugar, see Fig. 6.2). This linkage determines the polarity, sequence, and structure of the chain of molecules that compose nucleic acids, whether they be DNA or RNA (Fig. 6.5). It is interesting at this stage to note that for many years the macromolecular nature of DNA went unrecognized. Since only four major bases were evident from the hydrolysis of DNA, the compound was assumed to be a tetranucleotide and, as such, obviously lacked the capacity to be the genetic entity required even by the simplest of cells.

6.3 The genetic material

The DNA of most cells is double stranded. In the case of many bacterial phages and viruses, it is also circular. A polymer composed of nucleotide components with a 5'—3' polarity binds to another (complementary) polymer with a 3'—5' polarity to create the double-stranded DNA (Figs. 6.5 and 6.6). The recognition of the nature of the bonds that link one strand of a double-stranded DNA with its partner, and the fact that these bonds are very specific, provided the basis of the explanation of the mechanism by which DNA alone could encode genetic information. The groundwork for this important discovery came from analysis of the components released when DNA from a variety of sources was subjected to chemical hydrolysis. These experiments produced data which showed that although the base compositions, that is, the percentages of the various pyrimidines and purines, could vary enormously among species, a common relationship between bases was maintained such that the ratio of G:C or A:T always gave a figure that was about one. These data, together with X–ray crystallographic evidence that showed the regularity of the structures of DNA, led not only to the very important suggestion of the nature of the base pairing between strands of DNA and its specificity, but recognition by Crick and Watson of how this could explain the key biological role of DNA. A model of the 'double helix' that arose from these combined studies is shown schematically in Figure 6.6, wherein a C residue on one strand of DNA wherever it occurs is always 'paired' with a G residue on the opposite strand, likewise A with T (Fig. 6.7). The order in which the bases appear prescribes the genetic information. It is relevant to note that the bonds that link heterocyclic bases to sugars, and the latter to phosphates, are all covalent and as such very strong, requiring considerable energy to cleave. On the other hand, the so-called 'hydrogen bonds' (H bonds) that link one base residue to another to form double-stranded DNA are by their nature very weak bonds (less than 3 kcal of energy is generally sufficient to cleave a hydrogen bond as compared with more than 10 times this for the weakest covalent bond). The strength of the attachment between strands of DNA is in large part thus a consequence of the fact that many such H bonds are involved in the interaction between strands of DNA.

Biologically of great relevance is the fact that when, during mitosis, the strands of DNA separate and each single strand is then copied to reproduce double-stranded DNA, the specificity of base pairing ensures that a faithful, albeit complementary, replica of the coded DNA is made and the fidelity of the gene for future generations is maintained. If mistakes occur, however, as they do from time to time, normal cells have a variety of important functions that recognize individual errors and make the necessary repairs.

Following on the discovery of the mode by which fidelity of genetic information can be maintained was the elucidation of the mechanism by which the sequences of bases on any particular region of a strand of DNA could specify the sequence of amino acids in a corresponding

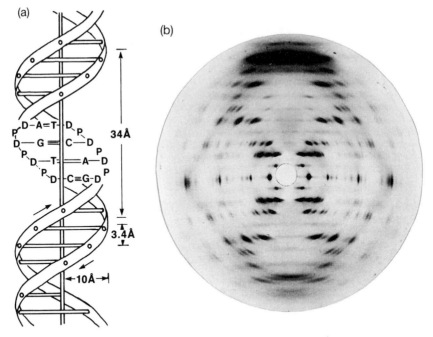

Fig. 6.6 (a) Schematic representation of the B form of double-stranded DNA, together with its dimension as derived from X–ray crystallographic analyses, and (b) its corresponding X–ray diffraction pattern (courtesy of Dr A. G. W. Leslie). Complementary bases (A and T, G and C) in opposing strands are held together by hydrogen bonds as shown (Fig. 6.7). This structure produces grooves of two different sizes in DNA, designated 'major' and 'minor', which can act as sites of entry to DNA by chemicals, enzymes, etc. (D represents the deoxyribose moiety, P phosphate, and A, G, T, C the respective heterocyclic bases).

protein, that is, how the genetic information is actually encoded within the DNA. The colinear relationship between DNA, RNA and proteins is such that (except in the case of retroviruses) a gene containing an 'anti-sense' version of information maintained in DNA, is faithfully copied into a complementary 'sense' version of a species of RNA known as a messenger (or mRNA) using the specific base pairing discussed above (that is, for example, CAT in DNA would specify AUG in mRNA). RNA messenger, using blocks of trinucleotide sequences as its code, in turn specifies the amino acids and their order in a protein. Why a 'triplet' code? There are only 20 essential amino acids and four distinct nucleotides, so a doublet code would be inadequate, whereas a triplet could specify 64 amino acids, or more than enough. The precise nature of the code, as worked out with mixtures of synthetic oligonucleotides, is shown in Table 6.2. Certain amino acids, for example methionine (MET), are

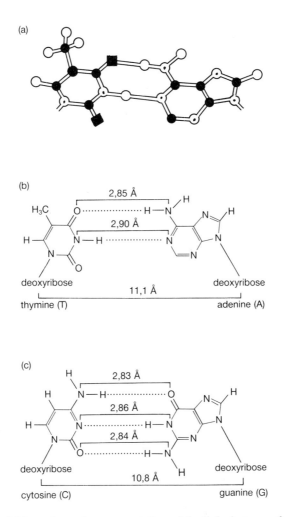

Fig. 6.7 Panel (a): a schematic representation of the links between the pyrimidine, thymine, and its purine complement, adenine. Panels (b) and (c): the hydrogen bonds formed between the base pairs T/A and C/G, respectively, and the distances found between the base links in double-stranded DNA. In general, the strength of a hydrogen bond is proportional to its distance. Here it is seen that not only are there three such bonds in the C/G partnership, but also that they are generally shorter. The energy required to separate these complementary bases is thus greater than that required for T/A base pairs. Hydrogen bonds determine the specificity that exists in DNA and can be considered the 'watchdogs' of fidelity during DNA replication or transcription of RNA.

Table 6.2 The genetic code

	U	C	A	G	
	PHE	SER	TYR	CYS	U
U	PHE	SER	TYR	CYS	C
	LEU	SER	STOP	STOP	A
	LEU	SER	STOP	TRP	G
	LEU	PRO	HIS	ARG	U
C	LEU	PRO	HIS	ARG	C
	LEU	PRO	GLN	ARG	A
	LEU	PRO	GLN	ARG	G
	ILE	THR	ASN	SER	U
A	ILE	THR	ASN	SER	C
	ILE	THR	LYS	ARG	A
	MET	THR	LYS	ARG	G
	VAL	ALA	ASP	GLY	U
G	VAL	ALA	ASP	GLY	C
	VAL	ALA	GLU	GLY	A
	VAL	ALA	GLU	GLY	G

The first letter of the triplet is in the left hand vertical column, the second in the horizontal axis and the third in the right hand vertical column.

only encoded (specified) by one particular triplet (in this case AUG). In other cases, the coding is 'degenerate' and more than one triplet can specify a given amino acid. For example, proline (PRO) is encoded with two C residues and a third base which can be either C, U, A or G. This degeneracy, together with the three triplets (UAG, UGA and UAA) that specify the termination of translation of a nucleotide triplet into an amino acid, is such that all 64 potential triplet codons play some role in the specification of protein structures. Although the frequency of usage of individual codons appears to be species specific, all are used. The universality of this code has only been challenged fairly recently with the discovery that triplets which normally specify translational 'stops' are used as coding sequences in some species, such as certain mito-chondrial DNA. The exceptions would appear to be rare however.

Space filling models of DNA usually represent it in its most stable (B) form. The dimensions of B form (Fig. 6.6) are derived from X–ray diffraction studies (similar studies suggest RNA exists in a less compact, or A form, type of helix). As far as is known, B DNA structurally repre-sents most of the DNA in a cell, and almost certainly that which is 'coding' (specifying proteins). However, for reasons not yet resolved, much of the DNA in a mammalian cell would appear to be not only non-coding but possibly irrelevant (or 'junk') DNA. Biologically, this is a difficult concept to accept with regard to highly conserved, and conservative, organisms. It seems more probable that such DNA, although not directly related to coding, has a function yet to be recognized. In this regard, it is interesting that experimental data suggest that certain specific DNA sequences, such as regular repeats of purines and pyrimidines, may specify alternative structural forms of DNA, which in turn might play roles in regulation of gene expression or other cellular functions which might be modulated by DNA, as well as in intracellular DNA recombination.

Before turning to other aspects of DNA, two further topics should be briefly noted. One concerns the remarkable solubility of this highly polymeric species. Since water solubility is not a common property of most highly polymerized materials, the explanation for the great solubility of DNA must lie in its capacity to form specific interactions with water. The phosphodiester bond generated by the interaction of phosphoric acid with hydroxyl groups of sugar residues in nucleosides creates not only the backbone for DNA, but leaves a single acidic residue on the phosphate moiety that at the normal pH of a cell should be negatively charged (Fig. 6.5). *In vivo*, this charge is neutralized by cations, such as Mg^{++}, to generate a macromolecular version of a 'salt' which is capable of interacting both electrostatically as well as via hydrogen bonding with water. In support of this notion, DNA isolated from cells is neutral and contains many molecules of water of hydration.

The second point is that DNA in the nucleus of a cell is not 'naked'. Rather, it is found in association with histones and other proteins to produce a characteristic and fairly regular chromatin structure (Fig. 6.1). Further organization of chromatin produces the highly ordered chromosome whose structures are specific and unique within each individual organism. It is interesting to note that the DNA of some viruses also appears to be organized as 'mini-chromosomes', which nonetheless have regions that do appear to be 'naked' and act as origins of DNA replication. Whether the same is true for higher organisms with regard to areas relevant to the initiation sites of DNA replication remains to be seen.

6.4 DNA damage

As earlier mentioned, many of the agents that produce mutations in DNA do so by altering the tautomeric form of a base (Fig. 6.3) such that inaccuracies occur during DNA replication, which may be reflected in the transcription of DNA into RNA. In many cases, these mutations may be 'silent' in that they occur in the 'wobble' allowed at the third base (degenerate) position of some of the triplet codons (Table 6.2). In other positions within a codon, mutations could lead to an alteration of protein structure which, if function were not thus impaired, might be allowed. In fact, such alterations can even lead to mutants with selective advantages over the 'wild type' species. Other alterations could be positively harmful and, if not repaired, ultimately lethal either to the cell or, in the case of cancer causing lesions, if such there are, to the whole organism. In addition to mutations produced by exogenous agents, such as certain organic and inorganic chemicals, X irradiation (see Chapters 7 and 8), etc., there is always a background level of mutation in a cell produced by the hydrolytic interaction of water itself with DNA. Such damages include hydrolytic cleavage of the glycosidic bond resulting in depurination (Fig. 6.8) or depyrimidination, and ultimately in strand breaks, or deamination of exocyclic amino groups. For example, cytosine converted to deoxyuracil (an abnormal base in DNA) by deamination would produce a 'mismatch' during DNA replication which could lead ulti-

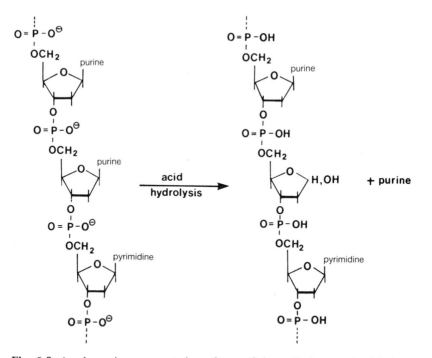

Fig. 6.8 A schematic representation of one of the well characterized lesions of DNA, that of depurination. Loss of a purine (or pyrimidine) base, if not repaired, can lead subsequently to DNA chain breaks.

mately to the concomitant alteration of the structure of protein. It has been calculated that the rate of release or purines from double-stranded DNA occurs at a rate of about $10^4/\text{day}/10^{10}$ bases (in rat liver cells), whereas depyrimidination occurs with slightly lower frequency (about $5 \times 10^2/\text{day}/10^{10}$ bases). Deamination proceeds marginally slower than depyrimidination. Were normal cells not endowed with a variety of mechanisms to combat such lesions, it can be seen that water alone could pose a serious threat to the accurate survival of genetic information. Hydrolysis could also lead directly to phosphodiester bond cleavage, disrupting the DNA backbone itself. Although theoretically possible, this mode of damage is not thought to be of great physiological relevance, although the alkylation of a phosphodiester (to a phosphotriester) could create a more labile substrate for hydrolysis. The role of phosphotriesters in DNA damage of mammalian DNA is only beginning to be investigated and its effect assessed.

Most cells have a limited capacity to correct lesions produced in DNA by exogenous or endogenous reagents. A variety of different repair processes have been identified, and some of them well characterized, at least in bacteria. There is no compelling evidence to suggest that higher organisms do not have repair processes comparable in type and in effect to those found in the better studied *E. coli.* In normal individuals, these processes must effectively compete with the background levels of mutations in DNA. It is obvious, however, that in individuals deficient (or defective) in one or more of the repair processes and probably in ageing individuals in general, this delicate balance can be disturbed, with deleterious consequences.

Many mutagens are also carcinogens (see Chapters 7 and 8). Some of the best studied agents that act on DNA are the simple alkylating agents, whose biological effect can be directly related to their site of action (Fig. 6.9). Some of the most damaging agents, which can be shown in animal models *in vivo* to induce tumour formation, are those that modify the oxygen moiety at the 6–position of guanine and lead to the creation of an unusual tautomeric form of this base in DNA. This modification alters two of the sites normally used in forming base pairs with cytosine, and can lead to a site specific error during DNA replication. Significant, and certainly of great biological importance for the individual, is the fact that by far the site most reactive to alkylating agents in DNA is, however, the N–7 position of guanine; lesions at this site, fortuitously, are essentially harmless since they have little effect on hydrogen bonding. Nonetheless, it can be seen how the build up of such lesions in DNA, by creating multiple positive charges, could be deleterious in other ways, and efficient repair pathways exist to remove N–7–methylguanine from DNA.

It has been shown by a variety of methods that during evolution trans-

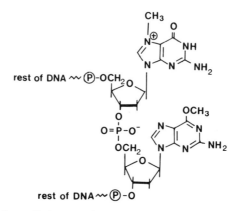

Fig. 6.9 Two of the well characterized lesions produced at guanine sites in DNA by simple alkylating agents. Modification of the N–7 position (on the 5 membered heterocyclic ring) generates a positively charged species, but is essentially 'silent' since it has no effect on base pairing in DNA. Conversely, methylation at the O–6 position of the 6 membered ring, if not repaired, is a dangerous lesion, being both mutagenic and carcinogenic.

forming (or tumorigenic) retroviruses arose by incorporation of cellular DNA into the genome of weakly or nontransforming viruses. A most interesting recent finding is that in one instance, at least, the difference between a viral oncogene and its normal cellular counterpart is the presence of mutations in the former, which lead to simple amino acid alterations in the protein specified by the respective genes (see Chapter 10). One of the most promising aspects of the high technology that now attends the analysis of DNA is that it provides the tools for investigating alterations in potentially normal functions that accompany malignancies. It would be surprising if such changes were not fairly widespread.

6.5 DNA manipulation

The fact that mammalian DNA can be amplified by recombinant DNA technology and (potentially) expressed in both prokaryotic and eukaryotic systems makes many experiments possible that would hitherto not have been feasible. This should engender a sense of optimism, and even adventure, in those interested in exploring the cellular and molecular biology of cancer. It has, for example, already allowed, *inter alia*, a sequence homology to be observed between some of the normal growth factors of cells and those of viral and cellular 'oncogenes', implying a function for the latter in uncontrolled cell growth (see Chapter 12).

Many vector systems for generating recombinant DNAs that can be amplified by replication in bacterial systems, and even expressed in bacteria or mammalian cells, have been generated.

A detailed description of nucleic acid molecular biology used for this purpose is beyond the scope of this Chapter; however, a brief account may be given here to explain some of the terminology and methods employed. The applications are discussed elsewhere in this book. Perhaps one of the most important tools comes from the discovery of enzymes known as restriction endonucleases in many bacteria. The restriction enzymes recognize specific sets of DNA sequences in double-stranded DNA and cut both strands of DNA at or near these sequences. In some instances, the enzymes cut through both strands at a single point generating blunt–ended molecules, whereas with others the cuts are at precisely spaced points along the two strands and generate overlapping ('sticky' or overhanging) ends. Various other enzymes are available for filling in or cutting back at these ends. These techniques allow unrelated DNA molecules to be joined together (ligated); in particular this is of use for propagating sequences from eukaryotic organisms in prokaryotic hosts such as bacteria. For example, the entire genetic information (genome) of the human chromosomes can be ligated to bacteriophage (bacterial virus) DNA, giving rise to a 'library' of human DNA. These molecules are more readily produced (and reproduced in large quantities), can be isolated as homogeneous clones, and can be manipulated further (e.g. for nucleotide sequence analysis, for mutagenesis experiments, for gene expression studies, etc.). One of the most common techniques is to isolate a specific clone of interest and to label it with a radioisotope so that it can be used as a probe to examine the gene in various DNA or RNA preparations. One example has already been described in Chapter 3 (see Fig. 3.4) in which human DNA was cut with a restriction enzyme; the fragments of DNA were separated by size by electrophoresis through a gel, and then transferred to a filter. The filter was then exposed (hybridized) to a radioisotopically labelled probe for an immunoglobulin locus and the specific binding (hybridization) was measured by exposure of the filter to X–ray film. In the specific example shown, the study examined whether the immunoglobulin locus had been arranged compared to the germ line sequences, as a measure of differentiation of B lymphocytes. Similar techniques have been applied to the study of cellular oncogenes (see Chapters 10–12).

Such genetic manipulations are as yet in their infancy, and not wholly without pitfalls, as is beginning to be recognized. For example, genes expressed in heterologous systems may produce functions that are without activity in their normal hosts, possibly as a consequence of incorrect or incomplete protein modification that could result in aberrant folding or unusual instability. Further, gene functions expressed at abnormally high levels, even in homologous systems, can lead to unexpected effects, including cell death. 'Dose response' may prove a difficult problem to solve, at least in terms of defining underlying mechanisms of gene action within a cell. Another basic problem for biotechnology appears to be the expression of genes in the wrong cellular compartment following introduction of DNA into cells (transfection). The critical problems for DNA, or gene, manipulation now appear to be not how to 'clone' and express a particular part of DNA, or even a particular gene, but how to introduce it into a cell and regulate its expression so as to obtain *in vitro* data that are meaningful in terms of *in vivo* responses.

Essentially what is implicit in the above discussion is the fact that all the 'rules of the game' have not yet been determined, although great progress has been made. It is significant that the need for regulation of gene expression is now being widely recognized. With this in mind, vectors have been developed that allow control of DNA replication and many of them contain RNA polymerase promoters that can be additionally regulated by such external agents as temperature, hormones or heavy metals.

One of the other basic problems in gene manipulation and expression arises from the fact that in mammalian cells mRNAs are often not colinear with respect to genomic DNA. Rather, they reflect the fact that enzymic processes have occurred in the cytoplasm, subsequent to transcription, which have 'spliced' together non-adjacent regions of RNA to produce the functional messengers for proteins. For expression of such genes *in vitro*, the messenger itself must first be isolated and reversibly transcribed into DNA, before the latter can be introduced into suitable vector systems and studied. This process is both tedious and frequently unsuccessful, particularly in the case of mRNAs present in low copy numbers in cells, and/or unstable. In attempts to circumvent this, interesting new classes of vectors have been developed. These are hybrid DNAs with elements derived both from plasmid and viral sources, such that for expression they can be 'shuttled' between bacteria and mammalian cells, and even packaged as retrovirus particles, thus allowing recovery of input material. Since they contain all the signals for retrovirus transcription, these vectors provide the capacity for correctly splicing, in an *in vitro* system, the input DNA. Thus the latter should be re–isolatable as a reversibly transcribed copy of its message.

Gene manipulation is the basis of a new approach to medicine designated 'gene therapy'. For example, if 'cancer genes' can be identified and defined, they should be subject to manipulations (for example, controlled site specific mutagenesis) that could render them inactive and even possibly subjects for 'gene therapy', if corrected genes could be substituted for the aberrantly expressed ones. Such problems for the future at least deserve thought. An interesting alternative approach just beginning to be explored involves the use of complementary (antisense) sequence of mRNAs which, upon being introduced into cells, should at least theoretically be capable of combining with the messenger and thereby rendering it inactive. This potentially fruitful avenue will no doubt be widely examined in the near future, with particular regard to the prevention of expression of aberrant genes.

6.6 Conclusion

This historical approach to DNA has been presented because it shows how many scientific disciplines have been, even indirectly, involved in taking us to a point where we can begin to approach the problem of human cancer in a non-empirical manner. At the moment it seems ironic, and paradoxical, for example, that one of the few human cancers that has been firmly associated with a viral infection (e.g. Burkitt's lymphoma with Epstein Barr virus) is still preferentially treated with massive doses of cyclophosphamide, a nitrogen mustard and potent carcinogen (indeed cyclophosphamide is a drug of choice in the therapy of many human tumours). The aim of understanding at a molecular level the pathological processes defined broadly as 'cancer' is obviously to be able to control them. Ideally such containment should come about by a less empirical manner than that presented as an example above, where although the disease is initially eradicated, the patient is undoubtedly left with many undesirable lesions (indeed, in a large proportion of Burkitt's lymphoma cases, the tumour reappears and notably is no longer susceptible to treatment).

At least one success story can be cited, that is the control of herpes simplex by the drug Acyclovir, as arising from application of the scientific method. Among others, patients immunosuppressed prior and subsequent to transplant therapy become immediately susceptible to the effects of reactivation of herpes viruses. Once the existence of a thymidine kinase gene was identified in herpes simplex virus, specific antagonists of the kinase enzyme were sought. The drug, Acyclovir, a nucleoside analogue, was developed; it blocks a vital step in the enzyme pathway and thus counters the reactivation of herpes simplex viruses, and provides protection for the patient. If cancer(s) can be related to specific sequences of DNA, it should be possible, in a similar fashion, to search for their control.

Further reading

Alberts, B., Bray, D., Lewis, J., Raff, M., Roberts, K., and Watson, J. D. (1983). *Molecular biology of the cell.* Garland Publishing Inc, New York.

Cepko, C., Roberts, B. E., and Mulligan, R. C. (1984). Construction and applications of a highly transmissible murine retrovirus shuttle vector. *Cell* **37**, 1053–62.

Glover, D. M. (ed.) (1985). *DNA cloning. A practical approach.* IRL Press, Oxford.

Gluzman, Y. (ed.) (1982). *Eukaryotic viral vectors.* Cold Spring Harbor Laboratory, Cold Spring Harbor, New York.

Hnilica, L. S. (ed.) (1983). *Chromosomal non-histone proteins.* **i.** *Biology.* CRC Press, Boca Raton, Florida.

Lindahl, T. (1979). DNA glycosylases, endonucleases for apurinic/apyrimidinic sites, and base excision-repair. *Progress in Nucleic Acid Research and Molecular Biology* **22**, 135–92.

Singer, B., and Grunberger, D. (1983). *Molecular biology of mutagens and carcinogens.* Plenum Press, New York.

7

Chemical carcinogenesis and precancer

CAROLINE WIGLEY

7.1 The role of chemical carcinogens and mutation in human cancer

As outlined in Chapter 1 and considered in detail in this and subsequent Chapters (8, 9, and 10) carcinogenesis is a multistage process and each stage may be influenced by different factors. From epidemiological data and animal studies, and most recently from molecular analysis of tumours, there is little doubt that chemical agents are involved at some stage, although there are many other contributing factors. Many potentially carcinogenic agents are present in our diet and environment. There is convincing evidence that the site of action of these agents is the genetic material in cells; many known and suspect chemical carcinogens cause mutations. Even so, it is not entirely clear whether a change in DNA sequence is needed. We include in our definition of mutation gross DNA changes such as rearrangements and should bear in mind that heritable changes in gene expression, whilst not mutational events at the sequence level, might have similar effects on the cell phenotype.

7.1.1 *Epidemiological evidence*

This is discussed in Chapter 4 but a few examples illustrate the situation. The classic example was described in 1775 by Percival Pott who noted that chimney sweeps had a high incidence of cancer of the scrotal skin attributed, quite correctly, to chronic contact with soot—a mixture of chemicals including polycyclic hydrocarbons which were later shown to be carcinogenic in animals (see on). β–napthylamine and other aromatic amines have been linked to bladder cancer in workers in the dye industry, whereas industrial exposure to nickel and some chromates has been strongly implicated in the causation of cancers of the respiratory system. There are also naturally-occurring carcinogens which may be present in the diet. A good example is a substance present in bracken fern which may cause tumours in the alimentary tract in animals and possibly in man in areas where fern hearts (fiddles) are eaten as a delicacy. Other intestinal carcinogens may be formed in the gut by the action of intestinal micro–organisms on substances in the diet or in the bile. Better known but less well defined is the chemical carcinogen(s) in tobacco smoke associated with lung cancer (see Chapter 4). A list of potentially carcinogenic chemicals is published by the International Agency for Research on Cancer (see Table 7.1).

We now know that almost all chemicals implicated by epidemiologists as human carcinogens can cause cellular mutations in the conventional sense, i.e. localized base changes in DNA, but there are a few exceptions. Asbestos causes cancer of the pleural cavity (see Chapter 4) but is not mutagenic in test systems. Diethylstilboestrol, a synthetic steroid hormone, was given in the past to prevent miscarriage in pregnant women; later it was found to cause vaginal tumours in the offspring at puberty, by a mechanism which does not seem to involve DNA mutation in the strict sense.

There are some instances where there may be an increased tissue susceptibility to the tumour inducing activity of carcinogens. In some rare conditions an inherited trait predisposes affected members of a family to develop a particular cancer (see Chapter 5). This led Knudson and others to propose that the first event in carcinogenesis involved DNA mutation and that this mutation could, in rare instances, be transmitted in the germ cell line from parent to offspring. As a rule, this first or initiating mutation occurs after birth, in a target somatic cell. One heritable cancer predisposing condition, xeroderma pigmentosum (XP), is one of the best understood of a group of conditions about which

Table 7.1 Chemicals with proven carcinogenic activity in humans

Chemical (or industrial process)[1]	Main type of exposure[2]	Main route of exposure[3]	Target organ(s)
Aflatoxins	Environmental, occupational	Ingestion, inhalation	Liver
4-aminobiphenyl	Occupational	Inhalation, ingestion, skin contact	Bladder
Arsenic compounds	Occupational, medicinal, environmental	Inhalation, ingestion, skin contact	Skin, lung, liver[4]
Asbestos	Occupational	Inhalation, ingestion	Lung, pleural cavity, gastrointestinal tract
Auramine manufacture	Occupational	Inhalation, ingestion, skin contact	Bladder
Benzene	Occupational	Inhalation, skin contact	Haemopoietic system
Benzidine	Occupational	Inhalation, skin contact, ingestion	Bladder
Bis(chloromethyl)ether	Occupational	Inhalation	Lung
Cadmium-using industries (cadmium oxide?)	Occupational	Inhalation, ingestion	Prostate, lung[4]
Chloramphenicol	Medicinal	Ingestion, injection	Haemopoietic system
Chloromethyl methyl ether (associated with bis(chloromethyl)ether?)	Occupational	Inhalation	Lung
Chromium (chromate processing industries)	Occupational	Inhalation	Lung, nasal cavities[4]

Table 7.1 —*continued*

Chemical (or industrial process)[1]	Main type of exposure[2]	Main route of exposure[3]	Target organ(s)
Cyclophosphamide	Medicinal	Ingestion, injection	Bladder
Diethylstilboestrol	Medicinal	Ingestion (acts transplacentally)	Uterus, vagina (in offspring)
Haematite mining (radon?)	Occupational	Inhalation	Lung
Isopropyl oils	Occupational	Inhalation	Nasal cavity, larynx
Melphalan	Medicinal	Ingestion, injection	Haemopoietic system
Mustard gas	Occupational	Inhalation	Lung, larynx
2-naphthylamine	Occupational	Inhalation, skin contact, ingestion	Bladder
Nickel (nickel-refining industries)	Occupational	Inhalation	Nasal cavity, lung
N,N-bis (2-chloroethyl)–2-naphthylamine	Medicinal	Ingestion	Bladder
Oxymetholone	Medicinal	Ingestion	Liver
Phenacitin	Medicinal	Ingestion	Kidney
Phenytoin	Medicinal	Ingestion, injection	Lymphoreticular system
Soots, tars and oils	Occupational, environmental	Inhalation, skin contact	Lung, skin (scrotum)
Vinyl chloride	Occupational	Inhalation, skin contact	Liver, brain,[4] lung[4]

[1] The precise chemical(s) responsible may not be known.
[2] The main types of exposure mentioned are those by which the association has been demonstrated; other exposures may occur.
[3] The main routes of exposure given may not be the only ones by which such effects could occur.
[4] There is indicative evidence for these organs.
Adapted from Tomatis *et al.* (1978) *Cancer Research* **38**, 877–85.

the defect is known. Individuals with XP suffer from a deficiency in their ability to repair DNA damaged by ultraviolet light in particular; this is demonstrated in cell cultures prepared from small biopsies of a patient's skin. The skin exposed to sunlight in XP patients is at risk of developing cancer, providing a very strong argument linking DNA damage (and, by implication, its faulty repair or lack of repair), mutation and cancer.

7.1.2 *Evidence from animal studies*

Considerable support for the evidence from epidemiological studies came when Japanese workers showed for the first time early this century that a number of potent hydrocarbon carcinogens cause cancer when applied to the skin of rabbits. Subsequently, many other suspected chemicals were shown to be carcinogenic by similar techniques. Nowadays, most drugs, food additives, etc. are tested on laboratory animals, usually rodents, for general toxicity and long term carcinogenicity (see on). Very many substances have now been shown to be tumour-producing in experimental animals. Some produce tumours at the site of application, e.g. on the skin. Others may produce tumours at the site of absorption, e.g. the bowel if given by mouth, or at the site of the breakdown (metabolism), e.g. in the liver, or in the excretory organ, e.g. kidneys or bladder (see Table 7.1). In some instances, a carcinogen may produce tumours in an entirely unexpected organ. For example, dimethylbenz(a)anthracene, when given by mouth, causes breast cancer in female rats, but it has to be given at a particular time in the development of the breast during puberty. There seems to be a critical sensitive period which depends on the hormonal status of the cells (see Chapter 13). Similar complex factors may operate in other tissues also, so that exposure to a carcinogen is necessary, but not sufficient, for cancer induction in these cases. Intensive long-term administration by several routes is essential if possible toxic and carcinogenic effects are to be excluded.

7.1.3 *Molecular evidence*

If cancer can be caused, partly or wholly, by chemical carcinogens inducing mutations in DNA, the powerful techniques of modern molecular biology can be used to detect differences between the DNAs of normal and tumour tissue from a single cancer. The cellular oncogenes (c-*oncs*) are one group of genes for which comparisons of DNA sequence have shown mutations in human tumours (Chapters 10 and 11). Members of the *ras* oncogene family, in particular, have been shown to be mutated, usually at one particular position, leading to the production of a protein altered at amino acid 12 in DNA from bladder carcinomas, colon carcinomas, neuroblastomas and sarcomas. We know that this highly specific mutation must affect the function of the c-*onc* because the mutant gene, but not its normal homologue, can dramatically alter the phenotype of cells in culture transfected with the tumour DNA (see Chapter 10).

Agents other than chemicals can cause mutations. Irradiation is known to damage human DNA (see Chapter 8), and some viruses may also be mutagens when they integrate into host cell DNA (see Chapter 9). We must turn to experimentally induced cancer in animals to find direct evidence that chemical carcinogens can cause mutations such as those in c-*onc* genes that have been linked to cancer induction in humans (see Chapter 10).

Perhaps the best example of this comes from the induction of breast tumours in female rats by nitrosomethylurea, a DNA alkylating carcinogen. All nine tumours in one experimental series contained an 'activated' *ras* gene (Ha-*ras*-1) and one of the genes which was isolated and analysed in detail showed that the same amino acid codon (at position 12 of the protein) was mutated as in the human cancers of unknown causation mentioned earlier. Convincing as this might seem, the other side of this picture is rather puzzling: only a minority of human tumours contain mutant oncogenes of the sort we have just described. Is it that the mutant gene is not necessary for the development of that cancer, although it may play a small accessory role in making up the complex cancer phenotype? Can other mutant genes, whose presence cannot yet be detected by currently available cloned probes, substitute in function for the c-*onc* genes? Or can c-*onc* genes be activated in ways which do not involve mutation in the widely accepted sense?

There is a separate line of evidence which suggests quite strongly that recessive mutations of genes, whose identities are less well characterized than the oncogenes, are involved in at least two rare malignancies of childhood: Wilms' tumour of the kidney (see Chapter 11) and retinoblastoma (see Chapters 5 and 11).

7.2 Experimental approaches to the study of carcinogenesis by chemicals

7.2.1 *The biology of cancer induction in animals—precancer and multistage models*

Studies on the experimental induction by chemicals of cancer in laboratory animals introduced several new concepts, particularly the multistage theory (see Fig. 7.1). Carcinogens fall into two groups, complete and incomplete. The former can produce tumours on their own, whereas the latter cannot and require subsequent exposure of the treated (initiated) cells to promoting agents, which are not carcinogenic in themselves.

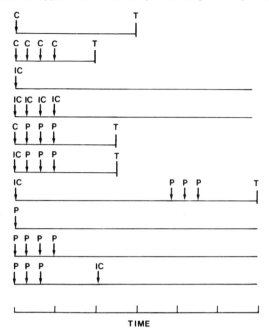

Fig. 7.1 Initiation and promotion in carcinogenesis. Schematic representation of various schedules of treatment of mouse skin with a complete or incomplete carcinogen and tumour promotor. Different combinations and sequences in time are shown horizontally. Tumours result after different latent periods only from schedules where 'T' is indicated. C=carcinogen; P=promoter; T=tumour; IC=incomplete carcinogen.

Promoting agents can also lead to the development of tumours when applied to tissue previously treated with a low dose of a complete carcinogen which would not in itself produce tumours. Polycyclic aromatic hydrocarbons and the nitrosamines are complete carcinogens and can act as initiators and promoters. The complexity of the situation is illustrated by urethrane, an incomplete carcinogen when applied to the mouse skin but a complete carcinogen in the foetal lung. Promoting agents are less well defined but seem to be specific for particular tissues. One group, the phorbol esters extracted from some plants, act as tumour promoters for hydrocarbons in skin.

During experimental carcinogenesis in various tissues, macroscopic and microscopic changes in the affected tissues which precede the appearance of tumours have been defined (see Chapter 1) as altered discrete focal areas within the carcinogen treated region. These focal areas of abnormal tissue are intermediate in character between normal and malignant. In time, further changes occur in these foci culminating in the development of overt cancer. The cells in the precancer foci have an increased risk of cancer development compared with normal tissue, i.e. they are precancerous. The different stages in the process of carcinogenesis have been detected in man and in animals and can now be analysed. I shall illustrate this by describing three experimental animal systems for inducing cancer of epithelial tissues in skin, liver and large bowel (colon and rectum). In the colon system, in particular, there are similarities to tissue changes in humans that, from epidemiological evidence, are considered to be precancerous. This suggests that the experimental models are a valid way of studying the disease and may provide clues to possible means of medical intervention.

Carcinogenesis in mouse skin is the classic model system in which two stages in the process of cancer development, initiation and promotion, were first described. A single application of a chemical carcinogen is applied to the shaved back skin and this results in the initiation of an unknown number of cells which, if they are left without further treatment, will persist for a very long time without showing any apparent changes. If a second class of chemical agent, a tumour promoter, is applied to the same area at any time, even a year later, and the treatment repeated regularly, benign tumours (papillomas) appear. They are believed to arise from some of the initiated cells in the carcinogen treated skin. A small proportion of these papillomas may develop into fully malignant tumours after further applications of promoter.

Something is known about the mechanisms by which the two classes of agent act. Initiating agents and complete carcinogens are almost always DNA-damaging (genotoxic) (see on) and it seems very likely that the initiating event involves some form of carcinogen-DNA interaction and subsequent damage. Initiated cells persist in the tissue long after the initiating agent has disappeared and the lesion produced is both stable and heritable, i.e. it has the characteristics of a mutation. Conversely, most promoting agents are not mutagenic although in some cases they may modify gene expression. It is now thought that promotion itself consists of several steps, some irreversible and some reversible, and that promoting agents too may be either complete, and able to perform all functions, or incomplete, and active at only one or a few stages. A third term, progression, is usually reserved for the process by which cells of a benign or malignant tumour acquire more and more aberrant characteristics—the bad to worse principle of tumour evolution.

Similar sequences of events occur in other tissues. Cancer of the liver can be induced by chemical carcinogens fed to rats. For example, aflatoxin B1, a mould product which may contaminate certain foods in the tropics, is one of the most potent liver carcinogens known. In all probability it contributes to the high incidence of human liver cancer in the tropics; it seems to act in combination with hepatitis B infection (see Chapter 9). One of the earliest effects of chronic aflatoxin B1 treatment is the appearance of nodules of hyperplastic precancerous liver cells. These nodules have a range of enzyme abnormalities distinguishing them from surrounding normal tissue. Iron is lost from the precancerous nodules but glycogen stores increase. In the liver, there seems to be an absolute requirement for cell proliferation before nodules can be induced. Aflatoxin is toxic and kills many liver cells. The tissue then regenerates to restore the lost mass. [The powers of regeneration in the liver are remarkable; in rats three quarters of the organ can be removed surgically (partial hepatectomy) and regenerative proliferation will restore the original tissue mass within weeks.] Partial hepatectomy can in fact act as a promoting stimulus in rat liver carcinogenesis, and tumours arise in the regenerated liver after an initiating, prehepatectomy treatment with a carcinogen. Neither chemical nor surgical treatment alone is sufficient for cancer induction in the adult animal. Interestingly, in young weanling rats, where the liver is growing rapidly during normal development, there is no need for a proliferative stimulus and an initiating dose of carcinogen alone will induce cancer.

Indeed, stimulation of cell division appears to be a necessary component of the promotion stages of carcinogenesis in most if not all tissues, but it is not usually sufficient. Some types of hyperplastic stimuli are more effective than others. Promotion is obviously a complex process which is only recently becoming better understood, particularly with the development of cell culture model systems for studying this aspect of carcinogenesis (see on).

Cancer induction in the colon induced by dimethylhydrazine injected into rats or mice shows well defined precancerous stages. A sequence of pathological changes (Fig. 7.2) can be observed before overt carcinomas develop, and the type and amount of altered colon epithelium depends on carcinogen dosage as well as length of treatment. Submucosal glands become abnormal (dysplastic), and benign polyps (adenomas) arise with increasing incidence with both dosage and time. Histologically, carcinomas can be shown to develop directly from polyps and, more rarely, from abnormal glands, indicating that these are precancerous stages in colon carcinogenesis. This is precisely the conclusion reached by pathologists from observations on human colon cancer. In families with familial polyposis coli (see Chapter 5), affected members develop multiple polyps of the colon and rectum at an early age and at least one polyp will almost certainly become carcinomatous within about 10 years. Usually, the entire colon is removed surgically before this time. This

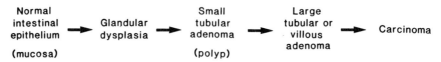

Fig. 7.2 Flow diagram showing the presumptive precancerous stages between normal and malignant tissue, identifiable histologically in human colorectal epithelium. Note: arrows indicate the direction of increasing potential for malignant change, not that cells necessarily pass through all of the precancerous stages between normal and malignant tissue.

offers the pathologist a unique opportunity to study the precancerous lesions which in other circumstances would escape clinical detection. Most pathologists agree that, in polyposis patients, focal areas of carcinoma develop almost invariably from pre–existing polyps (or more rarely from microscopic glandular abnormalities) and that the polyps represent a precancerous stage. The adenomas themselves can be classi-fied according to their potential for malignant change. Size (above 1 cm^2) and the presence of a particular histological pattern (villous) is accom-panied by a statistically increased chance of cancer developing from a particular polyp. Thus there may be additional, more advanced pre-cancerous stages in the multistage sequence, but these are less well defined (see Fig. 7.2). It is thought that, in the general population, precancerous polyps may also occur but are few in number and arise later in life and sporadically, preceding the cancer by a similar 10 or 15 year interval. The animal carcinogenesis model of colon cancer is thus especially suitable for the study of factors (including dietary com-ponents) suspected from epidemiological studies of being involved in the adenoma (or polyp) to carcinoma progression sequence. For instance, bile acids and their derivatives may have promoter like activity (see earlier); this has already been shown in animal experiments. In addition, a few laboratories are beginning to make use of cell culture techniques to investigate precancerous cells from polyps *in vitro* (see on).

7.2.2 *Mechanisms of carcinogen activation and action*

Until the late 1960s, some of the most potent carcinogens, the polycyclic aromatic hydrocarbons, were unable to mutate cells in culture. We now know that this is because many carcinogens need to be metabolized by cellular enzymes to a reactive derivative before they can be effective, and the test cells used were deficient in one or more metabolic functions and were unable to activate the chemical. Similarly, these (and most other) chemicals must be metabolized to electrophilic derivatives before they are carcinogenic. In animals, metabolism usually happens in the target cells from which the cancer will develop; most reactive metabolites have short half lives in solution in body fluids. Occasionally, activation may occur in the liver. The capacity for metabolism is genetically determined and may be species specific. For instance, the guinea pig lacks a critical enzyme for the activation of acetylaminofluorene (AAF) to its active metabolite, N-hydroxy-AAF, and is thus resistant to its carcinogenic effects. There are also differences between tissues in the extent of metabolic activation of a particular chemical and in the relative extents of deactivation (or detoxification) and activation to the ultimate carcinogenic derivative.

Figures 7.3 and 7.4 show the main routes of chemical activation and sites of binding to DNA of two potent carcinogens. These polycyclic compounds, suspected of being human carcinogens, are both activated initially by a complex of enzymes associated with intracellular membranes, the cytochrome P450-associated mixed–function oxidases (MFO). Aflatoxin B1 is metabolized by MFO to several products including the 2,3–epoxide derivative shown in Figure 7.3. Here an oxygen bridge has been introduced enzymatically across a carbon–carbon double bond, producing an unstable intermediate proximate metabolite. This then reacts preferentially with the 7-position of guanine residues in DNA and forms one of the two major carcinogen-DNA adducts found in rat liver. The MFO are also responsible for metabolizing the polycyclic hydrocarbon carcinogens; benzo(a)pyrene is a good example. The 7,8-position double bond is opened enzymatically and the epoxide is formed, as with aflatoxin B1. The compound is a substrate for a number of enzymatic and non-enzymatic reactions but the important one for carcinogenicity involves soluble enzymes (not bound to membranes) called epoxide hydrases. The 7,8-epoxide is converted to the

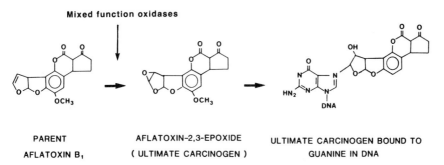

Mixed function oxidases

| PARENT | AFLATOXIN-2,3-EPOXIDE | ULTIMATE CARCINOGEN BOUND TO |
| AFLATOXIN B₁ | (ULTIMATE CARCINOGEN) | GUANINE IN DNA |

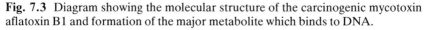

Fig. 7.3 Diagram showing the molecular structure of the carcinogenic mycotoxin aflatoxin B1 and formation of the major metabolite which binds to DNA.

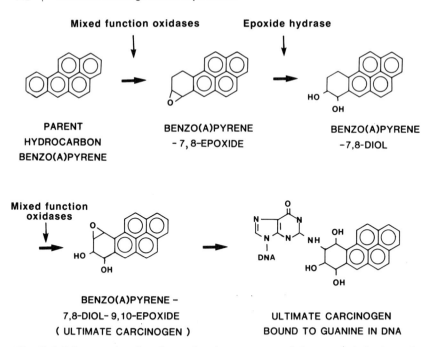

Fig. 7.4 Diagram showing the molecular structure of the aromatic hydrocarbon carcinogen benzo(a)pyrene and formation of the major metabolite which binds to DNA.

7,8-diol and this now forms a good substrate for, amongst other reactions, a second epoxidation of the 9,10-position as shown in Figure 7.4. DNA binding occurs through this epoxide to the 2-amino group of guanine and this is the major adduct found in mouse skin under conditions where carcinomas would be expected after an appropriate latent period. Metabolism of other recognized or suspected carcinogens, the aliphatic N-nitrosamines, for instance, may involve less complicated metabolic routes of activation, culminating in the alkylation (formation of ethyl or methyl derivatives) at specific sites on DNA bases.

7.2.3 DNA repair

What then happens to DNA which has been modified by alkylation or by the formation of nucleic acid adducts with large bulky hydrocarbon molecules? Are there mechanisms by which a cell detects and repairs such lesions so that its DNA sequence of bases is faithfully restored? In bacteria, this is certainly so and there is a considerable amount of knowledge about the precise pathways of repair and the enzymes involved in recognizing, excising and repairing the carcinogen induced damage. Much less is known about mammalian cells but it seems certain that inefficient or faulty (error prone) repair of DNA is important in some types of cancer. The classic example of this is the induction of skin cancer by exposure to the ultraviolet component of sunlight in individuals suffering from XP (see above and Chapter 5). Exposure to ultraviolet light also leads to skin cancer in normal individuals but only if excessive, i.e. in Caucasians in the tropics, but the XP patients' skin is particularly sensitive because of the underlying genetic biochemical defect in their cells. This is known to involve part of the DNA repair mechanism so that their cells are deficient in repairing ultraviolet induced DNA damage. This can also be shown in cells cultured from patients' skin biopsies. There are other cancer prone conditions which are thought to involve defects in DNA repair, but these are less easily explained. For instance, ataxia telangiectasia (AT), Fanconi's anaemia and Bloom's syndrome are thought of as chromosome breakage syndromes. AT cells are sensitive to agents such as X-rays which cause gross chromosome breakage due to deficient repair of this type of damage. As well as having many other clinical defects, AT patients are susceptible to cancers of lymphatic tissues and leukaemias, but the relationship between this susceptibility, DNA damage and faulty DNA repair is still unclear.

In summary, most carcinogens need to be activated metabolically to be converted to the ultimate carcinogen that binds to DNA, modifying accessible DNA bases in a precise way throughout the genome, to an extent which depends on the dose and extent of metabolic activation. It is likely that small errors in repairing this damage or, on a larger scale, complete chromosome breakage, perhaps due to lesions on both DNA strands in the same vicinity, are important. Thus, mutations at the DNA sequence level or those involving gross changes such as large deletions and translocations (see Chapter 11) are strongly implicated in the mechanism of carcinogen action.

7.2.4 *Cellular transformation* in vitro

Transformation is a term used for changes seen in tissue culture, whereby more-or-less normal cells become altered to resemble cancer cells. This can happen spontaneously as a rare event whose frequency depends on a variety of factors and on the species. Cells from some rodents, e.g. mouse, transform spontaneously in culture whereas human and avian cells rarely (if ever) do. Physical agents (see Chapter 8), chemicals, and viruses (see Chapter 9) can transform cells *in vitro*. In many cases where the cell transformation system is well defined, near normal, diploid cells can be converted with reasonable efficiency into cells which can grow into invasive tumours if they are put back into a suitable animal host. The converted or transformed cells in culture are then said to be tumorigenic and the process by which they became so can be studied as a model for carcinogenesis *in vivo* (spontaneous or induced).

Many different culture systems for studying transformation have used mesenchymal or 'fibroblast' cells (see Chapter 1) which rarely give rise spontaneously to malignant tumours in man or laboratory animals. They probably do not provide a very good model system for studying the relationship between cell differentiation and neoplasia, but they are easy to grow and manipulate in culture and they have certainly provided us with ways of studying some fundamental aspects of carcinogenesis. For instance, the system devised by Heidelberger and his group used a clone of mouse embryo fibroblast cells called C3H/10T$\frac{1}{2}$. One parameter of transformation that correlates well with tumorigenicity in this cell system (as it does in many others, but not invariably) is the appearance of a property known as anchorage independent growth (AIG). Normal cells need to be anchored to and spread on a solid substrate before they can divide and form a colony or clone from a single cell. Some cancer cells are able to grow and form colonies when suspended in a semisolid medium such as soft (0.33 per cent) agar. If untransformed C3H/10T$\frac{1}{2}$ cells are treated with a chemical carcinogen, a small proportion of the cells will grow in soft agar and these cells are also usually tumorigenic. The frequency of transformation to this phenotype can be measured after correction for the proportion which survived the carcinogen induced toxicity. The efficiency with which certain carcinogens transform cells to AIG has been used by some scientists as a rapid screening test for chemicals which might cause cancer (see on) but it is not as reproducible as other tests and is not widely used. There are many other changes which can be induced in cell culture by carcinogens and for which there is evidence of a link with the cancer cell phenotype. Changes in components of the filamentous cytoskeleton of cells is one such example. Since none of these markers of transformation in culture is invariably associated with cancer cells, their role in carcinogenesis remains an area of active investigation and dispute.

As mentioned earlier, some aspects of carcinogenesis cannot be studied in simple fibroblast cell systems, namely those concerned with differentiation and tissue homeostasis (the balance between cell renewal by division and cell death in a defined population)—a key abnormality in cancer. Some aspects of these properties can be investigated in specialized systems such as in differentiated epithelial cell cultures. Methods have been established for growing some of these more fastidious cell types from rodent and human tissues, but so far they are in the early stages of experimental development. It has been shown conclusively that chemical carcinogens, such as the hydrocarbons, benzo(a)pyrene, and dimethylbenzanthracene, can induce transformation and eventually tumorigenic potential in epithelial cells treated with the carcinogen in primary culture, i.e. cells grown directly from animal tissues. Various types of rodent cells have been used, including skin keratinocytes, salivary gland duct cells, epithelium from the respiratory system, and urinary bladder cells. All of these epithelial systems demonstrate one feature particularly clearly: transformation, like carcinogenesis, is a multistage process. There is a relatively long period of time between treating normal cells with a chemical, sometimes just for a single short exposure, and the eventual emergence of cells which will grow as tumours in an appropriate animal host. During this long latent period, more or less discrete precancerous stages occur wherein the cells appear altered in a characteristic way but are not yet capable of forming tumours in an animal. There are good grounds for believing that these inter-mediate stages are equivalent to the precancerous stages in carcino-genesis observed *in vivo* (see above). Amongst the properties which frequently alter during the precancerous stages in transformation are chromosome number (which usually increases, and often nearly doubles, the normal complement), loss of dependence on growth stimulating factors in serum (see Chapter 12), increased ability to grow clonally from single cells (clonogenicity) or at least at a reduced cell density, and the acquisition of a prolonged or indefinite lifespan in culture (immortality—an escape from senescence). We know very little about the factors which govern progression through these precancerous stages. Further studies will investigate the effects of tumour promoters, identified from animal experiments, and other known modifiers of gene expression which do not conform to the carcinogen/mutagen category of initiating agents.

7.2.5 *Precancerous cells* in vitro

Human cells of all types and, in particular, normal epithelial cells which give rise to the common human cancers, are extremely resistant to trans-formation induced by chemicals in culture. The reasons for this are poorly understood. It is now possible to culture epithelial cells directly from some tissues which are already precancerous. The early stages of transformation in these cells, especially the stage(s) leading to immor-tality and the capacity for indefinite propagation *in vitro*, have already taken place. We can now study such cells and try to identify the factors which lead to the development of more malignant cell properties or conversely, those that induce reversion to a more normal state.

This approach is most useful where the precancerous tissue is readily available, usually through surgical procedures. In patients with familial polyposis coli, diseased tissue is removed surgically. Polyps from these surgical specimens have been cultured successfully in our laboratory and immortal cell lines have been derived from about one specimen in five which survived the initial preparation procedure and remained uncontaminated by intestinal microorganisms.

The uterine cervix, oral tissues, oesophagus and trachea also provide suitable precancerous tissue from biopsies, but work using these tissues is in its early stages.

7.3 Screening for carcinogens

7.3.1 Animal carcinogenicity tests

Most known human carcinogens and many other chemicals will produce tumours in experimental animals under appropriate, although sometimes very artificial, conditions. In fact, it is required by law that any new chemical introduced for use in or by humans (as medicines, cosmetics, food additives, weed and pest killers, agricultural fertilizers, household cleansing products, to give a few examples) must be tested in laboratory animals for their long-term effects. This is enormously costly in time and expenditure so it is vital that tests should be carefully planned and informative. This requires a knowledge of the way in which chemicals are metabolized (see above) and excreted in different species and whether these characteristics are appropriate to the human situation. For instance, the guinea pig would be inappropriate for testing AAF since it lacks the enzyme necessary to convert this chemical to its active, carcinogenic form. In practice, most tests are done on rats and mice, male and female, which are exposed for a long period to the maximum tolerated dose, often one to two years. The route of administration usually depends on the likely mode of human exposure, by inhalation, in the diet or drinking water, or via skin contact. After the necessary length of time, animals still surviving are examined for tumours which can be confirmed as malignant by a pathologist.

As discussed earlier, human cancers are thought to take many years to evolve after the initiating event in a susceptible target cell. This can range from about 10 years up to almost the total lifetime of an individual. This fact alone poses a very real problem for the experimenter who wants to confirm the safety of a potentially useful chemical. Animal studies still form the main acceptable evidence for Food and Drug Safety authorities throughout the world, and yet they are very time consuming and expensive. As an example, to test one compound thoroughly for carcinogenicity in two species (rats and mice) costs approximately £300 000 and takes up to three years. As it became apparent that most compounds with proven carcinogenic activity were genotoxic, a number of more rapid tests were developed as first-order screens for large numbers of chemicals at between 1 and 10 per cent of the cost of animal experiments, depending on the type and number of rapid tests used.

7.3.2 *Rapid screening tests*

A large number of different tests have been put forward over the last few years as potentially useful indicators of carcinogenic activity. After a series of comparative trials, the authorities in most countries reached agreement on the type of evidence which would be acceptable. This requires a compound to have been tested in assays measuring mutation (both in bacteria and in mammalian cells in culture) and for their ability to cause chromosome breakage both *in vivo* (in the animal) and *in vitro* (in cell culture). The results of a battery of about four rapid screening tests selected from within these categories should, if the results are unequivocal, provide information on the potential carcinogenicity of a chemical which would be accepted by safety authorities in lieu of long-term animal data.

The most well known and widely publicized rapid test for chemical carcinogens takes the name of its originator, Bruce Ames. This test assesses the mutagenicity of chemicals, with or without metabolism by activating enzymes (from a crude subcellular fraction, S9, of rat liver, a rich source of membrane-bound enzyme activity including the MFO) in a range of specially selected strains of *Salmonella* bacteria. These bacterial strains have each been constructed in the laboratory to detect mutations of a specific kind. For instance, one strain is able to indicate a particular nucleic acid substitution which alters one base pair to another in bacterial DNA after exposure to a DNA damaging agent. Another strain detects chemicals able to cause frameshift mutations (whereby addition or deletion of one or more nucleic acids other than a multiple of three causes the whole reading frame of the triplet code to be thrown out of phase), and the encoded protein is drastically altered. The bacteria used as test strains are themselves mutants and are unable to make a particular amino acid essential for their growth, such as histidine. The test then detects whether a particular chemical can cause the specific base pair substitution or frameshift mutation needed to revert the mutant bacteria to their wild type capacity for synthesizing the essential amino acid. This is done because the investigator can most easily score the number of bacterial colonies which do grow on an incomplete nutrient agar substrate (one which does not supply the particular amino acid). Most carcinogenic chemicals induce a wide range of mutations which may kill the bacteria, so it is important to test a chemical at a dose giving an acceptable level of toxicity that can be measured separately under non-selective conditions. Obviously a positive result is one in which a chemical induces a significant increase in reverted (auxotrophic) bacteria

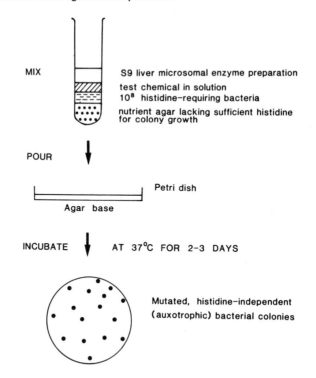

MIX

S9 liver microsomal enzyme preparation
test chemical in solution
10^8 histidine—requiring bacteria
nutrient agar lacking sufficient histidine
for colony growth

POUR

Petri dish

Agar base

INCUBATE AT 37°C FOR 2-3 DAYS

Mutated, histidine—independent
(auxotrophic) bacterial colonies

Fig. 7.5 Diagram showing the basic Ames' test procedure for detecting muta-genicity of chemicals in bacteria. A panel of similar tests is generally used, each designed to detect different chemical activities and types of mutation in order to predict carcinogenic potential.

capable of forming colonies on a selective (deficient) nutrient agar sub-strate where the unaffected bacteria cannot grow (Fig. 7.5).

The Ames test is probably one of the least expensive and most rapid tests available (taking only a couple of days) to detect a property, namely mutation, common to most human carcinogens. However, there are some drawbacks to the test which mean that the results obtained with it should be considered suggestive rather than conclusive evidence for or against the carcinogenicity of a suspect chemical compound. First, the complete spectrum of enzymes involved in metabolizing a variety of carcinogens is not present in the particular liver microsome fraction (S9) component of the assay mixture. This means that although mutagenic derivatives of a chemical may be generated by the microsomal enzymes, they may not be the ones produced by an intact cell or in the body, and so present a different picture of the chemical's potency. It is even possible that a false positive or negative result might be obtained for similar reasons. In practice, the Ames test, using a battery of four *Salmonella* strains each designed to detect a particular type of mutation, has achieved greater than 90 per cent accuracy in predicting both carcinogens and non-carcinogens in 'blind' trials. However, the relative potency of the chemicals was predicted less accurately in quantitative comparisons between different classes of chemicals.

Because mammalian cell DNA is more complex than bacterial DNA, mutation tests in mammalian cells *in vitro* must also be performed, even though they are rather more complicated to do and take longer to produce results. The mutations most commonly used are deficiencies due to DNA sequence modification in either hypoxanthine guanine phosphoribosyl transferase (HGPRT) or thymidine kinase (TK) activity, enzymes involved in nucleic acid synthesis (see Fig. 7.6) or to a mutation which reduces the capacity of the drug ouabain to bind at the cell surface and block membrane transport. The most commonly used mutation is resistance to HGPRT (HGPRT⁻) because, although recessive, it can be induced at relatively high frequency due to its location on the X chromosome, i.e. inactivation of the single gene copy in male cells is

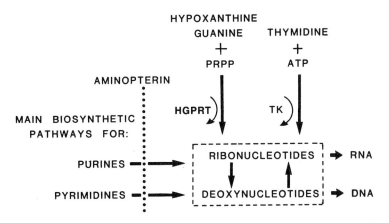

Fig. 7.6 Diagram showing the biochemical pathways utilized in the synthesis of nucleic acids. The biosynthetic (*de novo*) pathway can be blocked by aminopterin and the alternative salvage pathway can be abolished by mutation in hypoxanthine guanine phosphoribosyl transferase (HGPRT) or thymidine kinase (TK) genes. This is detected by cellular resistance to the cytotoxic base analogue drugs 6-thioguanine (or 8-azaguanine) and bromodeoxyuridine respectively. Mutation in a forward direction (HGPRT⁻ or TK⁻ phenotypes) or reversion of mutants to the wild type (resistance of aminopterin) are increased in frequency by many chemical carcinogens.

sufficient for expression of the mutant phenotype. The assay procedure involves treating suitable mammalian cells (often Chinese hamster fibroblasts) with a suspect chemical, with or without activation by the S9 rat liver cell enzyme fraction. The treated cell population is assessed (i) for its ability to grow from single cells to form clones as a measure of the degree of toxicity of the chemical (reduction in clone formation compared with untreated cells), and (ii) for the number of mutations in a given number of cells cultured in the presence of the drugs 6-thioguanine or 8-azaguanine. Unaffected cells take up the selective drug, incorporate it into nucleic acid and are thus killed. Mutated cells fail to do so because they lack HGPRT and cannot utilize base analogue drugs. They depend solely on the alternative biosynthetic pathway and are spared. They grow to form clones of mutant cells which can be stained and counted after one to two weeks, and their numbers expressed as a mutation frequency within the surviving fraction (after correction for toxicity of the suspect chemical). Relative to the control 'background' level of mutation in untreated cells, an elevated mutation frequency would indicate that the suspect chemical has potential carcinogenic activity.

Chromosome mutations, i.e. aberrations such as chromatid breaks (see Chapter 11) caused by chemicals, are also good indicators of carcinogenic activity and this property forms the basis of the second pair of rapid screening tests. The *in vivo* assay relies on the living animal to activate the test chemical, if this is necessary, after it has been fed or injected, and metabolism may occur in the liver or in the target cells. In this test, target cells are usually from the bone marrow where blood cell precursors are dividing rapidly and are highly sensitive to DNA damaging agents. At several times after injecting the chemical, samples of bone marrow cells are prepared for chromosome analysis (see Chapter 11). Chromosomes in the metaphase part of the cell cycle, just before cell division, are condensed and relatively easy to see. Many metaphase chromosome spreads are analysed and the average numbers of breaks, or discontinuities, in the chromatid arms of each chromosome are counted. Significant increases above the spontaneous background level indicates that the chemical may be carcinogenic. The same kind of analysis may be performed on cells in tissue culture, which can either be human blood lymphocytes in short term culture or permanent cell lines of human or rodent origin. These are treated with the chemical *in vitro*, with or without the metabolizing enzyme S9 preparation, and chromosomes prepared at two or three times thereafter to find the peak of chromosome breaking activity; this may vary, but is generally at 24–48 hours.

7.4 Prospects

7.4.1 *Early diagnosis of precancerous conditions*

With most precancerous lesions, there are no problems for the patient who is probably unaware of their presence. In rare circumstances, a large adenoma of the bowel for instance may cause obstruction or bleed chronically and require surgery, but generally the lesions are asymptomatic. These situations are distinct from some other clinical conditions, such as ataxia telangiectasia and Down's syndrome, where obvious multiple abnormalities exist, including an increased risk of particular cancers to which the clinician will already be alerted.

The main clinical problems in cancer usually arise when metastasis to distant parts of the body occurs (see Chapter 2) so that local surgical excision or radiation therapy is no longer feasible. By definition, precancerous tissues of epithelial origin have not invaded the underlying stroma (see Chapter 1) although the individual cells may be highly abnormal in other respects. There can only be the possibility of metastasis once invasion has taken place. In some tissues, such as breast, this may take place when the cancer is very small but cancer cells must at least have penetrated vessels in the stroma. Is there any way of detecting abnormal precancerous tissues before invasive properties are acquired? In some cases there may be. Again, I will use an example from precancerous colon tissue. The haemoccult test used to detect cancer of the colon and rectum relies on the fact that many cancers ulcerate and bleed chronically and blood can be detected biochemically in the faeces. Thus a simple screening test can often help in diagnosing cancer (or help rule it out) in individuals with bowel problems, when malignancy is suspected. In fact, many precancerous adenomas of the large bowel, particularly the more advanced ones, will also be detected with this test, and can be removed surgically. In the near future, it should be possible to use a similar approach to detect in faecal samples more specific products of premalignant colon cells either actively secreted into the bowel lumen or shed from dead cells. The problem is whether this type of test will be practical for the population as a whole, perhaps over a certain age, or just for high-risk individuals with a family history (see Chapter 5). Similar principles could theoretically apply to products of abnormal tissues released into other body fluids. Screening for cervical precancerous lesions using a smear from the cervix to look for abnormal cells is a well known example of a different technique used to identify potential cancers before the risk of invasion and metastases arises. Apart from these examples, screening for overt cancer of various tissues and organs presents a great problem, with little chance at present of finding precancerous lesions by current, insensitive and, for the most part, non-specific methods. It is in this area of clinical cancer research that much effort is needed, particularly where clinicians and scientists in the laboratory can combine efforts and devise sensitive diagnostic procedures. Monoclonal antibody technology will undoubtedly have a major influence in this area (see Chapters 18 and 19).

7.4.2 *Understanding and preventing tumour progression*

Very little is known about the factors that govern the fate of precancerous lesions and determine whether or not a cancer develops and progresses. Some clues have come from epidemiological studies, but information is sparse. There is evidence that dietary factors, such as the amount of fat we eat, can play a role in the later stages of colon cancer development, that hormones influence progression in breast cancer patients, that components of cigarette smoke probably act as promoters and influence late stage lung tumour progression, which can be retarded by stopping smoking—however long ago the habit was established (see Chapter 4). In liver cancer, particularly in the Third World, hepatitis B virus infection and chronic hepatitis may also act as a promoting influence by creating tissue damage and stimulating regeneration, a situation which is known from animal experiments to allow expression of chemical carcinogen induced genetic changes, culminating in cancer.

If we had clearer, more reliable evidence for the nature of major factors which promote tumour progression, even at the very late stages in the development of the common human cancers, we should be able to arrest the process, or slow it sufficiently for the disease to cease to be a life threatening one.

Further reading

DeCosse, J. J. (1983). Precancer. *Cancer Surveys* **2**, 347–518.

Farber, E., and Cameron, R. (1980). The sequential analysis of cancer development. *Advances in Cancer Research* **31**, 125–226.

Freeman, A. E. (1980). Induction of mammalian cell transformation by chemical carcinogens: basic considerations. In: *Mammalian cell transformation by chemical carcinogens* pp. 37–45 (eds. N. Mishra, V. Dunkel, and M. Mehlman). Senate Press, Princeton, New Jersey.

IARC mongraphs. Supp. 2 (1980). *Long term and short term screening assays for carcinogens: a critical appraisal.* IARC, Lyon.

Moolgarkar, S. H., and Knudson, A. G. Jr. (1981). Mutation and cancer: a model for human carcinogenesis. *Journal of the National Cancer Institute* **66**, 1037–52.

Slaga, T. J. (ed.) (1983–4). *Mechanisms of tumour promotion.* **I–IV.** CRC Press, Boca Raton, Florida.

Sukumar, S., Notario, V., Dionisio, M-Z., and Barbacid, M. (1983). Induction of mammary carcinomas in rats by nitroso-methylurea involves malignant activation of H-*ras*-1 locus by single point mutations. *Nature* **306**, 658–61.

8

Radiation carcinogenesis

G. E. ADAMS

8.1 Introduction

8.1.1 *The problem*

Although mankind has always been exposed to natural background ionizing radiation, there is considerable doubt whether in the past such exposures have had any significant role to play in the aetiology of human cancer. Radiation carcinogenesis is a twentieth century problem, as indeed are the problems of carcinogenic risk from other hazards to which society is exposed. Cancers induced by ionizing radiation are indistinguishable from most cancers arising from other causes and their occurrence can only be identified by a statistical analysis of excess incidence over the 'natural' incidence. Much of our information on human radiation carcinogenesis is derived therefore from epidemiological sources. Studies of occupational exposure of diagnostic radiologists, uranium miners and workers in the nuclear industries, for example, have provided some information. Much more, however, has come from analyses of cancer incidence in patients exposed to radiation for medical purposes, either for diagnosis or for treatment of non-malignant conditions.

Another major source of information has been the long-term follow up of survivors of the atomic bombs dropped in 1944 on Nagasaki and Hiroshima. This Life Span Study has been in progress since 1950 and has achieved a remarkable level of precision particularly in regard to the dosimetry. In many cases, the precise location of the individuals and the shielding effect of buildings and other structures is now known accurately.

Studies on radiation carcinogenesis in experimental animals have addressed problems such as the pathogenesis of the various cancers that have been identified, inter-species variation, the relationships between cancer induction and cell mutation and other cellular phenomena, dose relationships and, most important of all, the validity or otherwise of animal experiments for assessing radiation risk in human populations. While such studies have provided much information on the biology of radiation carcinogenesis, estimates of radiation risk in humans still rest heavily on the data from epidemiological studies. As in other fields of carcinogenesis, knowledge of events at the cellular and molecular level is essential to an understanding of radiation carcinogenesis, a complex multistage process that extends from the very early physical, chemical, and cellular changes initiated by the absorption of radiation to the delayed effects that only appear many years later.

The energies of photon or particulate radiations emanating from radio-nuclides, X–ray sets and particle accelerators are vastly in excess of those of the chemical bonds in biological molecules. Ionization, i.e. electron ejection from atoms with which the radiation interacts, is there-fore the primary initial event. The time scale over which energy is imparted to the atom is governed by the speed of the particle (usually at or near the velocity of light), the dimension of the atom and the extent of energy loss. A quantum of γ radiation, or an energetic α particle, will pass through a small molecule and deliver energy to it, in a time between 10^{-17} and 10^{-18} sec. The subsequent physical, chemical, and biological processes that follow this event are only expressed as an induced cancer perhaps 30 years or more later. Thus, it is not surprising that the inter-pretation of radiation carcinogenesis in terms of the primary physical and molecular events is a complex undertaking.

8.1.2 *The temporal stages of radiation action*

It is convenient, though not rigorously precise, to classify the many processes of radiation action into four stages, namely, physical, chemical, cellular, and tissue effects (Table 8.1).

8.1.2.1 *The physical stage.* Radiation deposits its energy in discrete pack-ages. Their magnitude and spatial distribution depend on factors such as

Table 8.1 The temporal stages of radiation action

1. *The physical stage*	
10^{-18}–10^{-17} (secs)	Fast particle traverses small atom or molecule
10^{-16}	Ionization: $H_2O \rightarrow H_2O^+ + e^-$
10^{-15}	Electronic excitation: $H_2O \rightarrow H_2O^*$
10^{-13}	Molecular vibrations: dissociation
10^{-12}	Rotational relaxation: $e^- \rightarrow e^-aq$
2. *Physico-chemical and chemical stage*	
10^{-10}–10^{-7}	Reactions of e^-aq and other free radicals with solutes in radiation tracks and spurs
10^{-7}	Homogeneous distribution of free radicals
10^{-3}	Free radical reactions largely complete
Seconds, minutes, hours	Biochemical changes (enzyme reactions)
3. *Cellular and tissue stage*	
Hours	Cell division inhibited in microorganisms and mammalian cells; reproductive death
Days	Damage to gastrointestinal tract (and central nervous system at high doses)
Months	Haemopoietic death; acute damage to skin and other organs; late normal tissue morbidity
Years	Carcinogenesis and expression of genetic damage in offspring

the energy of the radiation, the nature of the absorbing medium, and particularly the type of radiation. The 'densely ionizing' radiations (i.e. α particles, protons and neutrons) lose energy over a much shorter distance than do the 'weakly ionizing' X and γ rays. The biological effectiveness of the particulate radiations in cell killing, mutagenicity, cell transformation, and carcinogenic potential are substantially greater than the weakly ionizing or low 'LET' radiations (LET or 'Linear Energy Transfer' is a measure of the rate at which energy is imparted to the absorbing medium per unit distance of track length).

Interaction of radiation with an atom ejects an electron, or electrons, in less than $\approx 10^{-16}$ sec. The ejected electrons have energy greatly in excess of atomic ionization potentials and cause many more of the secondary ionizations responsible for the subsequent chemical changes which lead to biological damage. The secondary electrons lose energy by collision and eventually undergo dipole interaction. This involves electrostatic interaction between the negative charges of the secondary electrons and the slight positive charge associated with the hydrogen atoms in water. This polarization in water is due to the higher electronegativity of the oxygen atom compared with that of hydrogen. The inter-action in aqueous media is complete in about 10^{-12} sec ('the dielectric relaxation time'). The trapped electron or, as it is called 'the hydrated electron' (e^-aq), has, in many respects, the properties of many free radicals. It can diffuse considerable distances and can undergo rapid reaction with many diverse types of chemical structures including those present in most biological molecules. Its formation marks the transition to the chemical stage of radiation action.

8.1.2.2 *The chemical stage.* The chemical stage of radiation action is concerned mainly with the formation and reaction of molecular frag-ments such as free radicals and excited molecules. Roughly speaking, radiation energy deposited in the cell is partitioned according to the relative proportions of the constituent atoms (at least for the low atomic number elements normally represented in biological tissue). This is known as 'the principle of equipartition of energy' and implies that about 80 per cent of the overall energy deposited in the cell by ionizing radia-tions initially occurs in the aqueous component. This is why so much attention in the past has been devoted to the study of the radiation chemistry of water and aqueous solutions.

The hydroxyl radical (OH), an oxidizing species of high reactivity, is formed very quickly from the ionized water molecule, H_2O^+, by inter-action with neighbouring water molecules and by rapid dissociation of excited H_2O molecules. The reactive hydrogen atoms and hydrated electrons are the corresponding reducing equivalents so that, overall, water radiolysis is described by the simple equation

$$H_2O \rightarrow H(+e^-aq) + OH$$

Some of the radicals interact together to form molecular hydrogen and hydrogen peroxide. The remaining radicals diffuse away from the radia-tion track and react with other molecules in the environment. There is much evidence that damage to biological molecules caused by free radicals contributes to loss or change of cellular function following irradiation. The problem that remains is to identify those reactions that are relevant to the observed cellular response to radiation. The time scales for these reactions are very short and most will be complete in times much less than a millisecond. Others, however, will take longer.

8.1.2.3 *The cellular stage.* Ultrastructural changes in cells can sometimes be observed a short time after irradiation. Local protrusions of the plasma membrane, for example, can be observed within minutes of exposure of cells to a relatively high dose of radiation. Within a few hours these changes are followed by membrane distention and later by invagination of the nuclear membrane. These effects are accompanied by changes in the permeability of the membrane and loss of essential enzymes. However, the more important effects (i.e. the loss of, or changes in, cellular function that occur at much lower radiation doses) can only be observed after longer periods. Loss of reproductive capacity is only evident when the cell fails to divide and chromosomal changes or cellular mutations are observable only after sufficient cell divisions have taken place to allow the analyses of aberrant cells in the total population. Similarly, measurement of changes in the repair capacity of irradiated cells, a process which is normally complete within a few hours of irradiation, usually requires clonal analysis of irradiated populations. Nevertheless, the stages in the cell cycle when radiation damage is most critical are now known. Mammalian cells are usually most radiosensitive during mitosis and very early in the G_1 phase and usually at their most resistant in early S phase, although this is very dependent on radiation quality. Cellular sensitivity to low LET radiation is usually much more variable than it is to high LET radiation.

8.1.2.4 *The tissue stage.* The response times of mammalian tissues to radiation exposure vary widely as do their sensitivities. The observation that mammalian cells show maximum sensitivity to radiation during mitosis predicts firstly, that the fertilized mammalian egg cell (zygote) would be highly sensitive to radiation, and secondly that, in the animal, the most radiation sensitive tissues would be those that turn over rapidly. This is indeed the case. The rapidly dividing proliferating stem cells of the haemopoietic system and the intestinal epithelium are particularly sensitive and respond more quickly than do the moderately sensitive tissues such as lung and the basal layer of the skin. Cells that do not normally divide except after an appropriate stimulus, i.e. parenchymal cells of the liver and connective tissue, are less sensitive still, and cells that divide only during embryonic development are the least radiosensitive. The time of onset for normal tissue damage and mortality depends on the radiation dose.

8.2 Radiation and human cancer

8.2.1 *Radiation dose and radiation risk*

Radiation dose to tissue is expressed in terms of absorbed energy per unit mass as the gray (Gy), which is 1 joule/kg. The older unit, the rad, still in common use, is equivalent to 100 ergs absorbed per gram of tissue and is equal to 0.01 Gy. Carcinogenic potential depends upon absorbed dose and is greater per unit dose for high LET radiations than for low LET radiations. The latter type becomes less effective per gray as the dose falls which is not the case for high LET radiation. This means that, for example, neutrons that are five times more effective than gamma rays at a given dose may be relatively much more effective than gamma rays over a lower dose range. This dose dependence of relative biological efficiency (RBE) is a problem in assessing risk following exposure to a mixture of radiation qualities. This has been encountered in the analysis of the atomic bomb data from Japan.

Estimates of cancer risk may be made in various ways. *Additive* risk expresses the number of *excess* cases per unit of time per unit of dose in a given number of exposed individuals. The *multiplicative* or relative risk model expresses the ratio of the risk in the irradiated population to that in a non-irradiated control group. Additive risk has the advantage of specifying the number of individuals involved and is the approach favoured by UNSCEAR (United Nations Scientific Committee on the Effects of Atomic Radiations) in the Absolute Risk Model. For example, a risk of 10^{-4} implies one excess cancer over a given period, in a population of 10 000 individuals each of which has received an average dose of 1 gray.

8.2.2 *Radiation epidemiology*

Numerous long-term studies are in progress on human populations that have been exposed to radiation. These studies ask questions about overall cancer incidence, excess of individual cancers, latency periods and, where possible, dose response relationships in groups of individuals exposed to radiation arising from occupation, the environment and diagnostic or therapeutic medical procedures (UNSCEAR 1977, and 1982; BEIR 1980).

8.2.2.1 *Occupational exposure.* Excess lung cancers have been observed in underground workers including uranium miners, fluorspar miners in Newfoundland and some Swedish zinc and iron ore miners. The cancers are due to α particle radiation from inhaled radon gas emanating from radium present in the ores. Risk estimates are complicated by the long average latency period of 20 years, difficulties of assessing dose, and the evidence that heavy cigarette smoking substantially increases the risk.

Painters of luminous watch dials have been exposed to radiation through ingestion (by brush licking) of substantial quantities of radium[226] and radium[228]. These isotopes concentrate in the bone matrix and emit short range α particles. Results from a large US study have revealed 62 bone sarcomas and 32 carcinomas of the mastoid and paranasal sinuses in a total of about 2000 female dial painters. No more than one case would have been expected.

8.2.2.2 *Environmental exposure.* Exposures to *natural* sources of radiation are very low. It has been estimated, for example, that the average US citizen has accumulated by the age of 65 the equivalent of only 0.12 Gy from all natural sources and 0.04 Gy from man-made sources. Attention has been drawn to possible risks arising from the use in the building industry of natural materials containing radionuclides. Radon can slowly emanate from granite and other rocks used as infill in the foundations of houses. In earlier times, radon levels were very small due to normal ventilation. More recently, concern about energy savings has led to more efficient insulation in dwellings and this can result in a substantial increase in the indoor radon levels.

Although the *average* individual dose from man-made sources of environmental exposure is very low, substantial exposure has occurred in some select groups of individuals. For example, exposure to short and long lived radioisotopes of iodine in the fall-out from atmospheric weapons testing is responsible for excess thyroid cancer found in a small group of 240 female Marshall Islanders. Estimates of thyroid doses vary between 0.15 and 15 Gy.

The main source of data in the field of exposure to man-made environmental radiation is the Life Span Study on survivors from the atomic bombs dropped on Japan. This study has followed about 80 000 survivors who were briefly exposed to the radiation. Cancer incidence in this population is compared with that in 26 500 age matched, non-irradiated controls. A total of 180 excess cancer deaths occurred over the period 1950–74, corresponding to an increase over control of about 5 per cent, although this figure is misleading since a large proportion of the irradiated population received low doses relative to the remainder. First, excess cancer has occurred mainly in the groups receiving a whole body dose of 1 gray or greater and, secondly, the excess will undoubtedly increase after total life time follow up. A further four–year follow up has shown that the *total* cancer mortality from all causes has increased by 24 per cent. Figure 8.1 shows the *relative* risk of cancer mortality for various sites over the 1950–78 period. The excess leukaemia prominent over the first 20-year period is obviously still present although analysis has shown that it is no longer significant over the last four year period. Conversely, there is now evidence of increased rates for cancer of the stomach, lung, breast and urinary tract and, for the first time, excess risk of colonic cancer and multiple myeloma. These data clearly illustrate the remarkably long latent period in some types of radiation induced cancers. Final risk estimates will have to await the entire post-irradiation life span. Calculation of risks is also complicated by factors such as age at irradiation, sex, variation in dose response relationships for different cancers,

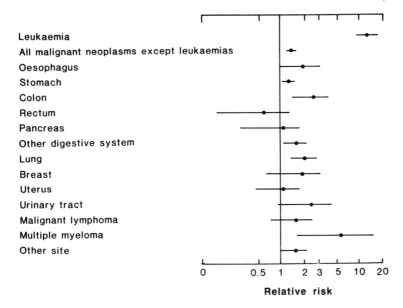

Fig. 8.1 Life Span Study: relative risk of mortality (90 per cent confidence intervals) for specific types of cancer (1950–78) (Kato and Schull, 1982).

and differences between incidence and mortality which can be influenced over a protracted period by improvements in therapy.

8.2.2.3 *Medical exposure.* The evidence for cancer induction by radiation used for various medical treatments for non-malignant conditions is too substantial to review here, but a few general points can be made. Excess thyroid cancers have been observed in children and young adults treated with X-rays for enlarged tonsils, enlarged thymus and naso-pharyngeal disorders, and ring worm of the scalp. There is equivocal evidence of excess cancer in patients treated for hyperthyroidism with iodine[131] (which is concentrated by the thyroid) probably because the epithelial cells are killed by the high local doses of radiation.

Excess cases of leukaemia and cancers of the uterus, kidney and bladder have occurred in women treated with pelvic irradiation for non-malignant gynaecological disorders. Leukaemia incidence, for example, in one group of patients had a two to three-fold increase over that expected. Excess breast cancer has also been reported in women who received fairly high doses of X-rays for treatment of mastitis during the period 1940–55, or during fluoroscopic examinations.

Two large current epidemiological studies are particularly significant.

From 1935–54, some 14 000 patients were given a fractionated course of X–rays to ameliorate the painful symptoms of ankylosing spondylitis, a disease which affects the spine. The estimated *average* dose to the bone marrow in the vertebrae was 3.4 Gy although the irradiation was not uniform. Thirty-one leukaemias were reported compared with 6.5 expected based on age- and sex-matched controls—a five-fold increase. Excess cancer of the oesophagus, stomach, lung, ovaries, and central nervous system, as well as multiple myeloma and lymphoma, were also observed at about the same rate as that in the Life Span Study of the bomb survivors.

There is much concern over the risks arising from the ingestion of radionuclides such as radium and plutonium. These isotopes, which concentrate in the bones, decay by emission of energetic, short-range α particles which can irradiate various regions of the bone matrix. Relevant to this are the results of studies on patients who, over a period of months, were given multiple intravenous injections of radium[224]. This isotope is short-lived (half-life of 3.6 days) and therefore decays while still on bone surfaces. One study involving 680 adults and 218 juveniles has shown respective incidences of bone sarcomas of 18 and 35 where only an 0.2 incidence rate would have been expected.

The induction of acute myeloid leukaemia (AML) has also been observed in experimental animals treated with such radionuclides. Deposition of the isotope on bone surfaces can lead to heavy irradiation of the marrow. Figure 8.2 is a neutron autoradiograph of plutonium[239] in trabecular bone and marrow of the mouse lumbar vertebrae. A thin section of bone is mounted on plastic sheet and placed in a nuclear reactor. Neutron induced fission fragments of the plutonium and other fragments damage the plastic. After etching of the plastic, the fission fragment tracks show as black lines. Irradiation of the bone marrow is clearly evident.

8.2.3 *Dose response relationships*

Radiation dose response relationships can be complex. It is a striking fact that in the huge number of patients successfully treated with radical radiotherapy for carcinoma of the uterine cervix, there is no evidence of a significant increase in the incidence of leukaemia despite the irradiation of normal bone marrow in the pelvic bones during treatment. Conversely, however, there is such evidence from the epidemiological study referred to above of patients treated with *lower* radiation doses for non-malignant gynaecological conditions.

The epidemiological data on radiation induced leukaemia generally, its relatively short latency period, and the substantial evidence available from experimental laboratory studies, combine to make leukaemia the

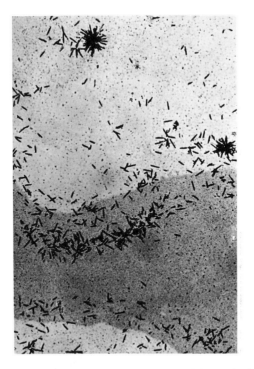

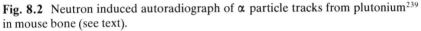

Fig. 8.2 Neutron induced autoradiograph of α particle tracks from plutonium²³⁹ in mouse bone (see text).

most suitable model for studying dose response relationships. Such information is essential for an understanding of the molecular and cellular aspects of radiation carcinogenesis as well as the calculation of risk for radiological protection purposes.

Figure 8.3 compares the dose response for mortality from all forms of leukaemia as observed in the ankylosing spondylitis study with that for induction of acute myeloid leukaemia in male CBA/H mice. The more precise experimental data clearly show an initial rise with increasing dose followed by a decrease at even higher doses. The human data are consistent with this type of response, as indeed are data for several other radiation induced human and animal tumours. The overall response curve is influenced by two factors. The probability of a malignant transformation at the *cellular* level rises with increasing dose. However, when the dose is sufficient to sterilize (kill or prevent cell division) some cells, the number that survive, and are therefore capable of transformation, *falls* with increasing dose. The counterbalancing of these two effects results in the overall dose response for cancer induction. This model,

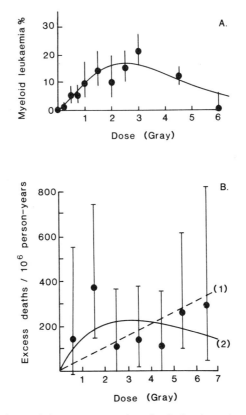

Fig. 8.3 Comparison of dose response data for induction of myeloid leukaemia in male CBA/H mice after brief exposures to 250 kVp X–rays (Fig. 8.3A) (Mole *et al.* 1983. *British Journal of Cancer* **47**, 285–91) with excess mortality rate from leukaemia (as a function of mean bone marrow dose) in irradiated spondylitic patients (Fig. 8.3B) (Smith and Doll 1982 *British Medical Journal* **284**, 449–60).
Line 1 Linear dose response relationship.
Line 2 Linear dose response relationship with cell killing component included.

suggested by Gray in 1965, adequately explains, for example, the lack of excess leukaemias following high dose radiotherapy to the pelvic region for treatment of carcinoma of the cervix referred to earlier.

Various empirical expressions have been used in attempts to describe the overall dose response relationships for human cancer induction although the lack of accurate data on radiation dosage is often a problem. For the experimental AML data in CBA/H mice, the curve fits reasonably well the expression $P = \alpha D^2 e^{-\lambda D}$ where P is the probability of induction, D is the radiation dose, and α and λ are constants. Knowledge of the response relationship for inactivation of the cells at risk would permit derivation of the response relationship for neoplastic transformation.

8.3 Cellular and molecular processes

8.3.1 *Cell inactivation*

A radiation dose of about 1 Gy leads to about 2×10^5 ionizations within the mammalian cell, of which approximately 1 per cent occur in the genomic material. A primary consequence is breakage of DNA strands. Of the 1000 or so strand breaks that occur, almost all disappear within a few hours, either by spontaneous rejoining, or by enzyme mediated repair (see Chapter 6). Some breaks remain, possibly as aligned double-strand breaks, and these are the major cause of loss of viability of some cells. Nevertheless, at this dose, some 40 per cent of the irradiated cells retain the capacity for growth despite the large amount of chemical damage sustained by the cells. Much of the initial chemical damage caused by the radiation is therefore of no consequence to the fate of the cell. Only a very small part of the damage, caused perhaps by the fairly rare local deposition of a large amount of energy near critical molecular sites, is important.

Useful information has been obtained from studies of the relative cytotoxic, mutagenic and transforming abilities of radiations of different LET. Figure 8.4 shows typical dose response 'survival' curves for cells in

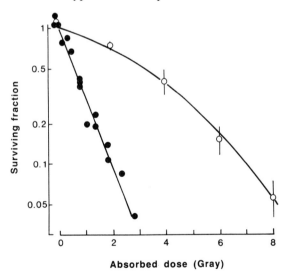

Fig. 8.4 Survival curves for V79 cells irradiated with low LET γ rays (○) and high LET α particles (●) (from Thacker *et al.* 1982 *Radiation Research* **92**, 343–52).

tissue culture irradiated with either low LET X–rays or high LET α particles. High LET radiations invariably are more effective and frequently show an exponential dose relationship (linear on the semi-log plot in Fig. 8.4). In contrast, low LET dose responses are curved when plotted similarly although, in some instances, the initial curvature observed at lower doses is followed by an exponential response. The LET differences in response are due to the very different spatial patterns of the initial atomic and molecular damage. Figure 8.5 shows schematically the energy deposition tracks for high LET α particles and typical low LET X–rays traversing a segment of the DNA helix. Some typical α particles deposit energy at the rate of about 100 keV per micron track length, which means that many ionizations will occur when the particle track passes through the DNA. The energy deposition rate is very much less for X–rays. There is a greater probability of double strand break formation from a single α particle track than there is from either a single X–ray track or from the alignment of two single strand breaks arising from two X–ray tracks. Many physical models based on such processes have been proposed to account for the shapes of dose response curves based on the 'accumulation' of damage or 'interaction' of sub-lesions. There are, however, alternative explanations.

Cells irradiated at low dose rates or with intermittent radiation show reduced inactivation. The effect of such treatments on the shape of dose

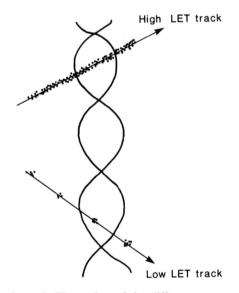

Fig. 8.5 Simple schematic illustration of the different patterns of energy depositions arising from low LET and high LET radiation tracks traversing a section of the DNA helix.

response curves has been explained on the basis of enzyme mediated 'restoration' or 'repair' processes. There is direct evidence that single strand breaks are much more readily repaired than double-strand breaks and therefore repair processes should be more efficient for low LET irradiation. The presence of a shoulder on low LET and survival curves is consistent with the existence of repair mechanisms which become inactivated, or more probably saturated, at higher doses.

8.3.2 *Chromosome damage and cell mutation*

8.3.2.1 *Chromosomal aberrations.* Radiation causes a variety of structural aberrations in mammalian chromosomes only some of which are lethal. Most of these aberrations appear to result from interactions between two or more lesions and can be conveniently grouped as exchanges (interchanges, intra-arm intrachanges and inter-arm intrachanges) and breaks or discontinuities. Not all such aberrations lead to cell death nor do those that are transmissible necessarily have detectable genetic consequences. The position of the cell in its cycle (or its status in regard to DNA duplication) leads to two types of aberration observed at metaphase (see Chapter 11). These are *chromosome type*, where both sister chromatids are involved in exchange for a given locus, and *chromatid type* where only one is affected. Radiation produces both types of aberration in contrast to most chemical chromosome damaging agents which cause only the latter type of aberration, as a rule.

Since cell sterilization and chromosome aberrations involve damage at the DNA level, one might expect some common types of behaviour in radiation dose response relationships. The efficiency of aberration induction for low LET radiations falls at low dose rates and for intermittent, or fractionated, radiation. Figure 8.6 compares the efficiencies for the formation of asymmetrical interchanges (dicentric aberrations) in human lymphocytes irradiated with single doses of either γ rays or fission neutrons. As for cell inactivation, the high LET neutrons are substantially more effective than the low LET γ rays on an equi-dose basis.

8.3.2.2 *Single gene mutation.* The scale of the initial radiation chemical lesions and that of the chromosomal aberrations observed at the light microscope level are separated by several orders of magnitude. The considerable length of nuclear DNA associated with the nucleosomes is duplicated and packaged in a very precise configuration in 25 nm fibres which are themselves folded and coiled into the structure of the metaphase chromosome (see Chapter 6). The small scale molecular changes which reveal themselves as major changes in chromosomal structure must involve considerable amplification. Further, it is likely that modification of some of the initial molecular changes will occur long before

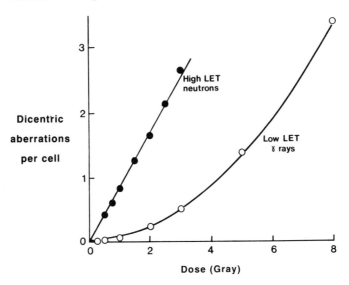

Fig. 8.6 The different efficiencies of high LET fission neutrons and low LET γ rays in causing dicentric chromosome aberrations in human lymphocytes (combined data of Lloyd *et al.* 1975, 1976, *International Journal of Radiation Biology* **28**, 75–9; **29**, 169–82).

these chromosomal changes are observable. Studies at the single gene level provide a much higher degree of resolution.

There are various examples in the literature of close correlations between the dose responses for radiation induced single gene mutation and radiation induced lethality. In general, the efficiency of mutation decreases with increasing dose, but when corrections are made for those cells that are killed by the radiation (and cannot therefore exhibit a mutational change) the correlations are revealed. An example is shown in Figure 8.7 for the radiation induction of thioguanine resistance in three types of mammalian cells. Resistance is due to reduction in activity of hypoxanthine guanine phosphoribosyl transferase (HGPRT), an enzyme which permits cells to incorporate purines from the growth medium (see Chapter 7). The coding gene is located on the X chromosome and therefore only one gene alteration is required to reveal the mutant behaviour. This allows elevation of mutation frequencies to be observed at reasonably low radiation doses. The plot of mutation frequency against the log of the surviving fraction is linear (Fig. 8.7) irrespective of variations in the shapes of the individual radiation dose response curves for both mutation and cell kill between the different cell lines. Surprisingly, the slopes are similar for the three different cell types. It is difficult to reconcile this behaviour in terms of two *independent* lesions leading

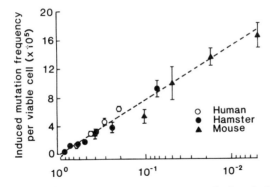

Fig. 8.7 Mutation survival relationships for the radiation induction of thio-guanine resistant mutants of cells from different species (from Thacker, 1979).

either to cell death or mutation. Thacker has argued that the repair process used by the cell in attempting to deal with the initial radiation damage is not entirely error free. If the probability of the repair system for *changing* the genetic material relative to that for *elimination* of the lesion in order to give non-mutant survivors is fixed, this would explain the constancy of the slope for the data in Figure 8.7. To what extent such behaviour holds for high LET radiations is not yet fully explored but it is significant that, like radiation lethality, the efficiency of radiation muta-genesis increases at high LET.

8.3.3 *Radiation transformation*

There are clear dose response inter-relationships for radiation induced cell inactivation, chromosomal changes and single gene mutations. Are such inter-relationships of value in understanding mechanisms of radia-tion carcinogenesis? *In vitro* models of carcinogenesis are now available to assist in answering this (see Chapters 1 and 7).

Neoplastic transformation can be induced in some cells in culture by various agents including radiation. These cells can induce tumours when reimplanted into the animal from which they were originally derived or when transplanted into other immunologically compatible hosts. Trans-formed cells often display other characteristics including loss of anchorage dependence and contact inhibition, or changes at the DNA sequence level. All such systems have limitations but some allow an accurate quantitative examination of radiation dose response relation-ships. The first observation of radiation induced oncogenic transforma-tion at the cellular level was made by Borek and Sachs in 1966 using short-term cultures of Syrian hamster embryo cells. Transformation is readily detected by the appearance of piled up colonies of cells on the culture plates. The system was used to establish a dose response relationship for radiation induced transformation at the cellular level. Another quantitative assay system involves the C3H10T$\frac{1}{2}$ mouse cell line. These fibroblast like cells show normal contact inhibition when growing in a confluent monolayer culture but treatment with radiation (or other agents) causes a morphological change in some cells. The cells give rise to colonies which overgrow the confluent cell layer and can induce fibrosarcomas after inoculation into the appropriate animal host. Transformation efficiency can be expressed as a frequency per cell *exposed* to the carcinogenic stimulus or per *surviving* cell. The distinction is important in interpreting dose response data. The major disadvantage of this system is that the cells are less stable than the cells of the short-term hamster embryo cell system, and spontaneous transformation may occur.

Studies with this and other transforming systems show decreased transformation efficiency with decreasing radiation LET in line with the trends for cell lethality, chromosomal aberrations and gene mutation described earlier. Similarly, transforming efficiency decreases for low dose rate radiations, an effect also explicable in terms of an error free repair component. Interestingly there is evidence of a *reverse* trend for low doses (< 2.0 Gy) of fission neutrons and it has been proposed that this is due to a mis-repair, or 'error prone' repair phenomenon.

Dose response curves for γ irradiated 10T$\frac{1}{2}$ cells are consistent with the bell shaped curves sometimes observed in experimental and human carcinogenesis (Section 8.2.2 and Fig. 8.3). This is illustrated by the transformation data of Elkind and co-workers reproduced in Figure 8.8 for 10T$\frac{1}{2}$ cells exposed to cobalt γ radiation. Correction of the bottom curve, which is expressed as transformants per exposed cell to take account of the surviving fraction of cells for each dose, gives the transformation curve for the fraction of cells at risk.

8.3.4 *Virus and oncogene activation by radiation*

Radiation leukaemia virus (RadLV) is a class of retroviruses (see Chapter 9) first isolated as a 'leukaemogenic activity' in cell free extracts from radiation induced thymic lymphomas in mice. Fractionated whole body irradiation with X–rays can produce up to 100 per cent lymphoma incidence in C57BL/Ka mice. These tumours express the virus in the primary tumour and in serial syngeneic transplants. Injection of cell free extracts intrathymically gives rise to identical tumours in the same strain of mouse. The induction of myeloid leukaemia in RFM/Vn mice following irradiation is also associated with retrovirus infection.

Oncogene activation has been demonstrated in radiation induced thymic lymphomas in mice. Transfection of NIH 3T3 cells with DNA

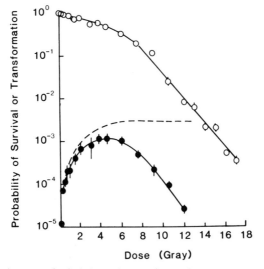

Fig. 8.8 Radiation survival (○) and transformation (●) data for 10T½ cells exposed to cobalt⁶⁰ γ rays (1 Gy/min) (from Elkind *et al.* 1983). Transformation frequency corrected for cell loss due to inactivation is represented by – – – –.

fragments from these lymphoma cells gives rise to activation of the *ras* oncogene.

Virus and oncogene activation are discussed in detail in Chapters 9 and 10.

8.3.5 *Some free radical aspects of radiation carcinogenesis*

Radiation carcinogenesis is a multistage process conveniently divided into *initiation* and *promotion* phases. Free radical processes are involved in both. The initial intra-cellular chemical damage caused by radiation must be mainly free radical in nature since the local energy deposition is greatly in excess of the normal bond energies of all the affected molecules. Many radiation chemical studies on DNA systems *in vitro* have led to a fairly complete knowledge of the various types, structures and reactions of DNA free radicals produced by radiation action. The fundamental problem that remains to be solved, a problem common to the molecular action of other types of carcinogens, is the identification of the *specific types* of free radical chemical damage critical to the onset of the multistage process of carcinogenesis.

8.3.5.1 *Radioprotectors.* It has long been established that various types of molecules containing the reactive sulphydryl group, –SH, influence radiation response. The effects include protection against: (i) cell lethality and mutagenesis *in vitro*, (ii) acute radiation morbidity *in vivo*, and (iii) late effects including radiation induced life shortening. There is much evidence that these protective effects are directly due to the relative weakness of the sulphur-hydrogen bond in the sulphydryl compounds. Free radicals produced either by the radiation or in subsequent chemical reactions can be 'restored' or 'repaired' by transfer of a hydrogen atom from the sulphydryl group of the protector. Such processes have been observed directly in various radiation chemical model systems using fast response pulse radiolysis techniques i.e.

$$X^{\cdot} \quad + \quad RSH \quad \rightarrow \quad XH + RS^{\cdot}$$
$$\text{(free radical)} \quad \text{(protector)}$$

Sulphydryl compounds can also inhibit radiation induced carcinogenesis. The effect is complicated however by the protective effect of these agents against cell lethality and life shortening. The reduction in the number of potential tumour cells and the shortening of the time in which late tumours can be expressed influences their radiation induced incidence. Protection against both these effects can lead to an apparent *increase* in incidence and this has been observed for some tumours. However, there is more consistency in the data for radiation induced thymic lymphomas. Figure 8.9 shows the protective effect of a mixture of radioprotective compounds (most containing sulphydryl groups) on the incidence of thymic lymphomas in irradiated C57 mice.

8.3.5.2 *Superoxide dismutase.* Evidence that free radicals are involved in the promotional phases of radiation carcinogenesis comes from studies with the enzyme superoxide dismutase (SOD). This enzyme is a powerful

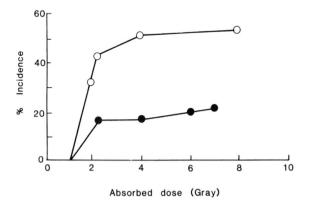

Fig. 8.9 Incidence of thymic lymphoma in C57BL male mice irradiated with 650 R X–rays (○). Protective effect of a mixture of radioprotective agents (●) (from Fry 1983).

catalyst for the removal of the superoxide radical-anion (O_2^-) ultimately formed in many cellular electron transfer processes. It has been proposed that this radical (or its reaction products, e.g. the hydroxyl radical) is highly damaging to the cell and that SOD has evolved as a natural cellular defence mechanism against free radical injury. There is evidence that this enzyme inhibits radiation transformation in the $10T_2^1$ and in the hamster embryo systems but, interestingly, does not need to be present at the time of irradiation. It does require, however, *prolonged* post-irradiation exposure. The hypothesis that free radicals are involved in the promotional phase of radiation carcinogenesis is supported by transformation experiments using chemical promoters and SOD. The phorbol ester tumour promoter, TPA for example, substantially increases radiation induced cell transformation but the effect is completely eliminated by treatment of the cells with SOD. The mechanisms of inhibition of free radical processes involved in tumour promotion are obscure but a plausible explanation may lie in the ability of SOD to inhibit free radicals involved in lipid peroxidation in cellular membranes.

8.3.6 *Interaction of radiation and chemical carcinogens*

Of particular concern in the field of radiological protection and the assessment of risk is the question of possible interaction between radiation and environmental carcinogens. Many experimental *in vivo* studies have been carried out to assess interactions between radiation and chemical carcinogens. Overall, the evidence is equivocal. A complicating factor is the life shortening effect of radiation which may mask any interactive influence of a chemical carcinogen. Nevertheless, there are experimental data indicating positive interactions particularly after foetal exposure. The carcinogen ethylnitrosourea (ENU) can act transplacentally in inducing various tumours in the offspring of mice treated with the chemical before birth. Leukaemia incidence is greater after both ENU and X irradiation than with each agent alone. Interestingly, the incidence of radiation induced ovarian tumours is also increased by exposure to ENU even though no such tumours were observed when ENU was administered without radiation. While such studies may highlight possible additional risks associated with combined exposure to radiation and chemical carcinogens, progress in understanding the mechanisms of such interactions must ultimately derive from the cellular and molecular approach.

Notwithstanding their limitations, the *quantitative* cellular transformation systems currently available have provided some information (see collected papers in *Radioprotectors and anticarcinogens* 1983, for a general discussion). Radiation transformation *in vitro* can be potentiated by various chemical agents including some drugs used in cancer chemotherapy, tumour promoters such as TPA, thyroid hormone extracts, and particularly, pyrolysates of protein foods such as Try-P-2 (3-amino-1-methyl-5H-pyrido-4,3-b-indol). The transforming efficiency of 1.5 Gy of X irradiation in hamster embryo cells, for example, is increased twenty-fold by the addition to the medium of only 0.5 µg/ml Trp-P-2.

Information on the potentiating effects (and indeed inhibiting effects) of various other chemical agents on radiation induced cellular transformation is steadily accumulating. The major problems in applying such information to the problems of human radiation carcinogenesis are the limitations of the *quantitative* transformation assay systems currently available. Established rodent cell lines of fibroblastic origin may not be appropriate models for investigating human radiation carcinogenesis since human tumours arise mainly from epithelial cells. Transformed human epithelial cells can behave quite differently from transformed cells of rodent origin. Nevertheless the rapid accumulation of knowledge on the various stages involved in the transition of a normal primary cell to a frankly malignant phenotype will eventually lead to the establishment of an assay system that is sufficiently quantitative for studies in radiation carcinogenesis. When that point is reached, there will be a much firmer basis for assessing radiation risk in the human population.

Further reading

BEIR (1980). National Research Council, Committee on the Biological Effects of Ionizing Radiation. *The effects on populations of exposure to low levels of ionizing radiation.* National Academy Press, Washington, D.C.

Elkind, M. M., Han, A., Hill, C. K., and Buonaguro, F. (1983). Repair mechanisms in radiation-induced cell transformation. In: *Proceedings of the 7th International Congress of Radiation Research* pp. 33–42 (eds. J. J. Broerse, G. W. Barendsen, H. B. Kal, and A. J. Van der Kogel). Martinus Nijhoff, Amsterdam.

Fry, R. J. M. (1983). Radiation carcinogenesis: radioprotectors and photo-sensitizers. In: *Radioprotectors and anticarcinogens* pp. 417–36 (eds. O. F. Nygaard, and M. G. Simic). Academic Press, New York.

Gray, L. H. (1965). Radiation biology and cancer. In: *Proceedings of the XVIII Annual Symposium on Fundamental Cancer Research* pp. 7–25. Williams and Wilkins, Baltimore.

Kato, H., and Schull, W. J. (1982). Studies of the mortality of A-bomb survivors. 7, Mortality, 1950–78. Part 1, Cancer mortality. *Radiation Research* **90**, 395–432.

Nygaard, O. F., and Simic, M. G. (eds.) (1983). *Radioprotectors and anticarcinogens.* Academic Press, New York. (Collected papers.)

Thacker, J. (1979). The involvement of repair processes in radiation-induced mutation of cultured mammalian cells. In: *Radiation Research Proceedings of the 6th International Congress of Radiation Research* pp. 612–20 (ed. S. Okada). Japanese Association for Radiation Research, Tokyo.

UNSCEAR (1977). (United Nations Scientific Committee on Effects of Atomic Radiation). Sources and effects of ionizing radiation: 1977 Report to the General Assembly, UN, New York.

UNSCEAR (1982). (United Nations Scientific Committee on Effects of Atomic Radiation). Ionizing radiation: sources and biological effects: 1982 Report to the General Assembly, UN, New York.

9

Viruses and cancer

J. A. WYKE

9.1 Introduction

Different forms of human cancer show marked geographic variations in incidence that mainly reflect social rather than genetic differences in the populations at risk. This suggests that variable environmental factors are responsible for a great deal of cancer (Chapter 4). These environmental risk factors comprise three categories: (i) physical agents (such as X-rays or ultraviolet light, Chapter 8), (ii) chemical agents (either directly carcinogenic or converted to carcinogens in the body, Chapter 7), and (iii) infectious agents. Of the infectious agents, bacteria, fungi, and parasitic animals have all been considered as potential carcinogens, but it is viruses that have received the most attention as risk factors in neoplasia of vertebrates. This has been justified for two major reasons. First, viruses are important causes of cancer in certain animals and they are being increasingly implicated in human neoplasia. Secondly, the laboratory study of tumour viruses has led to important insights into the mechanisms of carcinogenesis. These, however, are accolades conferred only with the benefit of hindsight and before we consider our present knowledge of virus associated cancer in more detail it is worth surveying the development of the subject. It is an instructive tale, demonstrating the stimulatory effects on research of advances in apparently unrelated areas as well as the stultifying influence of prejudice on the one hand and uncritical oversimplification on the other.

9.2 The history of tumour virology

9.2.1 *Pioneer days*

The first viruses were discovered towards the end of the 19th century as very small infectious agents, pathogenic for both plants and animals, that passed through filters capable of retaining the smallest bacteria. It was not long before comparable filtrable agents were found to cause tumours in animals. The first of these, discovered by Ellermann and Bang in 1908, induced erythroblastosis (erythroid leukaemia) in chickens. Interest in this finding was muted by contention over whether the disease was a true neoplasm or a hyperplasia, but it was soon shown by Rous in 1911 and Fujinami and Inamoto in 1914 that viruses could induce true tumours, sarcomas, in fowls. This too created relatively little interest in the scientific community at large, perhaps because the diseases of chickens were thought to have little relevance for those of man, and for 20 years the study of chicken tumour viruses was an esoteric pursuit.

Nonetheless, this period saw advances in other fields that would later become very significant. Selective breeding of laboratory mice produced some with high incidences of various cancers. This enabled Bittner in 1936 to show that the high incidence of mammary carcinomas in some strains was due to transmission of a filtrable virus. In the same decade, Rous, Shope, and others produced interesting studies on the virus induced papillomas and carcinomas of rabbits, and work with chicken viruses gathered momentum. The next major advance occurred in 1951 when Gross discovered the first mouse leukaemia virus. This early post-war finding was not the beginning of a new era in tumour virology but the end of an old one. By the beginning of the 1960s our views on tumour viruses were changing rapidly. The momentum behind this change had several sources, the main ones being our growing understanding of both viruses and neoplastic growth, and the development of techniques to advance this understanding by studies in tissue culture.

9.2.2 *The nature of viruses*

Viruses vary enormously in structure and complexity but they all share certain features that distinguish them from other forms of life. They do not have a cellular organization that is propagated by division of the whole entity, but can multiply only by replication of their genetic material (genome). The genome comprises either RNA or DNA and the proteins it encodes usually serve in genome replication or as structural components that protect the genome and facilitate its spread from host to host. Depending on the complexity of the virus, host functions may or may not be required to aid genome replication and transcription, but all viruses require host ribosomal functions for translation of their messenger RNA and thus they are all obligatory intracellular parasites. This enforced intimacy with their host can take many forms, ranging from cytolytic viruses that overwhelm host functions, replicate rapidly and kill the cell, to latent forms that seldom express their own functions and whose genome is replicated, in concert with that of the cell, by the host's own machinery. As we shall discuss later, this close symbiosis is also the reason why some viruses can cause cancer.

Some important human diseases are caused by viruses and there have been strong incentives to understand, and act against, these pathogens. Such stimuli led to the development of laboratory systems for detecting, growing and quantifying viruses, notably the use of tissue cultures to examine virus cytopathic effects (CPE). An important development was a virus assay, based on CPE, in which virus spread was limited and localized plaques of dead cells were thus produced on a layer of tissue culture cells. When similar assays were tried during the 1950s with certain tumour viruses, it was found that, instead of plaques of CPE, the viruses induced focal areas of piled up and morphologically altered cells (Fig. 9.1). Such behaviour was not entirely unexpected, for in the late 1930s it was shown that chicken sarcoma viruses could produce comparable changes in organ explants and on the chorioallantoic membrane of eggs. This tissue culture cell 'transformation' by tumour viruses provided a ready means to examine and quantify the effects of tumour viruses on cells, and it proved a great impetus to further research.

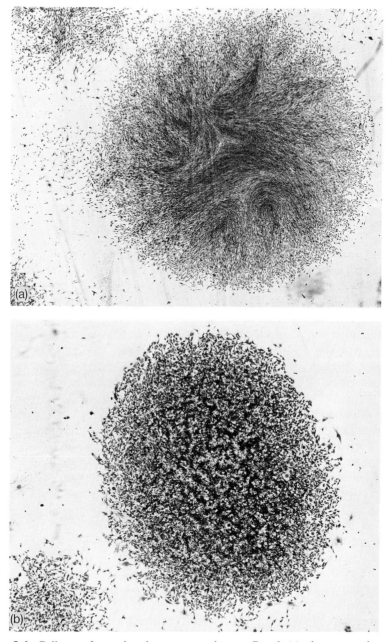

Fig. 9.1 Cell transformation by tumour viruses. Panel (a) shows a colony of uninfected cells of the Syrian hamster cell line BHK21/C13. The colony is flat and the cells are aligned in parallel array. In Panel (b) a colony of the same cell line is shown after transformation with the small DNA virus, polyomavirus. The cells are piled up and disorientated.

9.2.3 *Cell transformation—'tumours'* in vitro

The full significance of the discovery that some (by no means all) tumour viruses can transform cells *in vitro* can be appreciated by considering concepts then current on the nature of cancer. The availability of inbred laboratory animals, which facilitated the identification of some tumour viruses, also permitted experiments on the transplantation of tumours, and it was possible to show that with some tumours a single transplanted cell could cause a tumour in a previously normal animal. This focused attention on cancer as a disease of the single cell, a concept that accorded with a clonal origin of many cancers. Transplantation studies also demonstrated the stable heritability of the tumour phenotype and this, together with the knowledge that many carcinogens were also mutagens, emphasized the possibility that the initiating defect in cancer may often be a mutation in the genome of a somatic cell. The problem with this concept was demonstrating its validity. Every cell in a complex vertebrate contains tens of thousands of genes, so identifying the one or a few that are altered in cancer seemed a hopeless task.

Cell transformation by tumour viruses seemed to offer a way round this impasse. The speed and efficiency of this event suggested to workers in the 1960s that it resulted directly from the functioning of a virus gene. Thus, to find a gene whose activity led to cancer one had only to sift through the genome of a virus rather than that of a cell. Since some tumour viruses contained only enough nucleic acid to encode three or four genes, this simplified the quest over 10 000-fold, bringing its potential achievement within the ambit of the techniques then available. This reasoning encouraged many researchers to investigate the genetics and biochemistry of virus induced cell transformation and not only has this led to the discovery of a number of tumour inducing genes in viruses but studies on the nature of these genes have had enormous conceptual implications for the whole of basic cancer research (see on, and Chapter 10). It should be remembered, however, that these important advances had an element of serendipity in them for, as I shall discuss below, there are ways in which a virus might induce cancer that do not result directly from the action of one of its genes inside the tumour cell.

Work with tumour viruses is only one aspect of the use of tissue culture to study the behaviour of normal and neoplastic cells. Indeed, studies with cells explanted into the culture dish have pervaded all areas of modern biology and the very facility with which these techniques are applied have, from the outset, raised questions about the validity of the results they provide. Reservations about their application in investigating neoplasia centre around the problem of reproducing in culture all the cellular and humoral responses and topological restraints that influence tumour evolution in the whole animal. Conversely, some cells adapt readily to culture and the artificial environment of the culture dish may select characteristics of the cell that have little importance in the host. These considerations have stimulated many studies to identify the features of *in vitro* transformation that correlate most precisely with the ability to form a tumour in the animal. Unfortunately, no single characteristic of cells *in vitro* permits such a correlation. As we might have expected, the phenotypes of tumour cells and *in vitro* transformed cells differ in a complex, but not fully congruent, fashion from their normal counterparts. Studies *in vitro* will help to dissect this complexity but, for the time being, their full significance can only be assessed by continual reference to the behaviour of the cells in the whole animal.

9.2.4 *Modern concepts and questions*

Tumour virology still concerns itself with two broad questions: the role of viruses in clinical neoplasia, and the use of viruses in probing the mechanisms of carcinogenesis. We now understand enough about viral genomes and host cell functions to formulate ideas about how the former topic influences the latter (see on) and to relate these concepts to specific diseases. We also appreciate better the role of viruses as one component in what may be a multifactorial disease process, and this concept is taken into account when examining viruses as risk factors in human and animal cancer (see Section 9.3). Both these considerations are underpinned by the premise that cancer results from alterations in the structure or activity of a certain number of genes in the cell (see Chapter 10). Tumour virology, as a whole, can thus be regarded as a branch of molecular genetics.

9.3 Implicating viruses in experimental and natural cancers

How do we decide that an infectious agent is responsible for causing a given disease? The classic criteria were embodied in Koch's postulates of 1876 which stated that (i) the agent should be found in all cases of the disease, its location corresponding with the observed lesions, (ii) the agent should be capable of isolation from the lesions and growth in pure culture outside the body, and (iii) the culture, when inoculated back into an animal, should produce the identical disease.

It is apparent that many pathogenic bacteria, let alone viruses, do not fulfil Koch's postulates but, when satisfied, these criteria provide convincing proof of causality. Many viruses have been shown to cause tumours in laboratory and domestic animals in this way, with the proviso that 'culture outside the body' has, perforce, been done on living cells, not inert media. Any doubts this raises about purity of the organism could, in theory, now be answered by molecular cloning of viral genomes in bacteria, but this has not yet been considered a necessary precaution.

In contrast to the ease with which viruses have been implicated in animal tumours, their role in human disease has been extremely difficult to investigate. This explains why major efforts, during the 1970s, to identify viral causes for human cancer produced few clear leads, and convincing causal associations are only now becoming apparent. A major problem, of course, is the impossibility of ethically fulfilling Koch's third postulate; other animals can be used to test the oncogenicity of human viruses but the results they yield can be misleading. Attempts have been made to modify Koch's postulates by including evidence for the presence of viral genomes or proteins in the tumours (when infectious virus cannot be found) and by asking whether the person with a tumour shows a specific immune response against the candidate virus. However, even if positive, these tests only show that a virus is associated with a tumour, not that it is a cause. Good evidence for causality would, of course, be provided if elimination of virus infection (for instance by immunization) also eliminated the incidence of the tumour, but such evidence has not yet been provided for any major virus associated human neoplasm.

A further problem in implicating viruses in human neoplasia is the complexity of the disease in man. Many virus induced tumours in animals occur in a high proportion of the infected population, often at a relatively early stage of the animal's short lifespan and, in the case of laboratory animals, selective breeding has enhanced these features. The virus is clearly a major risk factor in the disease. Human populations, in contrast, are usually outbred with no marked inherited predispositions to cancer (but see Chapter 5) and the disease usually occurs towards the end of a long lifespan with a pattern of incidence that suggests a multi-factorial causation (Chapter 4). Indeed, the role of a virus in human neoplasia is often first hinted at by epidemiological data, the same data also showing that only a minority of the infected population develop tumours. Virus infection is thus usually one of a complex of interrelated risk factors that operate at different stages of development of a tumour, as shown in Figure 9.2. This figure depicts three main groups of risk factors: those relating to virus infection, those concerning the cellular alterations involved in neoplasia, and those affecting the host response to both viruses and tumour cells. Let us consider how they may operate at three arbitrary stages in the evolution of a virus associated neoplasm.

9.4 Risk factors predisposing to virus associated neoplasia

The risk factors are shown diagrammatically in Figure 9.2. In Stage 1 a virus must infect the host and, depending on the mechanism by which it

RISK FACTORS IN VIRAL CARCINOGENESIS

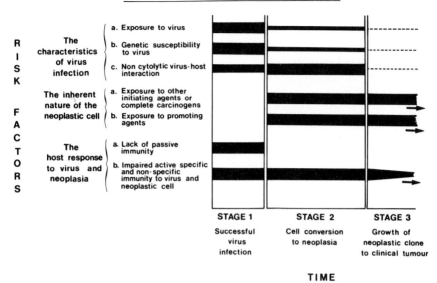

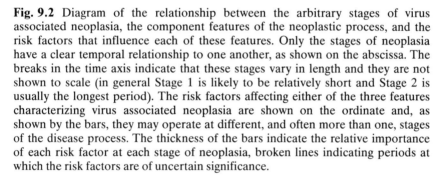

TIME

Fig. 9.2 Diagram of the relationship between the arbitrary stages of virus associated neoplasia, the component features of the neoplastic process, and the risk factors that influence each of these features. Only the stages of neoplasia have a clear temporal relationship to one another, as shown on the abscissa. The breaks in the time axis indicate that these stages vary in length and they are not shown to scale (in general Stage 1 is likely to be relatively short and Stage 2 is usually the longest period). The risk factors affecting either of the three features characterizing virus associated neoplasia are shown on the ordinate and, as shown by the bars, they may operate at different, and often more than one, stages of the disease process. The thickness of the bars indicate the relative importance of each risk factor at each stage of neoplasia, broken lines indicating periods at which the risk factors are of uncertain significance.

instigates neoplasia (see on), infection must lead to persistence of virus genetic material in the host or to some stable, virus induced alteration in certain cells. Infection-related risk factors important at this stage are exposure to the virus (dose of virus and route of infection) and whether or not the host cells are susceptible to virus penetration and growth. The acquired resistance of the host, either by passive or active immunity (see Chapter 15), is also crucial, as in any other virus infection.

The requirement for Stages 2 and 3 distinguishes the pathogenesis of virus associated neoplasia from that of acute cytolytic virus diseases. In Stage 2, the conversion of an infected cell to neoplastic growth, the important characteristic of virus infection is the need to establish a non-cytolytic virus cell association, since, obviously, only live cells can form

tumours (an exception to this requirement may be those instances where
the mechanism of virus oncogenesis is indirect, see on). Some tumour
associated viruses, such as the retroviruses and hepatitis B virus, can
replicate without causing massive cell death, whilst herpesviruses can
persist in latent, inactive forms in living cells. Other tumour viruses, however, can only convert a cell to neoplasia if full replication of the virus is
blocked, either because the host cell is unusual or the virus has some
defect. In either case, the infection that leads to neoplasia is unusual and
may be inapparent in other ways, yet another factor making it difficult to
link virus infection to neoplasia.

Futher complicating factors important at Stage 2 are the requirements
for (i) additional carcinogens or promoting agents (see Chapter 1), or
(ii) the action of agents that affect host immune responses. In many virus
associated tumours of man, such additional factors seem as or more
important than virus infection itself.

Stage 3 in this sequence is the multiplication and progression of a neoplastic cell to form a clinical tumour. Infection related risk factors are
probably of little importance to this late stage in tumour evolution,
although if expression of the virus persists it may serve as an antigenic
target for host immune respones. Co–carcinogens, on the other hand,
may remain important as tumour progression occurs (Chapter 7).
Impairment of the host immune response is also likely to remain
important. There is, in fact, a pervasive connection between host immune
deficiency and the development of virus associated tumours, particularly
in man, which may be summarized as follows.

1. Immune mechanisms, such as T cell mediated cytotoxicity, natural
killer cell activity and interferon, can reduce the growth of virus induced
tumours in laboratory animals (see Chapter 15).

2. Immune impairment is seen in many virus induced tumours in
animals. In some instances, as with agents that infect T cells (see Chapter
3) like Marek's disease virus and feline leukaemia virus, virus infection
itself is immunosuppressive. In other cases a co-carcinogen has this
effect, an example being the role of bracken fern in papillomavirus
associated alimentary carcinomas of cattle.

3. Human patients receiving immunosuppressive therapy show an
increased incidence of a limited range of tumours, many of which are
tumours in which virus infection has also been implicated. Indeed, so
striking is this overlap that it has been suggested that viruses may play a
role in all tumours whose incidence is increased in immune deficient
individuals. However, in only one type of therapy induced tumour has
virus been directly implicated so far: the immunoblastic 'lymphomas'
associated with Epstein Barr virus (EBV) (see Chapter 3).

4. Finally, immune impairment seems a risk factor in the natural

history of a number of virus associated human neoplasms. Notable among these are tumours linked to infection with the human T cell leukaemia/lymphoma virus (a retrovirus), certain papillomaviruses, hepatitis B virus and the herpesvirus, Epstein Barr virus.

9.5 Important tumour viruses of animals and man

The oncogenic viruses are a very diverse group. They include members of all the major families of DNA viruses that infect vertebrates, with the exception of the very small parvoviruses and the very large poxviruses. On the other hand only one family of RNA viruses, the retroviruses, can cause tumours. The tumour viruses vary greatly in the complexity of their genomes, in the types of neoplasms they induce and in the requirement for cofactors in tumorigenesis. What do they have in common?

One universal feature is the importance of a DNA stage in the replication of the viral genome. The retroviruses are unique among viruses whose free infectious forms contain RNA in that this genome is copied soon after infection into double-stranded DNA by an RNA dependent DNA polymerase enzyme carried in the virus particle. Moreover, this DNA 'provirus' is then inserted ('integrated') by a covalent linkage into the host cell DNA. Such integrations seem another frequent, but not invariant, hallmark of tumour viruses: whole or partial viral genomes are very often detected in tumour cell chromosomes. It is not clear why integration occurs so commonly since it is obligatory in only one of the mechanisms by which tumour viruses cause neoplasia (see on). However, it may serve mainly to ensure a stable association between viral and host genomes during the lengthy development of a neoplastic cell lineage. In this context it is interesting that a number of poxviruses can induce cellular hyperplasia and some apparently encode proteins related to growth factors (see Chapters 1 and 12), yet none of them induces stable neoplasia. Could this be because they complete their life cycles in the cytoplasm of the cell and do not enter the nucleus?

Various groups of tumour viruses are shown in Tables 9.1, 9.2, and 9.3. These lists are representative and not comprehensive, and for a fuller account the texts listed at the end of this chapter should be consulted. Entries in the tables have been chosen because of (i) their historical or research interest, (ii) an intrinsically interesting pathogenesis, (iii) their importance as pathogens of man and domestic animals, or (iv) their inclusion elsewhere in this Chapter.

9.5.1 *Retroviruses (Table 9.1)*

This is a family of small viruses with RNA genomes of 5–10 000 nucleotides. Only one subfamily, the oncoviruses, contains tumorigenic

Table 9.1 Some oncogenic retroviruses of animals and man

Virus genus	Viruses	Associated tumours	Other risk factors[1]
Type B oncovirus	Mouse mammary tumour virus	Mammary adeno-carcinoma	Pregnancy (altered hormone levels)
Type C oncovirus	Avian sarcoma-leukosis virus complex	Various sarcomas, some carcinomas, lymphomas and leukaemias	Genetic susceptibility affecting virus penetration, replication and spread
	Avian reticulo-endotheliosis virus complex	Lymphoma and leukaemias	
	Mouse leukaemia and sarcoma viruses	Various sarcomas, lymphomas and leukaemias	Genetic susceptibility affecting virus penetration, replication and spread
	Feline leukaemia virus	Leukaemia lympho-sarcoma (mainly T cell)	
	Bovine leukaemia virus	Lymphosarcoma leukaemia (B cell)	
	Primate leukaemia and sarcoma virus	Fibrosarcoma, myeloid leukaemia	
	Human T cell lymphotropic virus	Adult T cell leukaemia/lymphoma	

[1] Where known or suspected. The absence of listed risk factors does not imply that such factors are unimportant.

members and of the genera in this subfamily (classified according to virus particle structure) by far the most important is the Type C virus genus.

The retroviruses of chickens were the first tumour viruses to be discovered and, together with comparable viruses of mice, they have played a crucial role in the history of tumour virology. They retain the centre of the stage in our attempts to understand the molecular basis of neoplasia (see on and Chapter 10), and only one group of avian retroviruses, the causal agents of fowl leukosis, is of commercial importance.

Two other important retrovirus pathogens of domestic animals are feline leukaemia virus and bovine leukosis virus. The latter is of commercial importance in many parts of the world where it causes the most common malignancy in cattle. Leukaemia and lymphosarcoma are also the most frequent tumours of domestic cats but they account for only a fraction of the deaths attributable to feline leukaemia virus, which also causes anaemia, immunosuppression and related diseases, making it now the most frequent non-traumatic cause of death among cats in developed countries.

The diseases caused by these cattle and cat retroviruses provide interesting parallels for a disease complex in man associated with infection by a retrovirus group called human T cell leukaemia virus (HTLV). With all three agents the prevalence of infection in the population is greater than the incidence of neoplasia. Indeed, in the case of HTLV the associated tumour, adult T cell leukaemia/lymphoma, is rare and, even in areas where HTLV infection is widespread, only about one in 80 of the infected population develop the malignancy (presumably, unidentified cofactors are important in oncogenesis). Nevertheless, as with feline leukaemia virus, HTLV may induce diseases other than neoplasia. Two strains, HTLV–1, and –2, are associated with T cell malignancies whilst a third, HTLV–3, has been implicated in acquired immune deficiency syndrome (AIDS), a T cell deficiency. The effect of the HTLV complex is clearly finely balanced between stimulating and suppressing T cell growth.

9.5.2 *Small DNA viruses (Table 9.2)*

The most important human oncogenic viruses appear to be in this group. It is estimated that 200 million people, mainly in Third World countries, are chronically infected with hepatitis B virus and are at risk of developing cirrhosis (fibrosis of the liver) and primary liver cancer. This tumour at present probably causes more deaths worldwide than any other malignancy, with about 500 000 fatalities per annum. However, even at this level it is clear that only a minority of those infected with the virus develop the tumour and other risk factors, which may vary from area to area, must be important. Postulated factors include smoking, superinfection with another virus (the Delta agent), and consumption of alcohol or food contaminated with aflatoxin B1 derived from the fungus *Aspergillus flavus*. Very similar viruses cause liver tumours in rodents and these should provide a good model for studying this important human disease.

One genus of the Papovavirus family contains two important tools of the molecular biologist, polyoma and SV40, and two agents closely related to these that commonly infect man, BK and JC virus. These latter have not been associated with any human tumour but they are frequently detected in immunosuppressed individuals, they transform cells in tissue culture and they can induce tumours in rodents, so they are clearly still

Table 9.2 Some oncogenic small DNA viruses of animals and man

Virus family	Virus	Genome size[1]	Host of origin	Associated tumours	Other risk factors[2]
Hepadenavirus	Hepatitis B group	3 kb	Man, apes, rodents, ducks	Liver cancer	In man: alcohol, smoking, fungal toxins, other viruses
Papovavirus	Polyoma	5 kb	Mouse	Various carcinomas and sarcomas	
	SV40	5 kb	Monkey	Sarcomas (in rodents)	
	BK and JC	5 kb	Man	None in man; neural tumours in rodents and monkeys	
	Papilloma	7–8 kb	Man	Genital, laryngeal and skin warts, may progress to:	
				Cervical carcinoma	Smoking, herpes simplex viruses
				Laryngeal carcinoma	X-irradiation, smoking
				Skin carcinoma	Sunlight, genetic disorders possibly affecting immunity
			Cattle	Genital, alimentary and skin warts, may progress to:	
				Alimentary carcinoma	Possibly carcinogens and immune suppressants in bracken fern
				Skin carcinoma	Sunlight, genetic predisposition (lack of pigmentation)
			Other mammals	Papillomas, may progress to carcinomas	Experimentally, carcinogens such as methylcholanthrene

[1] In kilobases (kb); one kilobase is 1000 base pairs of nucleic acid.
[2] Where known or suspected. The absence of listed risk factors does not imply that such factors are unimportant.

The papillomaviruses, in contrast, have long been known to cause tumours in many animals—benign warts (papillomas). However, it is now clear that these lesions can become malignant, but they have a natural history that may be very complicated. For instance, molecular biology techniques have revealed well over 20 different papillomaviruses that infect man alone, and those types commonly associated with benign growths may not be the same as the types found in malignant lesions (the most important of which is carcinoma of the uterine cervix). Moreover, the progression from benign to malignant growth can depend on several other predisposing factors (see Table 9.2). One example gives a flavour of this complexity. The very rare human disease epidermodysplasia verruciformis shows some familial clustering (suggesting a genetic component) and usually arises in young patients with congenitally defective cell mediated immunity. It is characterized by disseminated skin warts of two main types from which can be isolated many different papillomaviruses. Carcinomas may later develop from one type of wart associated with a subset of these papillomavirus types. The carcinomas arise mainly in areas exposed to sunlight. Thus specific papillomaviruses, immune deficiency and a co-carcinogen (in this case UV light) all combine in the disease process. Factors of these three classes also operate in the genesis of alimentary carcinomas in cattle and, indeed, the triad of virus, co–carcinogen and immune impairment are a common motif in many of the tumours, particularly those of man, considered in this chapter.

9.5.3 Large DNA viruses (Table 9.3)

Of the two families considered here, the adenoviruses cause mild non-neoplastic diseases in man but the same strains can cause tumours in hamsters and, as a consequence, they have been studied intensively. There is no evidence that they play a role in human cancer, but these studies have been enormously fruitful for those interested in the basic molecular mechanisms of gene expression and regulation.

The herpesviruses are more significant pathogens. Marek's disease virus causes a commercially-important disease of chickens characterized by a T cell proliferation that infiltrates nervous tissue (hence the description, neurolymphomatosis). Three other herpesvirus types have been linked with human neoplasia. For two of these, the Herpes simplex viruses and cytomegalovirus, the evidence that they play a causal role in certain cancers (Table 9.3) is intriguing but not conclusive. For EBV the causal link is more persuasive. Not only does this agent cause the non-neoplastic infectious mononucleosis (glandular fever), a disease particularly common in young adults, but it is also a major risk factor in nasopharyngeal carcinoma, a common malignancy in some heavily populated parts of the world such as southern China. Once more,

Table 9.3 Some oncogenic large DNA viruses of animals and man

Virus family	Genome size[1]	Virus	Host of origin	Associated tumours	Other risk factors[2]
Adenovirus	30–50 kb	Types 2, 5, 12	Man	None in man; sarcomas in hamsters	
Herpesvirus	130–250 kb	Frog herpesvirus	Frog	Adenocarcinomas	Ambient temperature
		Marek's disease	Fowl	Neurolymphomatosis (T cell)	Genetic predisposition of unknown basis
		H. ateles and *H. saimiri*	Monkey	Lymphoma, leukaemia (T cell)	
		Epstein Barr virus	Man	Burkitt's lymphoma Immunoblastic lymphoma Nasopharyngeal carcinoma	Malaria Immune deficiency Salted fish in infancy, histo-compatibility antigen genotype
		H. simplex types 1 and 2	Man	Cervical neoplasia (?)	Papillomaviruses, smoking
		Cytomegalovirus	Man	Kaposi's sarcoma (?)	Immune deficiency, histo-compatibility antigen genotype

[1] In kilobases (kb); one kilobase is 1000 base pairs of nucleic acid.
[2] Where known or suspected. The absence of listed risk factors does not imply that such factors are unimportant.

however, we see the familiar pattern: infection is far more widespread than the incidence of the tumour, and other factors are clearly important. This is even more evident in the case of Burkitt's lymphoma, a B cell tumour of children in West Africa and New Guinea linked jointly to EBV infection and endemic malaria. A large proportion of children in these areas have experienced both known risk factors, yet only a small minority develop the tumour. What else is required for tumorigenesis? Specific chromosomal rearrangements seem an important prerequisite, but what favours such events and what are their biological consequences? These are discussed further in Chapters 10 and 11 but the answer can be given here—we do not know.

9.6 Prophylaxis and therapy of virus associated neoplasia

Although we are clearly ignorant of many aspects of the pathogenesis of virus associated tumours, the knowledge that a virus is implicated can be used in attempts to manage the disease at any of the three arbitrary stages of virus associated neoplasia described above and in Figure 9.2. In general these measures are more effective in veterinary medicine (where the health of the herd can override the survival of the individual) than in human practice.

9.6.1 *Preventing virus infection*
The level of oncogenic viruses in the hosts' environment can be reduced by hygiene and husbandry techniques, and by detecting and, if necessary, eliminating carriers. The latter approach has been used in managing diseases caused by the avian, feline and bovine retroviruses and it has some limited applications in man, for instance in detecting agents like hepatitis B virus and HTLV in donor blood intended for transfusion.

Increased genetic resistance to infection can be bred into domestic animals, an approach successful in developing chicken strains relatively resistant to both avian leukosis and Marek's disease.

However, in most cases acquired immunity to infection is the only option. Vaccines made from ground-up wart tissue have long been used as a prophylactic against papillomas in animals, but the first successful commercial vaccines against a neoplasm were produced against Marek's disease and are a great boon to the poultry industry. We may soon anticipate vaccines against feline leukaemia but, in contrast to veterinary problems, proposals to produce vaccines against human oncogenic viruses have long been controversial, for several reasons. (i) In many instances the role of the virus in the tumour is uncertain, (ii) tumour production may be a rare outcome of infection by a widespread and not very pathogenic virus, and (iii) since tumours may result from an aberrant virus cell interaction, a classic vaccine, based on inactivated or attenuated virus, may itself pose a health risk. This last objection may soon be obviated by using purified immunogens produced by genetically manipulated portions of viral genomes or synthesized in the laboratory.

However, the first two considerations suggest that the returns (in terms of improved health of the population) may not justify the outlay unless the virus causes significant disease in addition to its oncogenic potential (as is the case with hepatitis B virus), unless there are clearly defined, small, high risk populations or unless the virus is the only clearly defined risk factor in the genesis of a common tumour (as with EBV associated nasopharyngeal carcinoma). In other instances prevention of neoplasia may be better tackled by examining other risk factors.

9.6.2 *Preventing cell conversion to neoplasia*

Other potentially avoidable risk factors tend to operate at this stage. In man they include habits (notably smoking), dietary factors (which may be even harder to eliminate than smoking unless, like aflatoxin contamination, they are obviously undesirable) and other diseases. The most striking example of the latter is malaria, a risk factor in Burkitt's lymphoma in certain tropical areas but also a crushing disease problem in its own right in many parts of the world. Indeed, reducing or eliminating some of these risk factors would have benefits far beyond the reduction in cancer incidence, and this seems so evident that one doubts that the incentive of reducing cancer will work where other imperatives have so signally failed.

9.6.3 *Tackling clinical neoplasia*

Can a knowledge of tumour virology contribute to tumour diagnosis and therapy? So far such applications have been on a small scale but in principle a detailed understanding of the role of any given virus in cancer should aid diagnosis and prognosis by screening for characteristic viral genes or proteins, or a host response to them. It is harder to see how such knowledge could be applied to therapy but, curiously, there have been a few examples of regression of virus associated tumours in response either to viral antisera or to a 'vaccine' extracted from homogenized tumour. There is also the tantalizing example of interferon, a general antiviral agent produced by host cells after infection with many different viruses that also has an antitumour effect in a few cases that is, as yet, poorly understood.

Clearly, we will not advance much further with these considerations until we unravel the details of how a tumour virus subverts cell growth. Fortunately, as the next section describes, such understanding is beginning to take shape from the amorphous complexity of tumour virus behaviour.

9.7 The mechanisms of virus induced neoplasia

We have already seen that workers in the 1960s set out to identify viral genes that directly converted normal cells to neoplastic growth. However, the many variations of intracellular parasitism exhibited by viruses could, in theory, permit neoplasia by a number of other mechanisms. Indeed, as we identify more tumour viruses so we are compelled to invoke an ever widening spectrum of pathogenic mechanisms. In this section we will survey, with examples, these different modes of virus induced neoplasia (Table 9.4).

The two major categories of the disease process are, (i) that in which the tumour cell ancestry must at some stage have been infected by the

Table 9.4 Mechanisms of virus induced neoplasia

Pathogenic mechanism	Examples
Indirect	
Suppression of host immune system, impaired elimination of tumour cells	Marek's disease virus, feline leukaemia virus, HTLV
Stimulation of cell proliferation, increased 'targets' for other neoplastic changes	
(a) tissue regeneration after virus cytolysis	None yet known
(b) mitogenesis of immune competent cells	Possibly some mouse leukaemia virus
Direct	
'Hit and run': no crucial virus gene or structure whose persistence is essential. Viral DNA or viral functions act transiently as mutagens	Possibly some herpesviruses
Crucial parts of viral genomes persist in tumour cells; virus carries a gene whose product directly or indirectly initiates and/or maintains neoplasia	
(a) this is an *oncogene* descended from normal cell counterpart (*proto-oncogene*)	Rous sarcoma virus, acute leukaemia viruses
(b) this gene has no related normal cell counterpart	SV40, polyomavirus, HTLV
Insertional mutagenesis: virus DNA inserted in the host chromosome augments or destroys normal gene expression	Avian leukosis viruses, mouse mammary tumour virus

tumour inducing virus, and (ii) that in which the tumour cell ancestry need not be infected by the virus. Neoplasia in the first category is a direct consequence of infection whilst in the second category it results indirectly, from infection of other cells (the terms intrinsic and extrinsic have also been used to describe these two mechanisms).

9.7.1 *Indirect mechanisms: suppression and stimulation of cell proliferation*

Most virus infections kill cells and if the cells of the host's immune system are targets for viral infection then immune deficiency, particularly an impairment of cell mediated immunity, can result. The role of immune surveillance in cancer has been controversial (see Chapter 15) but, as we saw above, many virus associated neoplasms occur in hosts with immune deficiency and it is possible that tumour cells arising in these hosts by unknown mechanisms are simply not eliminated. Viruses such as avian reticuloendotheliosis viruses, Marek's disease virus, feline leukaemia virus, HTLV, and cytomegaloviruses are known to have immune suppressive effects, but in most instances they seem to have another, possibly direct, tumorigenic effect. One possible exception is HTLV–3, the putative cause of acquired immune deficiency syndrome (AIDS) in man. This virus can be considered oncogenic since many AIDS patients develop mesenchymal tumours such as Kaposi's sarcoma which may affect connective tissues in many parts of the body. However, unlike the other HTLV strains, HTLV–3 does not appear to act directly in tumour causation and its effect may be due solely to immune impairment and a consequent inability to kill tumour cells arising by other mechanisms.

Another possible consequence of virus infection is a reactive cell proliferation, the expansion of a cell population, increasing the chance of occurrence of a neoplastic change. This can take two forms, regeneration of tissue damaged by virus cytolysis, or mitogenesis of immune competent cells chronically stimulated by viral antigens. It was once suggested that liver tumours associated with hepatitis B virus infection might be due to the former mechanism, but this now receives little credence and there are no other likely examples of this phenomenon. Mitogenesis of immune competent cells may contribute to some retrovirus induced mouse leukaemias; in the examples studied the cells themselves seem infected and the mechanism appears direct, but there seems no a priori reason why this should always be the case.

9.7.2 *Direct mechanisms: the 'hit and run' hypothesis*

It is conceivable that transient cell infection induces a heritable neoplastic change in the cell lineage and the infecting virus is then lost. In practice this mechanism is indistinguishable from the indirect modes described above, but in other instances, such as some herpesvirus induced tumours, portions of the viral genome frequently persist. However, since neither the fragment of persisting virus, nor its location in the cell genome, show any discernible pattern, it is suspected that they represent the 'footprints' of an earlier 'hit and run' event whose significance cannot now be assessed. Since they are difficult to investigate, 'hit and run' and indirect mechanisms are usually only considered after failing to demonstrate tumour formation by one of the direct mechanisms we now describe.

9.7.3 *Direct mechanisms: transforming genes with cellular ancestors*

The viruses that most readily transform cells in culture (Fig. 9.1) and most rapidly induce tumours in animals are the chicken and mouse retroviruses that cause sarcomas and 'acute' (rapid) leukaemias and the polyomavirus group of the papovaviruses. Using cell culture, mutants of these viruses with defects in transformation were obtained (Fig. 9.3) and analysis of these mutants defined transforming genes in the viruses. These genes, as predicted by the pioneer workers in this field, encode proteins necessary to initiate and/or maintain transformed cell growth, and they comprise two classes.

The retroviruses mostly contain transforming genes that play no part in virus replication and have, indeed, usually replaced portions of viral replicative genes in the virus genome. These genes are related to sequences in normal host cells from which they are believed to have evolved after 'capture' of the cell gene by the virus in some ancestral infection (indeed, this evolution is apparently sometimes recapitulated when tumours are induced by certain chicken and cat leukaemia viruses). These transforming genes were named viral oncogenes and the cellular counterparts became known as cellular oncogenes or, since they presumably serve some crucial non-neoplastic function in the host, protooncogenes. These oncogenes, first brought to our attention by the retroviruses, are now central to studies on the molecular biology of cancer (see Chapters 10, 11 and 12).

9.7.4 *Direct mechanisms: transforming genes without cellular ancestors*

The second class of transforming gene is exemplified by those in polyoma and SV40 viruses. These genes play a part in the virus life cycle (albeit sometimes a rather peripheral role) and they are not obviously derived from cellular ancestors. Protooncogenes are thought to function in normal cell growth and behaviour, with the viral oncogenes representing perverted forms of these activities that tip the cell into neoplasia. Since the actions of papovavirus transforming genes have similar consequences for the cell as the functioning of the retrovirus oncogenes, we

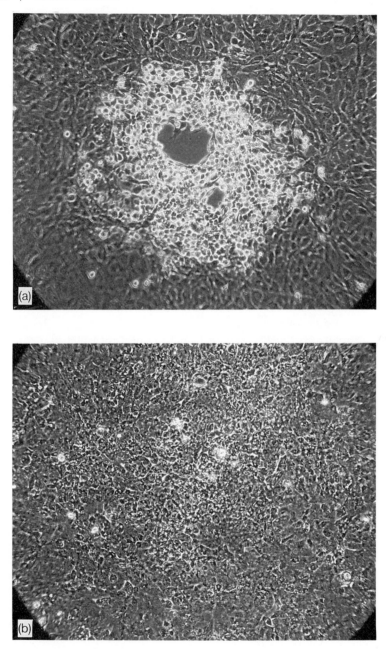

Fig. 9.3 Cell transformation by viruses with mutations in transforming genes. Some mutants of Rous sarcoma virus have 'temperature sensitive' defects in transformation. Infected cells grown at the 'permissive' temperature are trans-

can conclude that the former mimic functions in comparable regulatory pathways. They are 'analogues' to the retroviral oncogene's 'homologues' of cellular functions.

A few retroviruses also seem to possess genes whose provenance and activity are more akin to the papovavirus transforming genes than to retroviral oncogenes. Thus, a region of the HTLV genome that appears unrelated to any host sequence encodes a protein that may regulate the activity of cellular genes as well as its own genome. Some other retroviruses without oncogenes may induce neoplasia in a comparable fashion.

9.7.5 Direct mechanisms: insertional mutagenesis

It appears, however, that many retroviruses without oncogenes induce neoplasia by a different means. The majority of retroviruses contain only the genes needed for their own replication, they cannot transform cells in tissue culture, they induce tumours after a long latency, and tumour induction results from a direct effect of the viral genome rather than from the action of a virus-coded protein.

Avian leukosis viruses (ALV) are retroviruses of this type and studies on the lymphomas they induce provided the following clues to this mode of pathogenesis. All or most of the cells in a lymphoma contain ALV proviruses integrated at the same site in the host DNA. There are two explanations for this: either the provirus is obliged to integrate at one location or the tumour is a clone, all its cells deriving from a single ancestor. The former possibility is eliminated by showing that ALV can insert itself at many sites in the normal cells of the host. It follows that, although many cells in the bird are infected, in only a very small minority of these cells does an event occur that promotes the clonal neoplastic growth of the cell. When lymphomas from different birds are compared, ALV proviruses are found integrated in the same region of the host DNA in over 90 per cent of them, although many of these proviruses are incomplete. The conclusion, that the site of provirus integration is vital to tumorigenesis, led to the postulate that the provirus acts as a mutagen whose insertion disrupts host gene expression in that region. You should

formed because the viral transforming gene functions normally. At the 'restrictive' temperature the gene is inactive and the infected cells are normal. Panel A–A focus of transformed cells on a chicken embryo cell monolayer induced by infection with a Rous sarcoma virus temperature sensitive mutant and incubation at permissive temperature. The cells are rounded and detaching from the substrate, so that holes are appearing in the cell sheet. After photography the culture was incubated at restrictive temperature and four days later was photographed (Panel B). The cells are now flatter and more indistinct and the gaps in the cell sheet have been filled in. (Magnification × 100 in both.)

note that this is the only one of these postulated pathogenic mechanisms in which virus DNA integration is obligatory.

This concept of 'insertional mutagenesis' has been supported by studies very similar to those described above on other virus induced chicken tumours, on comparable tumours induced by some mouse leukaemia viruses and on adenocarcinomas caused by mouse mammary tumour virus. How does the virus exert its mutagenic effect? Does it destroy host gene functions, or stimulate them? In most cases host genes seem to be stimulated. Increased transcription of host DNA in the vicinity of an integrated provirus has often been detected, and this is generally ascribed to the action of elements in the provirus that increase transcription (such elements are required by the provirus to transcribe its own genes—see Chapter 10). Moreover, in a number of instances it has been shown that the proviruses have integrated in the vicinity of, and increased transcription of, host protooncogenes. This further implicates such genes in neoplasia, and where a provirus has not integrated near a known protooncogene it is suspected that its integration site pinpoints other genes that are important in tumorigenesis. We thus hope that new oncogenes will be identified in this 'guilt by association' process and this reasoning is pursued further in Chapters 10 and 11.

9.8 Conclusions

We have seen that viruses are important environmental carcinogens. In domestic animals they can be the predominant risk factors in some common and commercially important cancers. They are also implicated in some major human malignancies, although in man the interplay between viruses and other risk factors may be very complex. Prophylactic procedures against infectious diseases have been used efficiently for over a century and it was hoped that similar approaches might prove successful in eliminating virus associated cancer. However, the complexity of the disease process has frequently complicated such attempts and to improve management of these diseases we clearly need to understand more about the pathogenesis of virus induced neoplasia.

Such basic studies have, in fact, already spurred advances in other directions. Genes in small tumour viruses directly mediate the neoplastic growth of the cells they infect and such genes are analogous or homologous to genes in host cells. Tumour virology has thus provided the first glimpses of genes that become altered in cancer cells, no matter what the precipitating cause of the disease may be. Much modern cancer research now aims to widen this window, to identify the full panoply of these oncogenes, to detect the functions of their products, and to determine how these functions affect normal and neoplastic cell growth and behaviour. The development of this work is reflected in the next three Chapters and we will leave it with one final thought. At various stages in its history, tumour virology has been dominated by the precepts and techniques of different scientific disciplines. Beginning with observations on whole animals, the field has become sequentially the preserve of the pathologist, the cell biologist, and the molecular geneticist. Now with increasing emphasis on the products of oncogenes, the biochemist and protein chemist are coming to the fore. It is important that each of these disciplines realizes that it is looking at aspects of one biological question, and that it appreciates the accretion of understanding provided by its predecessors in the field. Only by such a breadth of view are we likely to close the circle and return to answer the questions that stimulated these studies—how do we prevent, diagnose or treat malignant disease in the whole organism?

Further reading

Brown, F., and Wilson, G. S. (eds.) (1984). Topley and Wilson's principles of bacteriology, virology and immunity. **Volume IV.** *Virology* 7th Edition. Edward Arnold, London. A general account of viruses.

Essex, M., Todaro, G., and zur Hausen, H. (eds.) (1980). Viruses in naturally occurring cancer. In *Cold Spring Harbor Conferences on Cell Proliferation 7.* More details on the clinical side.

Tooze, J. (ed.) (1980). *The molecular biology of tumor viruses: DNA tumor viruses.* 2nd Edition. Cold Spring Harbor Laboratory, Cold Spring Harbor, New York.

Weiss, R. A., Teich, N., Varmus, H., and Coffin, J. (eds.) (1982). *The molecular biology of tumor viruses: RNA tumor viruses.* 2nd Edition. Cold Spring Harbor Laboratory, Cold Spring Harbor, New York. The above are two tomes for reference only.

Wyke, J., and Weiss, R. (eds.) (1984). Viruses in human and animal cancers. *Cancer Surveys* **3**, 1–218. Relatively short and the best start for reading.

10

Oncogenes and cancer

NATALIE M. TEICH

10.1 What is an oncogene?

The term oncogene has been used in several of the preceding Chapters and will arise again in subsequent Chapters. In this section, we shall try to amalgamate current knowledge and hypotheses of this fascinating subject from a more functional view. The generic name 'oncogene' was coined to delineate a gene capable of causing cancer. Obviously, this may be an oversimplified concept as the previous Chapters have presented evidence that the genesis of a tumour is a complex issue involving multifactorial and/or multi-step processes.

10.1.1   *First encounter: retroviruses*

As discussed in Chapter 9, the family of RNA tumour viruses, *Retroviridae*, comprises a vast number of members from many animal species, with a wide range of pathogenic properties including neoplastic and non–neoplastic diseases. The most common oncogenic viruses (such as long latency leukaemia viruses and the murine mammary tumour virus) contain genes for their replication only, and cause tumours by mechanisms grouped as insertional mutations which may often take many months for clinical manifestation (see Chapter 9, Fig. 10.1, and below). However, about 50 virus isolates have the interesting property of being able to induce tumours in infected animals after very short latency periods (generally days or weeks) and furthermore often are capable of causing morphological alterations in cells grown *in vitro* (transformation, see Chapter 9). Dissection of the genomes of these viruses showed that most of them had lost genetic information coding for their replicative genes (and hence were known as replication defective, albeit transformation competent, viruses). New genetic information was inserted in place of the deleted material (Fig. 10.1). By a variety of genetic techniques, this new set of sequences was shown to be responsible for the short latency and transformation inducing capacities. Hence, the new sequences were designated as oncogenes, or *onc* genes. Nucleic acid sequencing and hybridization techniques revealed that the *onc* gene sequences of these 50 viruses were sometimes essentially identical and sometimes completely unrelated. Thus, approximately 20 different viral oncogenes (v-*onc* genes) were distinguished. Each of the separate v-*onc*s was given a different name, a three letter word to define the virus from which it was isolated which is italicized in type like other genes; this nomenclature is illustrated in Table 10.1.

The first important question to be asked was: where did the v-*onc* sequences come from? Again nucleic acid hybridization studies were used to demonstrate unambiguously that the v-*onc* sequences were almost identical to sequences in the cellular DNA of the animal species from which the virus was isolated so that cellular DNA contains genes which when 'transplanted' (transducted) into retroviruses are cancer causing genes. Moreover, it was shown that the *onc* sequences could be found in the DNA of every cell from virtually all higher vertebrate orders ('evolutionary conservation'). Thus, these sequences related to viral oncogenes are inherited from one generation to the next in the same way as one inherits genes for eye colour. It is clear, however, that these genes cannot be operating as cancer genes in cells (and indeed our own cells). How can we envisage this subtle but extremely important dichotomy? First, one could imagine that the genes were never turned on (expressed)

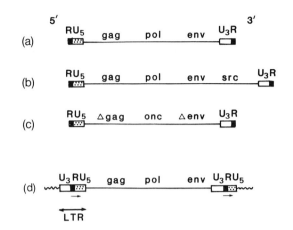

Fig. 10.1 Retroviral genomes. (a) Typical genome structure of a long latency leukaemia virus. The three replicative genes are shown: *gag*, the gene encoding the internal core structures; *pol* encoding the RNA dependent DNA polymerase enzyme known as reverse transcriptase; and, *env* encoding the envelope proteins inserted into the plasma membrane which becomes incorporated into mature virions. 5' and 3' denote the polarity of the molecule, as the RNA can serve directly as a mRNA molecule and be translated into protein (a positive strand genome). R denotes a short segment of RNA repeated at each end of the molecule. U_5 and U_3 denote noncoding unique sequences at each end that contain the regulatory elements (the promoter and enhancer sequences) for viral transcription. (b) The structure of the Rous sarcoma virus of chickens, the only retrovirus that contains all replicative genes and additionally an oncogene (*src*). (c) Structure of the acutely leukaemogenic or transforming retroviruses. These genomes generally lack all or part of one or more of the replicative genes, thus rendering them defective for replication. The deleted sequences have been replaced by cellular sequences that confer the oncogenic potential (generically called *onc* genes). The extent of replicative gene deletion and location of the *onc* gene are distinct for each viral isolate. (d) Structure of the integrated virus (DNA provirus). The mode of replication of retroviruses generates duplicated ends known as long terminal repeat (LTR) structures in which the U_5 region is duplicated at the extreme 3' end and U_3 at the 5' end. The LTRs are important for the integration of the provirus into chromosomal DNA and always generate a complete proviral DNA colinear with viral RNA. Another important feature is that the regulatory elements for viral transcription are now found also at the 3' end of the molecule and thus can serve as promoters or enhancers for adjacent cell genes (denoted by the wavy lines).

in animals. This is clearly not so, as messenger RNA (mRNA) molecules and also protein products of the genes can be found in different cell types, sometimes expressed in particular stages of the cell division cycle. Second, one could speculate that *onc* gene products were overexpressed when under viral regulatory signals, i.e. in their viral form, compared to

Table 10.1 Retroviral oncogenes

onc	Retrovirus isolates[1]	v-onc origin[2]	v-onc protein[3]	Virus disease	v-onc product activity[4]	v-onc product location	Human chromosome
src	RSV	chicken	pp60^{src}	sarcoma	PK(tyr)	inner side of plasma membrane	20q12-q13
	rASV	quail	pp60^{src}	sarcoma	PK(tyr)	inner side of plasma membrane	
fps	FuSV-ASV	chicken	P130$^{gag\text{-}fps}$	sarcoma	PK(tyr)	plasma membrane	15q24-q25
	PRCII-ASV	chicken	P105$^{gag\text{-}fps}$	sarcoma	PK(tyr)	plasma membrane	
	PRCIV-ASV	chicken	P170$^{gag\text{-}fps}$	sarcoma	PK(tyr)	plasma membrane	
	UR1-ASV	chicken	P150$^{gag\text{-}fps}$	sarcoma	PK(tyr)	plasma membrane	
	16L-ASV	chicken	P142$^{gag\text{-}fps}$	sarcoma	PK(tyr)	plasma membrane	
fes	ST-FeSV	cat	P85$^{gag\text{-}fes}$	sarcoma	PK(tyr)	plasma membrane	
	GA-FeSV	cat	P110$^{gag\text{-}fes}$	sarcoma	PK(tyr)	plasma membrane	
	HZ1-FeSV	cat	P100$^{gag\text{-}fes}$	sarcoma	PK(tyr)	plasma membrane	
yes	Y73-ASV	chicken	P90$^{gag\text{-}yes}$	sarcoma	PK(tyr)	plasma membrane	18
	Esh-ASV	chicken	P80$^{gag\text{-}yes}$	sarcoma	PK(tyr)	plasma membrane	
fgr	GR-FeSV	cat	P70$^{gag\text{-}actin\text{-}fgr}$	sarcoma	PK(tyr)	?	1p36
ros	UR2-ASV	chicken	P68$^{gag\text{-}ros}$	sarcoma	PK(tyr)	membranes	?
abl	Ab-MLV	mouse	P90-P160$^{gag\text{-}abl}$	pre B cell leukaemia	PK(tyr)	plasma membrane	9q34-qter
	HZ2-FeSV	cat	P98$^{gag\text{-}abl}$	sarcoma	PK(tyr)	plasma membrane	
ski	SKn-rASV	chicken	P110$^{gag\text{-}ski\text{-}pol}$ P125$^{gag\text{-}ski\text{-}pol}$	squamous carcinoma	?	nucleus	1q12-qter
erbA	AEV-ES4	chicken	P75$^{gag\text{-}erbA}$	?	?	cytoplasm	(1): 17p11-q21
	AEV-R	chicken	P75$^{gag\text{-}erbA}$	?	?	cytoplasm	(2): 17

Table 10.1 —*continued*

onc	Retrovirus isolates[1]	v-onc origin[2]	v-onc protein[3]	Virus disease	v-onc product activity[4]	v-onc product location	Human chromosome
erbB	AEV-ES4	chicken	gp65^{erbB}	erythroblastosis and sarcoma	truncated EGF receptor	plasma membrane	7pter-q22
	AEV-R	chicken	gp65^{erbB}				
	AEV-H	chicken	gp65^{erbB}				
fms	SM-FeSV	cat	gP180$^{gag\text{-}fms}$	sarcoma	?PK(tyr)	intermediate filaments, membranes	5q34
			gp140^{fms}		M-CSF receptor		
			gp120^{fms}				
fos	FBJ-MSV	mouse	pp55^{fos}	osteosarcoma	?	nucleus	14q21-q31
	FBR-MSV	mouse	P75$^{gag\text{-}fos\text{-}fox}$	osteosarcoma			
mos	Mo-MSV	mouse	P37$^{env\text{-}mos}$	sarcoma	PK(ser, thr)	cytoplasm	8q22^{5}
	Gz-MSV	mouse	?	sarcoma			
	MPV-MSV	mouse	p34^{mos}	sarcoma, erythroleukaemia, and myelo-proliferation			
sis	SSV	monkey	P28$^{env\text{-}sis}$	sarcoma	truncated PDGF (B chain)	membranes ? secreted	22q11-qter
	PI-FeSV	cat	P76$^{gag\text{-}sis}$	sarcoma			
	FT-FeSV	cat	?	sarcoma			
	TP2-FeSV	cat	?	sarcoma			
myc	MC29	chicken	P110$^{gag\text{-}myc}$	sarcoma, carcinoma, and myelocytoma	DNA binding	nucleus (P100 cytoplasmic)	8q24
	MH2	chicken	P100$^{gag\text{-}mil\text{-}myc}$	myelocytoma			
			p58^{myc}				
	CMII	chicken	P90$^{gag\text{-}myc}$	carcinoma			
	OK10	chicken	P200$^{gag\text{-}pol\text{-}myc}$	carcinoma			
	FeLV-*myc*	cat	?	granulocytic leukaemia			

Gene[1]	Virus/strain[1]	Origin[2]	Protein product[3]	Tumour	Function[4]	Subcellular localization	Chromosomal location
myb	AMV-BAI/A AMV-E26	chicken chicken	p45^{myb} P135$^{gag\text{-}ets\text{-}myb}$	myeloblastosis myeloblastosis and erythroblastosis	?	nucleus	6q22-q24
rel	REV-T	turkey	?p64^{rel}	reticulo-endotheliosis	?	?	?
kit	HZ4-FeSV	cat	P80$^{gag\text{-}kit}$	sarcoma	?	?	?
raf	3611-MSV	mouse	gP90$^{gag\text{-}raf}$ P75$^{gag\text{-}raf}$	sarcoma	PK(ser, thr)	?	(1): 3p25 (2): 4[5]
mil	MH2	chicken	P100$^{gag\text{-}mil\text{-}myc}$	see above for *myc*			
Ha-*ras*	Ha-MSV	rat	pp21^{ras}	sarcoma and erythroleukaemia	GTP binding GTPase	plasma membrane	(1): 11p13 (2): X[5]
	RaSV BALB-MSV	rat mouse	P29$^{gag\text{-}ras}$ pp21^{ras}	? sarcoma haemangiosarcoma			
Ki-*ras*	Ki-MSV	rat	pp21^{ras}	sarcoma and erythyroleukaemia	GTP binding GTPase	plasma membrane	(1): 6p32-q13[5] (2): 12p12-pter
	NY-FeSV	cat	?	sarcoma			
ets	AMV-E26	chicken	P135$^{gag\text{-}ets\text{-}myb}$	see above for *myb*		nucleus	11q23-q24
?	AEV-S13	chicken	gP155$^{env\text{-}onc}$	sarcoma, granulocytic leukaemia, and erythroblastosis	PK(tyr)	plasma membrane	?

[1] RSV=Rous sarcoma virus; ASV=avian sarcoma virus; FeSV=feline sarcoma virus; MLV=murine leukaemia virus; AEV=avian erythroblastosis virus; SSV=simian sarcoma virus; AMV=avian myeloblastosis virus; REV=reticuloendotheliosis virus; MSV=murine sarcoma virus. The other notations indicate specific viral strains.

[2] The origin denotes the species of animal from which the *onc* gene was transduced by a retrovirus. Note that in some cases the same *onc* gene has been transduced by retroviruses from different animals.

[3] The nomenclature has been standardized as follows: p=protein; pp=phosphoprotein; P=fusion protein between a retroviral replicative gene (*gag, pol* or *env*; see Fig. 10.1) and the *onc* sequence (note that this may influence the intracellular localization); gp or gP=glycoprotein. The numerals denote the molecular weight in kilodaltons, generally deduced from polyacrylamide gel electrophoresis.

[4] PK=protein kinase; tyr=tyrosine; ser=serine; thr=threonine; EGF=epidermal growth factor; PDGF=platelet derived growth factor; M-CSF=macrophage colony stimulating factor. See text for further details.

[5] These genes lack introns and are probably not transcribed (pseudogenes).

levels observed normally in cells. This possibility too has been ruled out for many of the cellular oncogene counterparts, but not for all. A third hypothesis is that the gene has cancer inducing activity if expressed in the wrong place or the wrong time. This theory is possible, there being at this time no evidence to rule it out definitively. A fourth alternative is that there are actual changes between the viral and cellular homologues. There is some evidence that such changes do occur, but again this does not apply to all oncogenes. Thus, both qualitative and quantitative changes may be responsible for oncogenic activity. For clarity, the term proto-oncogene is used for the cellular species; sometimes, the cellular counterpart may also be called a c-*onc* gene, but this term has a connotation that the gene is an oncogene, and it is best to distinguish it instead as one with only a *potential* oncogenic activity.

There is currently very active and widespread research to sort out the properties and functions of v-*onc* genes and protooncogenes, both similarities and differences, to understand what may cause the potential carcinogenic activity to become an actual one. Many of the problems have been tackled initially with v-*onc* genes which are more amenable to manipulation and dissection in the laboratory, and this will form the basis of the following sections.

The v-*onc* genes are useful for analysis of expression of the related protooncogenes in normal and tumour tissues. Messenger RNA preparations from different tissues, including embryonic tissues at different stages of development, were examined (in general, the technique known as Northern hybridization was used wherein mRNA molecules are fractionated by size during electrophoresis through agarose gels and then annealed to specific *onc* gene 'probes') to look for both the level of expression and the size of the specific mRNAs (transcripts). The most consistent finding was that most of these genes are expressed at some stage in some tissue; that is, they are regulated genes and participate in the cell's normal differentiation programme. It also became evident that the cellular *onc* genes may be abnormally expressed in certain tumours due to alterations in regulation, mutation, gene amplification or chromosomal translocation (see on, and Chapter 11).

10.1.2 *Second encounter: cellular oncogenes*

While the RNA tumour viruses have given us a handle on nearly 20 oncogenes, there are probably at least 20 others that have been determined from studies on tumours. These have been found by three major approaches (i) gene transfer, (ii) insertional mutagenesis mapping of virally induced tumours, and (iii) analysis of known chromosomal translocations or amplifications.

10.1.2.1 *Gene transfer.* The primary method of gene transfer is often known by the name DNA transfection. The DNA is isolated from tumour cells and introduced into recipient cells. It may be added as a calcium phosphate precipitate to assist uptake, taken up following an electric shock (electroporesis), or microinjected; the first is the most commonly used technique. The recipient cells are most usually the 'normal' immortalized mouse fibroblast line, NIH/3T3. The NIH cells have several advantages in this system (i) they are flat, contact inhibited cells in monolayer culture, and (ii) their DNA can be distinguished in hybridization experiments from DNAs of other species (thus allowing identification of donor DNA). The first property is the most important as the general goal is to examine the transfected cultures for the appearance of morphologically altered (transformed) foci due to the expression of an introduced oncogene. This procedure is represented diagrammatically in Figure 10.2. Although a lot of DNA is taken up by an individual cell, the majority of this material is degraded with time, and only a minority

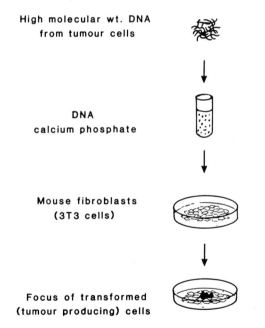

Fig. 10.2 DNA transfection. DNA isolated from tumour cells is introduced into recipient NIH/3T3 mouse cells. After several weeks, the monolayer is observed for foci of morphologically transformed cells. Repeated cycles of DNA transfection from transformed foci are generally performed. The transformed cells may be tested for tumorigenicity in nude mice. DNA from transformed cells is also examined for retention and identification of donor cell sequences.

becomes stably incorporated into the cellular genome. To identify the gene responsible for the cell's transformed phenotype, transfection of DNA from the transformed cells is carried out a second and third time; a procedure that eventually whittles down the amount of nonmurine DNA carried over.

One of the surprises from such analyses was that cellular genes related to the already known *ras* genes of retroviruses were found to be responsible for the transformed phenotype in about 20 per cent of human tumours tested. This could be due, at least in part, to the ability of NIH cells to respond morphologically to a given oncogene product, to the need for the gene to be genetically dominant (e.g. lack of expression of an inhibitor gene in the NIH cell), and to the need for the gene to be sufficient for the expression and maintenance of the transformed state. On second thought, perhaps it is not unusual to find that few genes other than *ras* related genes have been identified as being 'activated' (see on) in tumours. This may be due to the NIH cells being of the wrong lineage or species to respond to the effects of other genes. Or one may consider them to have a preneoplastic phenotype (see Chapter 7) as they already have the ability to grow continuously in culture, thus they may be more susceptible to genes whose effects are manifest during the later stages of tumour progression. Nonetheless, new oncogenes have been detected by this technique (Table 10.2).

10.1.2.2 *Insertional mutagenesis.* Retroviruses lacking v-*onc* gene sequences carry only the genes required for replication; after infection, a DNA copy of their genome is synthesized and becomes integrated within chromosomal DNA of the cell (the provirus, see Fig. 10.1). This event by definition is an insertional mutation and can have several consequences. The long terminal repeat (LTR) structures do not code for proteins but do contain the regulatory elements ('promoters' for initiation of transcription of mRNA molecules from the DNA, and 'enhancers' that may influence the levels of transcription of adjacent or distant genes) which permit transcription of the viral genes into mRNA molecules so that viral proteins are produced and incorporated into progeny virus particles. However, as shown in Figure 10.1, the replication and insertion of a provirus leads to the generation of two LTRs; one may be used for the production of progeny virus whereas the other may be used for promotion of an adjacent cellular gene ('downstream promotion'). The first example of this phenomenon came from the examination of B cell tumours induced in chickens by avian leukaemia viruses (ALVs) lacking *onc* genes. Hybridization of LTR probes to tumour RNA revealed not only transcripts expected from the proviral genome but also some that contained an LTR but no viral sequences; the remaining sequences were

Table 10.2 Nonretroviral oncogenes

Name	Tumour of origin	Method of detection	Human chromosome
N-*myc*[1]	Neuroblastoma	Amplification	2p23-p24
L-*myc*[1]	Lung carcinoma		
N-*ras*[1]	Neuroblastoma[2,3]	Transfection	1cen-p21
Blym	Burkitt's lymphoma[4]		1p32
dil	B cell lymphoma		
mcf2	Mammary carcinoma		
mcf3	Mammary carcinoma		
met	Chemically transformed osteosarcoma cells		7
neu	Neuroblastoma[5]		17
onc-D	Colon carcinoma		
ras related	Melanoma		
Tlym-1	T cell lymphoma		
Tlym-2	T cell lymphoma		
trk	Colon carcinoma		
tx-1	Mammary carcinoma		
tx-2	Pre B cell leukaemia		
tx-3	Plasmacytoma		
tx-4	T cell lymphoma		
bcl-1	B cell leukaemia	Translocation[6]	
bcl-2	B cell lymphoma		
bcr	Chronic granulocytic leukaemia		
tcl	T cell lymphoma		
T_kNS-1	Plasmacytoma[7]		
int-1	Mammary carcinoma	Insertional mutation[7]	12q14-pter
int-2	Mammary carcinoma	(all rodent)	11q13
Mlvi-1	T cell lymphoma		
Mlvi-2	T cell lymphoma		
Mlvi-3	T cell lymphoma		
Pim-1	T cell lymphoma		
Pvt-2	Plasmacytoma		
RMO-*int*-1	T cell leukaemia		

[1] Related to *onc* genes already known from retroviruses (see Table 10.1).
[2] Also in rodent tumours.
[3] See also Table 10.3 for mutated N-*ras* genes in other human tumours.
[4] Also in chicken B cell lymphoma.
[5] Rodent tumour. Related to the EGF receptor gene (c-*erbB*).
[6] These genes represent breakpoint regions; no oncogenic potential has yet been demonstrated for any genes in this region.
[7] Rodent tumours. No oncogenic potential has yet been demonstrated for the activated gene *per se*.

derived from cellular genetic material. Further analysis showed that the cellular gene was in fact the counterpart of the *myc* gene already identified in several avian viruses (Table 10.1 and Fig. 10.3). The integration event resulted in the use of the LTR as a promoter for transcription of the cellular *myc* gene, leading to inexorable production of *myc* RNA and protein. Upon analysis of many of these B cell tumours, it was found that there was no specific integration of the ALV provirus at a unique site upstream of the *myc* gene; the integration sites in individual tumours were often several kilobases different from one to another. ALV proviruses can integrate at a multitude of sites, even perhaps totally at random; however, the integrations near to *myc* presumably led to some selective advantage for the particular cell in proliferation, which might prime such cells for other neoplastic events to occur, or which might be oncogenic *per se*. Interestingly, the involvement of *myc* promoter insertions has also been observed in murine T cell leukaemias induced by murine retroviruses and in feline T cell leukaemias induced by feline retroviruses. Further, the previously known *erbB* oncogene (known as the counterpart of an oncogene isolated from avian erythroleukaemia viruses, AEV) has also been activated by promoter insertion by other strains of ALV in situations where they induced erythroleukaemia instead of B cell leukaemia. In many of these instances, the integrated provirus is no longer intact, i.e. one of the LTRs, as well as coding

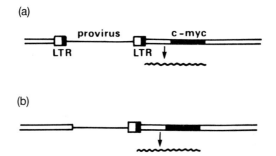

Fig. 10.3 Promoter insertion. In the example shown here, DNA from a B cell tumour (bursal lymphoma) of chickens induced by an avian leukaemia virus (ALV) has been examined for the site of provirus insertion. The provirus (shown as a single line bounded by LTRs) is located 'upstream' of the cellular gene known as *myc* and the viral LTR is being used as a promoter for the transcription of high levels of *myc* gene messenger RNA (mRNA), shown as a wavy line. For simplicity, the *myc* gene is shown as a contiguous element whereas it is actually composed of a 5′ untranslated exon and 3 coding exons separated by regions of noncoding sequences known as introns (the introns are also removed, 'spliced out', during the processing to mature mRNA molecules). (a) Provirus is intact. (b) Provirus shows deleted structure, lacking the 5′ LTR and some coding sequences.

sequences, may be lost, suggesting that the provirus itself is no longer required for maintenance of the neoplastic state.

A different phenomenon occurred when the integration sites for another retrovirus group, mouse mammary tumour viruses (MMTV, see Chapter 9), were mapped in a large number of tumours. As illustrated in Figure 10.4, there were apparently clusters of regions where proviruses inserted. However, the LTRs in most cases could not be used to promote transcription of downstream genes. In the majority of tumours, it turned out that there were regions bounded by the provirus insertions and that this central region contained a gene that was activated in the tumour and

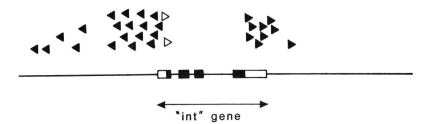

"int" gene

Fig. 10.4 Proviruses in mouse mammary tumour virus (MMTV) induced breast tumours. The integration sites of MMTV proviruses in a large number of tumours have been mapped chromosomally. Each site is denoted by an arrowhead and the direction of the arrow shows the direction of transcription of the provirus (5′ to 3′). Note that the activated gene is in a central region (designated *int* for integration) around which the proviruses cluster and that the polarity of the provirus is in an orientation such that downstream promotion cannot occur. There are at least two well characterized *int* loci, *int-1* and *int-2*; others may also exist.

silent in normal mammary tissue. The proviruses were oriented in a polarity that proscribed transcription of the central gene from the viral LTR, but presumably the enhancer element within the LTR was able to activate this cellular gene. In fact, (at least) two cellular genes may become expressed in this manner in different murine mammary carcinomas and have become known as the *int-1* and *int-2* loci. Thus, a second mechanism of insertional mutagenesis has been identified. Integration sites in other tumours have delineated further activated genes (Table 10.2). However, it must be stressed that these genes have not yet been shown to be oncogenes in a definitive test.

10.1.2.3 *Chromosomal abnormalities.* Various chromosomal abnormalities have been detected in tumours by karyotype analysis of metaphase chromosomes; some abnormalities seem specific for a distinctive tumour type (see Chapter 11). Because the *onc* genes mentioned above, whether originally identified in retroviruses or by gene transfer, all have cellular counterparts, each one can be mapped to a distinct region of a particular chromosome (Tables 10.1 and 10.2, and Chapter 11). These two observations were linked to ask two questions. First, did any of the known *onc* genes map in or near regions involved in abnormal tumour karyotypes? Second, could the abnormalities be used to discover new oncogenes?

The foreknowledge of promoter insertion of *myc* in ALV induced B cell tumours quickly played a role. Burkitt's lymphoma is a B cell tumour of humans in which both Epstein Barr virus and malaria are known co-factors (see Chapter 9). Additionally, it was previously known that tumour cells contained one of three chromosomal translocations (translocations refer to movement of genetic sequences from the normal chromosome site to another chromosome, see Chapter 11), involving part of the long arm of chromosome 8 becoming translocated to chromosome 14, 2 or 22 (the first occurring in approximately 90 per cent of tumours examined). The *myc* locus mapped to the long arm of chromosome 8 and it became obvious to examine whether it was translocated in these tumours. The simple answer was yes. Even more exciting was the finding that the *myc* locus translocated to regions containing different immunoglobulin loci (the heavy chain, κ and λ light chains, respectively, on chromosomes 14, 2 and 22). Mechanistically, this meant that the *myc* locus could now be found adjacent to a highly transcribed gene (an important function of mature B cells being that of immunoglobulin production, see Chapter 15). The generation of the translocation also tended to have another effect: the noncoding regulatory sequences of the *myc* gene were frequently 'decapitated' from the gene, thus leaving it to the controls of its new chromosomal milieu. In most instances the altered *myc* allele was shown to be transcriptionally active while the nonaltered one was silent. Moreover, the *myc* allele was sometimes located near the immunoglobulin enhancer element which could affect the level of *myc* transcription. Similar sorts of rearrangements also occur in immunoglobulin producing tumours (plasmacytomas) of mice and rats.

Another particularly well known translocation was the formation of the 'marker' Philadelphia chromosome in chronic granulocytic leukaemias (CGL, see Chapters 3 and 11) which represents a translocation between chromosomes 9 and 22 (although other variants are known which may involve segments from three different chromosomes). The net result is that the *abl* locus (known from retroviruses) becomes transferred from chromosome 9 to sequences on chromosome 22. The *abl* gene is located rather a long distance away from the site of the breakpoint (and hence is presumably not dissociated from its upstream regulatory sequences), but transcription of the gene is abnormal in that the *abl* mRNA molecules are much greater in size than normal.

Many other tumours contain recognizable translocations (see Chapter 11) and the translocation breakpoints of some of these have already been molecularly cloned. Although often listed as cellular oncogenes (e.g. some are included in Table 10.2), this remains a tenuous assignment until the sequences are shown experimentally to have neoplastic potential.

Another type of chromosomal abnormality seen in tumours is related to gene amplification and generally involves huge (100–1000 kilobases or more) DNA segments spanning many genes. The amplification may be observed as a homogeneously staining region (HSR) in which it occurs as a contiguous element in a chromosome, or as the formation of double minute (DM) chromosomes which are additional tiny mini-chromosomes (although they lack centromeres and therefore may be lost, or segregate, during cell division). The availability of v-*onc* gene probes proved useful in demonstrating that HSRs and DMs observed in cell lines derived from various tumours contained *onc* gene amplifications (e.g. Ki-*ras* in a mouse adrenocortical tumour cell line, *myc* in a human colon carcinoma line). Needless to say, these particular types of abnormalities require large degrees of gene amplification (large DNA segments repeated perhaps 50 or 100 times) to be detected by microscopic analysis of chromosomes. More sensitive techniques such as Southern blotting and hybridization (in which DNA is cut by endonucleases known as restriction enzymes, separated by size in gels, and transferred to nitrocellulose filters for hybridization to DNA probes) allow the detection of low levels of gene amplification or indeed the disruption or rearrangement of a single gene (Table 10.3).

One particularly interesting finding is the N-*myc* amplification in neuroblastomas. This property is observed only in those tumours histologically defined as grades III and IV and thus may be a reflection of tumour progression toward a more advanced malignant state. Similarly, *myc* amplification in cell lines derived from small cell lung carcinomas is correlated with an enhanced growth of the tumours when transplanted into nude mice.

Nonetheless, it should be remembered that large segments of DNA are reiterated in these amplifications and the *onc* gene may be merely a passenger in this event. Thus, other genes in the amplified regions could have significant consequences.

10.2 Identification of viral and cellular oncogene products

It is important to ascertain the physiological functions of oncogene products and to determine (or at least speculate) on how these products may lead to neoplastic changes within a cell. Such analyses include the subcellular localization of the gene product and deciphering biochemical

Table 10.3 Oncogene amplification

Gene	Human tumour	Degree of amplification
c-*myc*	Promyelocytic leukaemia[1]	20
	Colon carcinoma	40
	Small cell lung carcinoma	5–30
N-*myc*	Neuroblastoma[1]	5–1000
	Retinoblastoma[1]	10–200
	Small cell lung carcinoma[1]	50
c-*abl*	Chronic granulocytic leukaemia	5–10
c-*myb*	Colon carcinoma	10
	Acute myeloid leukaemia[1]	5–10
c-*erbB*	Vulval carcinoma	30
c-Ki-*ras*-2	Lung carcinoma[1]	
	Colorectal carcinoma[1]	4–20
	Bladder carcinoma[1]	
N-*ras*	Mammary carcinoma	5–10

[1] Primary tumour material.

functions associated with the expression of the product (see Table 10.1). To a large extent, these experiments rely on recombinant DNA technology, specific antisera, and luck.

10.2.1 src *and the tyrosine kinase family*

The Rous sarcoma virus (RSV) of chickens was one of the earliest retroviruses isolated and has turned out to be one of the most interesting from a genetic and biochemical standpoint. It is the only naturally occurring retrovirus with all replicative genes as well as an oncogene (see Fig. 10.1). The oncogene, v-*src*, was transduced from cellular DNA in such a way that the replicative genes of its presumptive parent virus (an avian leukaemia virus) remained intact with the new sequences appearing appended to the viral *env* gene. Early genetic experiments showed that inactivation of the v-*src* gene by mutations or deletions left a long latency leukaemia virus that could no longer cause morphological transformation of cells in culture.

With recombinant DNA technology, it was possible to obtain molecular clones of proviral DNA and the v-*src* (and subsequently cellular *src*) gene was characterized down to its last nucleotide. Comparisons showed that the nucleotide sequence of the cellular and viral genes were essentially identical. Two major differences could be noted however (i) the v-*src* gene lacks introns (some time during the process of transduction this occurs with all oncogenes picked up by retroviruses wherein the introns are 'spliced' out), and (ii) the last (carboxy terminal) 12 coding amino acids of v-*src* were different from those of cellular *src* (which is also 7 amino acids longer). Thus, transduction leads to splicing, truncation, and perhaps other sorts of recombinational events—a motif seen frequently in the derivation of the *onc* containing retroviruses.

The next important breakthrough came with the development of an antiserum that reacted specifically with the *src* gene product, obtained from an animal bearing an RSV induced tumour. The serum was used to show that the *src* gene product was located largely on the cytoplasmic side of the plasma membrane and was approximately 60 000 daltons in molecular weight. By metabolically labelling transformed cells with ^{32}P, it was shown that the protein was phosphorylated, and hence became known as pp60^{v-src}. The protein of the cellular gene also shared these properties and was called pp60^{c-src}.

One of the most interesting discoveries from this study was that the protein was apparently responsible for its own phosphorylation (auto-phosphorylation) and also that it had the ability to phosphorylate the immunoglobulin (Ig) molecule in the antiserum that was used to identify it. Further studies showed that the two proteins were phosphorylated on tyrosine residues and thus the oncogene product was identified functionally as a tyrosine protein kinase (cellular enzymes that phosphorylated serine or threonine residues were previously known, but this was the first time that a tyrosine kinase was characterized).

As further viral and cellular oncogenes were isolated, they were tested for a similar kinase function, and a number were found to be positive: *abl*, *fes*, *fgr*, *fms*, and *yes* (Table 10.1). Each represented the transduction of a distinct cellular gene, as the cellular homologues mapped to different chromosomes. Nucleotide sequence data confirmed this and also pointed out that there was a small region of sequence homology presumably related to the shared biochemical activity. The oncogene *erbB* also shares this sequence, but definitive evidence for tyrosine kinase activity is more difficult to establish (see Chapter 12). Two other oncogenes, *raf* (also called *mil*) and *mos*, show kinase activity but, in these instances, serine and threonine are the substrate sites rather than tyrosine. This large group of oncogenes sharing a related biochemical function became known as the protein kinase family.

There were two obvious questions at this stage. Do the cellular *onc* counterparts also display kinase activity? Could specific proteins in the cell be identified as target substrates? To the first question, the answer was generally yes, in that the *onc* proteins were capable of autophosphorylation, but often did not show any ability to phosphorylate Ig molecules. Answering the second question was more difficult. Levels of phosphotyrosine containing peptides in normal nontransformed cells are extremely low; thus, despite demonstrated kinase activity for c-*onc* gene products *in vitro*, their activity is virtually undetectable in cells. However, there is often a considerable elevation of phosphotyrosine in cells transformed with the kinase v-*onc* genes, suggesting that the v-*onc* products have greater activity. However, many different species of proteins seem to be affected rather than one or two specific target molecules.

Several of the proteins phosphorylated by *src* are of interest. One is the protein vinculin, a component of the cytoskeleton network of mesenchymal cells which is situated at areas of contact between cells or between a cell and a substrate (such as tissue culture dishes) known as focal adhesion plaques. The change in the phosphorylation pattern of vinculin could be responsible for some of the observable changes in transformed cells (rounding up, decreased adhesion to solid substrates, ruffling of the plasma membrane). Another interesting target is a protein known as p90 (so designated because it is 90 kilodaltons in molecular weight) which with another protein (p50) serves to transport pp60^{src} from its site of synthesis to the plasma membrane. While complexed with these two proteins, the *src* protein is neither phosphorylated nor does it exhibit kinase activity. The *src* product is also capable of phosphorylating lipids (i.e. it is a phospholipid kinase) such as phosphatidylinositol and diacylglycerol. These molecules are believed to function as 'second messengers' in response to growth factor stimulation, an important aspect of cell metabolism (see Chapter 12). Several enzymes of the glycolytic pathway are also targets for *src* kinase activity. Despite these identifiable changes, we are still a long way from demonstrating a direct link between these effects and the ultimate heritable change necessary for a cell to transform and develop into a neoplasm.

10.2.2 ras *and GTPase activity*

The *ras* oncogene was originally discovered in two murine retroviruses, known as Harvey and Kirsten murine sarcoma viruses (Ha-MSV and Ki-MSV). By nucleic acid hybridization, the *onc* genes of the two viruses were nonhomologous. This turned out to be due to the degeneracy of the triplet code of DNA because the *onc* gene products from the two viruses were virtually identical, p21^{ras}. Moreover, it was found that both Ha-*ras* and Ki-*ras* were each found at two separate chromosomal loci, although in each case, one locus appeared to be a pseudogene (a gene sequence lacking introns and thought to be untranscribed and thus not translated into protein, Table 10.1). Later, a gene showing homology to Ha-*ras* and

Ki-*ras* was detected in neuroblastoma DNA by transfection (see Table 10.2); this became known as N-*ras* and was mapped to yet another chromosome. These five different *ras* genes became known as the *ras* multi-gene family.

The viral p21^{ras} proteins were shown to have binding activity for guanosine triphosphate (GTP) and in fact enzymatically converted GTP to its di- and mono-phosphate forms. Thus, *ras* too is an enzyme, a GTPase. Comparisons of enzyme activity showed that p21^{v-ras} has less activity than p21^{c-ras}.

How did the change in activity come about? Nucleotide sequence analysis showed that in viral transductions (three separate isolates, the third being another capture of Ha-*ras*, see Table 10.1), the *ras* gene was intact, i.e. it was not truncated. But in each instance, there was one nucleotide change which in turn led to the substitution of a different amino acid compared to the cellular *ras* protein. The same event occurred in the neuroblastoma N-*ras* gene as well. These results, as well as those from other tumour transfections or site specific mutagenesis *in vitro*, showed that changes in the *ras* protein at amino acid residues 12 or 13, or residues 59–61 almost invariably led to a change in the oncogenic potential (Table 10.4, see also Chapters 3, 11, and 12). The easiest explanation is that these changes lead to major alterations in the conformational (three dimensional) state of the protein thereby diminishing its activity.

Another clue for *ras* function comes from studies on the yeast *Saccharomyces* which has two *ras* genes that stimulate adenylate cyclase. This finding led to the deduction that *ras* could be a regulator of adenylate cyclase similar to the known G proteins that transmit signals from cell surface receptors ('second messages', see Chapter 12). Binding of GTP is necessary for activation of G proteins and thus GTPase activity is a regulatory factor. The diminished GTPase activity of mutated *ras* proteins could lead to sustained effects on adenylate cyclase and the ensuing events in cell metabolism. The location of the *ras* protein on the cytoplasmic side of plasma membranes adds credibility to this hypothesis. Once again, how this leads to oncogenesis is unknown.

10.2.3 *sis and platelet derived growth factor activity*

The *sis* oncogene was originally found in a simian sarcoma virus and has a protein product, p28^{sis}, apparently found in the cytoplasm. The use of a computer database was the key to deciphering its physiological function. When the amino acid sequence of several tryptic peptide digests of the growth factor known as platelet derived growth factor (PDGF) was entered into the database, it was immediately obvious that the amino acid sequence was highly homologous to that of the putative protein product

Table 10.4 Mutated human *ras* genes

		Codon	
		12	61
c-Ha-*ras*-1[1]	Normal	gly	gln
	Bladder carcinoma	val	
	Lung carcinoma		leu
	Mammary carcinoma	asp	
c-Ki-*ras*-2[2]	Normal	gly	gln
	Lung carcinoma	arg	
	Lung carcinoma	cys	
	Lung carcinoma	lys	
	Lung carcinoma		his
	Colon carcinoma	val	
	Bladder carcinoma	arg	
	Neuroblastoma	cys	
N-*ras*[3]	Normal	gly	gln
	Neuroblastoma		lys
	Teratocarcinoma	asp	
	Fibrosarcoma		lys
	Melanoma		lys
	Lung carcinoma		arg
	Leukaemia	asp	
	Rhabdomyosarcoma		his

[1] Mutated c-Ha-*ras*-1 also detected in a human melanoma.
[2] Mutated c-Ki-*ras*-2 also detected in human pancreatic carcinoma, gall bladder carcinoma, rhabdomyosarcoma, ovarian carcinoma and acute lymphoblastic leukaemia.
[3] Mutated N-*ras* also detected in Burkitt's lymphoma, acute promyelocytic leukaemia, T cell leukaemia, acute myelocytic leukaemia and chronic granulocytic leukaemia.

of v-*sis*. Further experiments verified this observation, showing that v-*sis* represented a truncated form of the B chain of PDGF (this is discussed in greater detail in Chapter 12).

This observation was very exciting in regard to a central theme of tumours: continuous cell proliferation. Normally, PDGF is packaged in the subcellular blood components known as platelets which are released by the disintegration of blood megakaryocytes. The release is generally triggered as a response to a wound and the local delivery of PDGF stimulates, for example, endothelial or epithelial cells around the wound to proliferate and fill in the gap. Once healing has begun, platelets are no longer released, thus decreasing local PDGF concentrations; the net result is that the cells become quiescent again. However, if PDGF were to be continuously produced, the cells would be constantly stimulated to divide. So the function of v-*sis* in virally induced tumours might be envisaged in one of two ways (i) as an intracellular product that can still stimulate the specific PDGF receptor such that its 'signal' for cell division is transmitted to the cell nucleus (an autocrine mechanism), or (ii) as a secreted product interacting with specific PDGF receptors on its own, neighbouring (paracrine) or distant (exocrine) cells, thus stimulating cell growth.

Although PDGF (cellular *sis*) is overexpressed in at least one human osteosarcoma cell line, this does not seem to be a general feature of bone or other tumours so far examined.

10.2.4 erbB, neu *and* fms: *oncogenes with products related to growth factor receptors*

The computer database was again fundamental in showing high levels of homology between the putative protein product of the v-*erbB* oncogene (from avian erythroleukaemia viruses) and amino acid sequence derived from the receptor for the epidermal growth factor (EGF). As with v-*sis* and PDGF, the transduction of the cellular gene was a truncation event involving both the carboxyl and amino terminal coding portions of the gene. The v-*erbB* gene product is a faulty receptor; it lacks most of the external domain, including the binding site for ligand (EGF) and is also missing part of the intracytoplasmic domain (see Chapter 12). Interestingly, the EGF receptor is a protein that becomes modified by phosphorylation and possesses tyrosine kinase activity; both of these functional regions are retained in the v-*erbB* sequence (although as mentioned above, it has been difficult to demonstrate kinase activity in the viral product). Going back to the central *sine qua non* of cell proliferation, we can suggest that these modifications to the EGF receptor protein may be sufficiently important to its conformational state so that a continuous proliferation signal may be generated in the absence of the appropriate ligand (which it cannot bind in any case).

Malfunction of the EGF receptor molecule also occurs in nonviral human tumours. For example, a truncated version is produced in a cell line derived from an epidermoid carcinoma of the vulva due to gene amplification (and gene mutation presumably) as well as in several neurological tumours (for further discussion, see Chapter 12).

The oncogene *neu*, a transfectable gene from a carcinogen induced rat neuroblastoma, is related though nonidentical to *erbB* (see Chapter 12).

The pattern of mimicry of a receptor is also observed with the onco-gene v-*fms* (from a feline sarcoma virus). Although the normal cell gene has not yet been isolated, studies on ligand and antibody binding suggest that v-*fms* has been derived from the receptor gene for macrophage colony stimulating factor (M-CSF or CSF-1).

Oncogenes that could be other cell surface proteins as well as receptors (complete or truncated) include *abl* and *ros*.

10.2.5 fos, myb, myc, ets, *and* ski: *oncogenes with nuclear products*

Oncogene products located in the nucleus might be expected to have functions quite distinct from the *onc* proteins mentioned above. One of the most facile hypotheses would be that these oncogenes might be involved in direct regulation of gene expression, perhaps serving as DNA binding proteins to activate or inactivate transcription of a particular gene or set of genes.

The *myc* oncogene, isolated from four separate avian sarcoma viruses which induce sarcomas, carcinomas, and myeloid leukaemias, is perhaps the best characterized. One reason for heightened interest is its involvement in tumours caused by retroviruses lacking oncogenes as well as its translocation and increased expression in tumours lacking retroviruses (e.g. Burkitt's lymphoma, see above). The *myc* gene is also a multi-gene family with the cellular *myc* homologue of v-*myc* and two distinct but related genes detected in neuroblastomas and retinoblastomas (N-*myc*), and small cell lung carcinomas (L-*myc*) (see Table 10.2).

The *myc* gene is expressed in many cell types suggesting that its normal function is in a pathway shared by most cells. There is often more *myc* product in cells actively proliferating, although levels are also high in the most mature macrophages whose differentiation programme is nearing the terminal phase. It has been speculated that increased levels of *myc* transcription in tumour cells (in situations where the regulation is governed by new promoter or enhancer elements) may represent de-regulation of a negative feedback inhibition between the *myc* product and the *myc* gene, in situations where noncoding sequences have been removed or when the gene is amplified.

The *fos* gene may also work by direct feedback. The v-*fos* gene was originally isolated from two osteosarcoma viruses of mice, although cellular *fos* expression is relatively low in bone. One of the most exciting studies of *fos* has shown that it is actively transcribed within a few minutes of cells becoming exposed to appropriate growth factors and then transcription rapidly diminishes. Such experiments suggest that the *fos* gene product could be responsible for enhancing or activating genes for cell growth and/or differentiation. Interestingly, it appears that the normal *fos* promoter is the responsive element. However, more detailed studies on the cellular *fos* to v-*fos* derivation (which also includes the switch to use of the viral LTR promoter) show that v-*fos* is truncated within the carboxyl terminal coding portion of the gene, thereby changing the protein product as well as removing regulatory sequences at the 3' end of the gene. Because the v-*fos* gene is constitutively expressed at high levels and its protein product has a longer half life than that of cellular *fos*, it has been speculated that *fos*, like *myc*, may be involved in self-regulation by virtue of its carboxyl amino acid sequences interacting with the 3′ noncoding regulatory sequences. How this effect modulates expression of other genes is yet to be discovered.

The *myb* gene, first detected in two avian myeloid leukaemia viruses, appears to be the best example of a cell cycle dependent gene with levels highest during the G1 phase of growth. Whether this portends a role as an initiator or effector of cell division is as yet unknown, but intensive research in this area is under way.

Little is known about the *ski* oncogene detected in an avian carcinoma virus other than its size, chromosomal site and nuclear location. However, the latter would suggest that it may also be important in gene regulation.

The v-*ets* gene product is also located in the nucleus; however, because it is found in the virus as a protein fused to *myb* (see Table 10.1), it is as yet unclear whether the normal *ets* product is nuclear or not.

10.2.6 *Other oncogenes*

We have already seen that the cellular oncogenes may encode proteins that are growth factors, growth factor receptors, enzymes, and perhaps DNA binding proteins. Each new oncogene is examined for these properties and no doubt will be characterized, but oncogenes with other functions may yet be discovered. The major theme is that the normal gene counterparts are active, and presumably vital, to the functioning of cells, and abnormal properties may be attributed to mutation, truncation, amplification or deregulation.

10.3 Interactions between oncogenes

10.3.1 *Tripartite retroviruses*

Perhaps one of the most unexpected results from studying v-*onc* genes has been the discovery that a single virus genome often contained genetic information derived from two distinct cellular genes (often from two different chromosomes). The v-*src* gene of Rous sarcoma virus, as mentioned above, derives its carboxyl terminal sequences from outside the cellular *src* gene; these sequences are apparently from about 1 kb downstream of the gene. The FBR strain of MSV, in addition to *fos*, contains sequences called *fox* from another location which confer additional properties (see on). Similarly, the AEV strain, ES4, differs from strain H; the former contains *erbA* and *erbB*, the latter *erbB* alone. Both strains cause erythroleukaemias but erythroid cells transformed in culture show differences in growth requirements and differentiation capacity depending on the specific virus strain. The GR strain of feline sarcoma virus shows fusion of part of an actin gene with the transforming *fgr* gene. Finally, two viruses have shown acquisition of sequences from two genes, both of which have oncogenic potential on their own: the avian myelocytomatosis virus MH2 contains the oncogenes *myc* and *raf* (also called *mil*), and the E26 avian myeloblastosis virus contains *myb* and *ets*. The neoplastic potential of these viruses is expanded with regard to the types of tumours induced compared to viruses containing only one of the genes (see Table 10.1). In the case of v-*src* mentioned above, the unusual structure might have arisen by a large splicing event, but the others required more bizarre recombination. (However, it is still speculation whether transduction occurs at the DNA level between integrated provirus and adjacent cellular DNA, or at the RNA level between viral and cellular species, or by both mechanisms.)

10.3.2 *Co-operative transformation*

An old observation that primary rodent embryo fibroblasts, but not later passaged or established cell lines, were generally refractory to morphological transformation by transforming viruses was the basis of a new assay for oncogene activity. For example, the dual expression of the genes encoding the nuclear (large T) antigen and the membrane associated (middle T) antigen of polyomavirus (see Chapter 9) cause transformation whereas neither alone has this capacity, although large T confers longevity ('immortalization' to continued cell growth). A similar relationship was found between unrelated oncogenes, e.g. the mutated alleles of Ha-*ras*-1 (whether viral or cellular in origin) and *myc*. Eventually a pattern emerged of co-operation between a nuclear oncogene product and a cytoplasmic oncogene product (Table 10.5); the former also generally can immortalize nonestablished cells.

Co-operative transformation is not as stringent as described above; in a few cases, a single oncogene will suffice. Despite this, the discovery of co-operating oncogenes was particularly satisfactory given the multistage character of carcinogenesis, interweaving pathways of biochemical and physiological functions. But we have determined only the earliest step without generating clues to distinct targets or later cascades. Elucidation of the intermediate and final stages is necessary for both understanding and devising possible modes of intervention.

10.4 Other cellular genes that may be involved in oncogenesis

Apart from the oncogenes described above, there are some other cellular genes that display possible associations with oncogenesis.

One interesting protein, p53, was originally detected because it was

Table 10.5 Co-operating oncogenes[1]

Nonnuclear	Nuclear
Ha-*ras*-1[2]	v-*myc*
N-*ras*[2]	c-*myc*[3]
Polyoma middle T	Polyoma large T
Adenovirus E1b	Adenovirus E1a
	v-*myb*
	v-*fos*
	p53[4]

[1] Manifestation of the transformed phenotype requires one oncogene from the nuclear group and one from the nonnuclear group.
[2] Mutated allele.
[3] Normal and rearranged forms when supplemented with a strong promoter.
[4] p53 is discussed in Section 10.4.

immunoprecipitated from cells transformed by SV40 virus as part of a complex with the viral T antigen (see Chapter 9). The p53 product can be detected in normal cells as well, although it appears to have a shorter half life. This result suggests that the viral proteins stabilize p53 by formation of the complex. Further studies showed that p53 was present at above normal amounts in many different transformed and tumour cell lines including those not involving viruses. This nuclear protein has been observed in many different human tumours, and specific antibodies are detectable in a small but significant proportion of breast cancer patients. It also is capable of participating in co-operative transformation described above.

Two exciting results have been reported. First, microinjection of cultured cells in G1 with anti-p53 antibodies inhibits DNA synthesis; however, during other phases of the cell cycle the cells proliferate normally. This suggests that p53 could be a requisite rate–limiting protein for progression through the cell cycle. Second, a series of mouse leukaemias induced by the Abelson murine leukaemia virus (v-*abl*) have been established as cell lines; all were tumorigenic, but only one failed to metastasize. This exception was due to the integration of a 'helper' virus within the coding sequences of the p53 gene. Upon introduction of an intact p53 gene into these cells by transfection, the ability to metastasize was re-established.

A potentially analogous situation has been observed in another system. Tumorigenicity is conferred on NIH/3T3 cells following transfection with a mutated *ras* allele, but the tumours do not metastasize in immuno-competent histocompatible mice. Secondary transfection using DNA from a human metastatic cervical carcinoma cell line provided metastatic capability. This may not be a general phenomenon. The identity of the gene(s) responsible has not yet been established, but is eagerly awaited.

Another oncogene with other cell associations is *fos*. There have been two viral isolates of this gene, one in which *fos* alone was transduced and another in which other cell sequences (called *fox*) were also appended in the viral genome. The *fos-fox* fusion gene is more potent as a transforming agent in cultured cells (both in efficiency of transformation and in the range of cells susceptible to transformation). The precise role contributed by the *fox* sequences is as yet unclear. Additionally, immunoprecipitation assays to cells expressing v-*fos* or cellular *fos* show that the protein is always associated in a complex with a cell protein, p39. Neither antibodies to p39 or the gene itself have yet been obtained, but such reagents might shed light on the biological function of *fos*.

10.5 Protooncogene expression in normal development and differentiation

Although molecular clones to probe for oncogene expression are available for many of the genes described above, it is a rather daunting task to examine many different tissues. In some cases, it is also difficult to obtain sufficient amounts of homogeneous cell populations and thus one is not always able to make direct comparisons between a neoplasm and its normal counterpart. This has left large gaps in our knowledge of oncogene expression during embryonic development, differentiation stages, or cell cycling (Table 10.6), although eventually this knowledge will be available.

One well exploited system is the examination of mouse embryos at different days of gestation. Genes such as *raf*, Ha-*ras*, Ki-*ras* and *myc* are expressed throughout. The *abl* gene is highly expressed at day 10, corresponding to a period of foetal liver haemopoiesis, whereas *fos* peaks at later stages due to high levels in the extraembryonic membranes, particularly the amnion, and *fms* expression is observed in the chorion. Other genes are not present at detectable levels. It is not facetious to speculate that protooncogenes are vital to embryogenesis and that we may eventually know their specific roles.

To study changes with regard to cell cycling and proliferation, several methods have been used. Most rely on selecting cells in the same phase of the cycle using a cell sorter which measures levels of DNA or by synchronizing the cycle, usually by blocking the cells in a specific phase of the cycle by deprivation of specific nutrients or by chemicals. On removing the block, the cycle continues with many of the cells in the same phase. *In vivo* systems such as partial hepatectomy (where one lobe of the liver is removed) can be used to stimulate rapid regeneration of

Table 10.6 Protooncogene expression

Gene	High expression[1]	Abnormal expression[2]
abl	Mid-gestation embryo, testes, spleen, thymus	Chronic granulocytic leukaemia
*erb*A	Mid to late gestation embryo	
*erb*B	Mid-gestation embryo	Squamous cell carcinomas, glioblastomas
fes	Bone marrow	Myeloid and lymphoid leukaemia
fms	Macrophage, placenta	Mammary and renal carcinoma
fos	Amnion, chorion, mature macrophages, growth factor stimulated cells	Choriocarcinoma
mos	None	Plasmacytoma[3]
myb	Yolk sac, bone marrow, thymus	Myeloid and lymphoid leukaemia
myc	Ubiquitous	B cell lymphomas, promyelocytic leukaemia
raf	Ubiquitous	
ras	Ubiquitous	Numerous (see Table 10.3)
rel	Spleen	
ros	Kidney	
sis	Platelets	Osteosarcoma
ski	Cartilage, muscle, skin	
src	Spleen, macrophages, brain	Brain tumours
yes	Kidney	

[1] Most studies from experimental animals, principally mice.
[2] Human tumours or tumour cell lines.
[3] Rodent tumour only; gene activated by insertional mutagenesis (see Table 10.2).

cell number. Cell sorting has shown *myb* expression to be cycle dependent. Stimulation from quiescence shows *fos* to be activated within minutes followed by a rapid decline, whereas *myc* expression appears later but is less transient. The liver regeneration experiments show that the major nuclear oncogenes, members of the kinase family, and *ras* are expressed during the highly proliferative phase. Thus, these results recapitulate our awareness that oncogenes are involved in normal proliferative responses, but as yet do not explain how or why.

10.6 Lessons learned from oncogenes

It should be clear from the discussion above that oncogenes are expressed in a plethora of cell types. Even the truly tumorigenic v-*onc* genes do not answer our queries. For example, the murine *abl* containing virus causes immature B cell tumours in mice whereas the feline *abl* virus causes fibrosarcomas (Table 10.1). Is this due to differences in the nature of the fusion proteins (between *abl* and viral genes) or to some inherent properties of the two animal species? Site specific mutagenesis has shown that the *gag* portion of the mouse virus fusion protein is required for efficient transformation of cultured B lymphocytes though it is dispensable for fibroblast transformation which may explain in part this discrepancy. Furthermore, many strains of mice are genetically resistant to leukaemogenesis by the virus by a mechanism as yet unknown. We have to know more about the normal *abl* product. The highest level of *abl* mRNA in normal tissues occurs in the testes. Haemopoietic tissues also express high levels; is this significant in regard to aberrant transcription due to translocation in CGL? Other examples of these phenomena exist (see Tables 10.1, 10.2, and 10.6).

Understanding the role of the *myc* gene is certain to prove of central interest. The various v-*myc* genes are responsible for the induction of carcinomas, fibrosarcomas and myeloid leukaemias, whereas hyperexpression due to translocation or promoter insertion is observed in T and B cell leukaemias. Additionally, *myc* expression is apparent at low levels in most tissues, becomes elevated in cells responding to mitogens, and is very high in the most mature macrophages. There is also intriguing information from experimental manipulation of the gene. First, a new 'virus' was made by putting the cellular *myc* gene between viral LTRs from the MMTV genome and introduced into fertilized mouse ova. The use of LTRs ensured that the gene could be incorporated into chromosomal (and germ line) DNA and the mice (known as transgenic mice) were examined for abnormalities of development. However, it was only in adult female mice that a change was seen: the animals developed mammary carcinomas as a heritable trait. In a similar way, a construct containing *myc* and the enhancer element from an immunoglobulin gene (from a rearranged gene in a mouse plasmocytoma, see above) induced a high incidence of B cell leukaemias in the transgenic mice, whereas other enhancers from a leukaemia virus LTR or SV40 virus were less efficacious in inducing tumours and showed different target specificities (a T cell lymphoma with the former, and lymphosarcoma, fibrosarcoma and kidney carcinoma with the latter). These results emphasize the importance of specific promoter and enhancer elements of gene transcription in different cells and in neoplasia.

We are looking through a small window at what is going on in a cell. The viral oncogenes have called our attention to the cellular counterparts, and transfection assays and chromosomal aberrations have helped to identify further potentially important genes for neoplastic growth.

Genetic studies suggest that recessive changes or deletions may be contributory, but our present technology limits the means of detecting them.

Our sojourn into oncogenes has led to the conclusion that normal cellular genes can be diverted into neoplastic pathways by somatic mutations as diverse as single nucleotide substitutions to gross alterations involving translocations or amplifications. Underscoring these perturbations, there may be more subtle effects on expression in inappropriate cells, alterations in transcription rates or mRNA turnover, or stabilization of the gene products and, in turn, their target substrates within the cell.

Most of the changes observed have led to overexpression of the gene. But taking a cellular *onc* gene and putting it under the control of a strong promoter does not necessarily lead to oncogenic potential (indeed this works for *mos* but not for *src*). Overabundance of an *onc* gene product might also uncover cryptic activities normally absent when the protein occurs at some subthreshold dose.

Overall, cell metabolism and proliferation is an intricate and delicately balanced response to extracellular signals (e.g. mitogens), involving regulated transmission by effector molecules to the nucleus. Some of the known oncogenes already recapitulate a few stages of these mechanisms in their mimicry of growth factors and growth factor receptors. Others display functions suggestive of second messages or transmitters. And the nuclear oncogenes might be the ultimate effector molecules. Despite the formidable task ahead of identifying these interweaving pathways step by step, we have gained considerable insight within the last five years. Indeed, the studies on the first identifiable retrovirus oncogenes quickly aroused the interest of scientists in many areas of diverse research and showed how interrelated their endeavours had become.

In the final analysis, c-*onc* genes are just protooncogenes that march to the tune of a different trumpet.

Further reading

Bishop, J. M. (1985). Viral oncogenes. *Cell,* **42**, 23–38.

——, and Varmus, H. (1982). Functions and origins of retroviral transforming genes. In: *RNA tumor viruses* pp. 999–1108 (eds. R. Weiss, N. Teich, H. Varmus, and J. Coffin) **Vol. 1.** Cold Spring Harbor Laboratory, Cold Spring Harbor, New York.

——, —— (1985). Functions and origins of retroviral transforming genes. In: *RNA tumor viruses* pp. 249–356 (eds. R. Weiss, N. Teich, H. Varmus, and J. Coffin) **Vol. 2.** Cold Spring Harbor Laboratory, Cold Spring Harbor, New York.

Marshall, C. (1985). Human oncogenes. In: *RNA tumor viruses* pp. 487–558 (eds. R. Weiss, N. Teich, H. Varmus, and J. Coffin) **Vol. 2.** Cold Spring Harbor Laboratory, Cold Spring Harbor, New York.

Varmus, H. E. (1984). The molecular genetics of cellular oncogenes. *Annual Review of Genetics,* **18**, 553–612.

For detailed information on specific topics, consult the following specialized review series.

Advances in viral oncology. A continuing series of volumes published by Raven Press, New York (ed. G. Klein) covering the latest developments in viral oncology as well as oncogenes *per se.*

11

Chromosomes and cancer

D. SHEER

11.1 Introduction

The genetic basis of cancer was discussed in Chapter 5 in relation to both hereditary predisposition to cancer and DNA changes which occur in tumours themselves. In this Chapter I shall describe chromosome changes in tumours.

Most tumours have structural and/or numerical chromosome aberrations, some of which are consistently associated with particular types of tumours. Advances in gene mapping and recombinant DNA technology are now beginning to help us understand the nature of some of these aberrations. It is becoming apparent that sites of consistent chromosome rearrangements pinpoint genes which may be critically involved in malignant transformation, and that the rearrangements themselves can subvert the normal functioning of these genes.

Human somatic cells normally have 46 chromosomes; they are said to be diploid. Chromosome analysis is usually carried out on cells in mitosis (cell division), when the chromosomes become visible as distinct entities.

After identifying each chromosome in a cell by its characteristic size, shape, and staining properties, a karyotype displaying the full chromosome complement of the cell can be prepared.

The first specific chromosome abnormality observed in a human tumour was seen in Philadelphia in 1960 by Nowell and Hungerford who found an unusually small chromosome in the leukaemic cells of patients with chronic granulocytic leukaemia (CGL). This small chromosome was named the Philadelphia chromosome. The discovery of the Philadephia chromosome aroused considerable interest in cancer cytogenetics as it gave the first direct evidence for a consistent DNA-associated change in a tumour. The search for similar abnormalities in other tumours was hampered by the great variation in chromosome abnormalities from one patient to the next and by the finding of aneuploidy (abnormal chromosome numbers) and multiple rearrangements (abnormal breakage and rejoining of chromosomes) in many tumours. Furthermore, chromosome rearrangements could not be defined using staining methodology available then.

The introduction of chromosome banding techniques in 1970 revolutionized cancer cytogenetics. Consistent chromosome aberrations were shown to be associated with other types of tumours. Chromosome aberrations were shown to be related to one another within the different cells of a tumour, and further karyotypic changes were shown to occur during tumour progression. Short term culture methods to improve yields of dividing cells, and high resolution banding of elongated chromosomes now allow a more precise definition of rearrangements as well as the identification of previously undetected rearrangements. Using these techniques, most tumour cells can be shown to have some chromosomal defect.

Our current understanding of the significance of consistent chromosome aberrations in cancer will be reviewed below. Evidence that these aberrations are non-random has come from cytogenetic analysis of large numbers of human tumours. Haemopoietic tumours usually have rearrangements involving only a few chromosomes in an otherwise normal diploid karyotype. Solid tumours often have many more chromosome rearrangements with gross aneuploidy. For this reason, consistent or specific aberrations have been more easily detected in the haematological neoplasms, which are also easier to sample and have more dividing cells than solid neoplasms. This bias is reflected in the survey given below.

11.2 Methodology

Cytogenetic analysis of leukaemias is carried out on a bone marrow aspirate, or on a peripheral blood sample if the white cell count is high, by immediate processing (direct method) or after *in vitro* culture for 24–

72 hours. Solid tumours are more difficult to analyse since the cells have to be separated. Because of this, chromosome analyses of solid tumours have usually been done on cell lines derived from these tumours, or on pleural or ascitic fluid containing metastatic tumour cells.

As a rule, chromosomes are studied during or just prior to the meta-phase stage of mitosis when they become condensed and can easily be seen under the microscope. DNA replication occurs before mitosis so that each chromosome consists of two identical sister chromatids held together at the centromere. When making chromosome preparations, colchicine or a related agent is added to the tumour material to arrest cells in metaphase by disrupting the formation of the mitotic spindle fibres which normally separate the chromatids. The cells are then swollen in a hypotonic solution to make it easier to disrupt them and release the chromosomes. The cells are fixed in methanol-acetic acid, and meta-phase 'spreads' are prepared by dropping fixed cells onto microscope slides. Chromosomes are identified by staining techniques which produce a characteristic series of bands along the chromosomes. The two techniques most often used, G– and Q-banding, result in essentially the same banding patterns on the chromosomes. One method of producing G-banding is to treat the chromosomes with a weak solution of trypsin prior to staining with Giemsa stain; the preparation is then examined using conventional light microscopy. Q-banding is produced by treating the chromosomes with quinacrine-diHCl or quinacrine mustard; the preparation is then examined using fluorescence microscopy.

Until recently, cytogenetic techniques have produced karyotypes of normal human cells with approximately 300 bands (Fig. 11.1). It is now possible to obtain less condensed chromosomes earlier in mitosis. One method used is to treat the cultures with a drug, methotrexate, which blocks one of the metabolic pathways in DNA synthesis so that the cells collect at one stage before mitosis. The block is released by thymidine so that large numbers of cells in the same stage of mitosis are produced. These cultures are said to be synchronized. After a brief exposure to colchicine, high resolution karyotypes can be obtained with up to 1200 bands, thus allowing the delineation of previously undetected chromo-some aberrations. In the standard method these bands would normally coalesce as condensation proceeds during mitosis into fewer and thicker bands.

Our understanding of the molecular events occurring in chromosome rearrangements in cancer has been greatly facilitated by advances in gene mapping (localization of genes on chromosomes). This is done either by analysing human genetic markers present in human-rodent somatic cell hybrids (produced by whole cell fusions) which retain only a few human chromosomes, or by *in situ* hybridization of radiolabelled molecular probes directly onto metaphase or meiotic chromosomes.

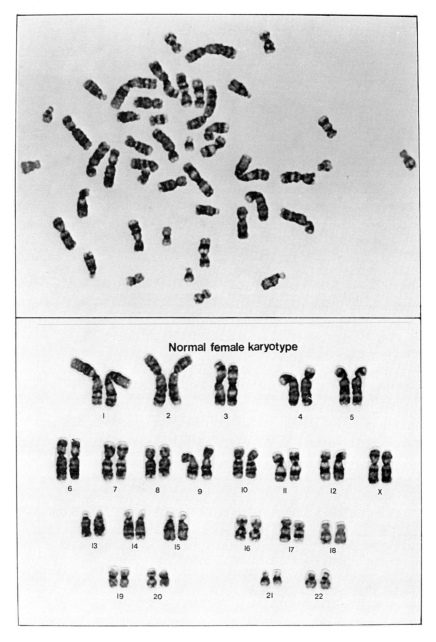

Fig. 11.1 G-banded metaphase spread (above) and karyotype (below) of normal female cell.

11.3 Terminology and types of chromosome aberrations in tumours

Karyotypes are described according to an International System for Human Cytogenetic Nomenclature. The total chromosome number is listed first, then the sex chromosomes, then gains and losses of whole chromosomes, and finally structural rearrangements. The short and long arms of chromosomes are represented by 'p' and 'q', respectively. Gains or losses of whole chromosomes are identified by a '+' or a '−' before the chromosome number. A gain or loss of part of a chromosome is identified by a '+' or a '−' after the chromosome number. 46,XY and 46,XX represent normal diploid male and female karyotypes. 47,XX, +8 represents a female karyotype with an extra copy of chromosome 8, which is the most common aberration in myeloproliferative disorders, while 46,XY,20q− represents a male karyotype with a deletion of the long arm of chromosome 20, which is present in 10–20 per cent of patients with polycythaemia vera. The most common structural rearrangement found in tumours is a translocation, in which segments of two or more different chromosomes are interchanged. Translocations are signified by a 't'; the chromosomes involved are enclosed within a first set of brackets and the translocation breakpoints are enclosed within a second set of brackets. For example, t(9;22)(q34;q11) represents a reciprocal translocation between chromosomes 9 and 22, with the breaks in the long arms of chromosomes 9 and 22 in bands q34 and q11, respectively. This translocation is present in most cases of chronic granulocytic leukaemia, and will be described in more detail below. Other structural chromosome rearrangements seen in tumours are inversions, deletions, and insertions. For example, inv(16)(p13;q22) represents an inversion within chromosome 16, with the breakpoints occurring in bands p13 and q22. This inversion has recently been described in acute myelomonocytic leukaemia with abnormal eosinophils. Finally, an isochromosome is derived from the loss of either the long or short arm of the chromosome with the duplication of the other arm. Thus, an iso(17q) or i(17q) consists of the duplicated long arm of chromosome 17. This aberration is frequently present in the acute phase of chronic granulocytic leukaemia. Only clonal chromosome aberrations will be reviewed below. These are defined as occurring within at least two cells within a tumour for structural rearrangements, or within at least three cells for the same numerical aberrations.

11.4 Leukaemias and lymphomas

11.4.1 *General survey*

Myeloid malignancies—acute myeloid or non-lymphocytic leukaemias (AML) and chronic granulocytic leukaemia (CGL)—are located primarily in the bone marrow, while lymphoid malignancies—acute lymphocytic and chronic lymphocytic leukaemias (ALL, CLL) and lymphomas—are found in the spleen, thymus and lymph nodes, as well as in the blood (see Chapter 3). Nomenclature of acute myeloid leukaemias, published by the French, American and British (FAB) Co-operative Group in 1976 is of particular relevance to cytogenetic studies, and is summarized in Table 11.1.

Table 11.1 FAB classification of AML

Description	Code
Acute myeloblastic leukaemia without maturation	M1
Acute myeloblastic leukaemia with maturation	M2
Acute promyelocytic leukaemia	M3
Acute myelomonocytic leukaemia	M4
Acute monoblastic leukaemia (poorly-differentiated)	M5a
Acute monocytic leukaemia (well-differentiated)	M5b
Erythroleukaemia	M6

Leukaemias and lymphomas usually have few chromosome rearrangements and chromosome numbers in the diploid range (other than Hodgkin's lymphomas which usually have chromosomes in the triploid– tetraploid range). These rearrangements have therefore been relatively easy to define, especially with high resolution chromosome banding. This technique has also enabled the definition of subtle rearrangements in different subtypes of AML (see on). A summary of consistent chromosome defects in leukaemias and lymphomas, and in the myeloproliferative disorder polycythaemia vera in which there is an increased production of red blood cells and their precursors, is presented in Table 11.2.

Trisomy is in some cases the only aberration observed in leukaemias and lymphomas, particularly trisomy 8 in AML and trisomy 12 in B cell CLL. However, translocations are the most common structural aberration. Translocations involving the same pairs of chromosomes recur within particular malignancies to varying extents. For example, the Philadelphia translocation, t(9;22), is present in the leukaemic cells of virtually all patients with CGL, whereas t(8;21) is present in the leukaemic cells of only 10–20 per cent of patients with AML–M2. The degree of specificity of different translocations is also variable. For example, a t(9;22) which appears identical to the Philadelphia translocation also occurs in AML–M1 and is the most frequent rearrangement in non-B,

Table 11.2 Consistent chromosome aberrations in leukaemias and lymphomas

Malignancy	Chromosome aberration
Leukaemias	
Chronic granulocytic leukaemia	t(9;22)(q34;q11)
Acute myeloid leukaemia	
M1	t(9;22)(q34;q11)
M2	t(8;21)(q22;q22)
M3	t(15;17)(q22;q12–21)
M4 with abnormal eosinophils	inv(16)(p13;q22)
M5a	t(9;11)(p22;q23)
M1, M2, M4 with increased basophils	t(6;9)(p23;q34)
M1, M2, M4, M5, M6	del(5)(q22;q23)
	del(7)(q33;q36)
	trisomy 8
Chronic lymphocytic leukaemia	t(11;14)(q13;q32)
	trisomy 12
Acute lymphocytic leukaemia	t(9;22)(q34;q11)
	t(4;11)(q21;q23)
	t(8;14)(q24;32)
Lymphomas	
Burkitt's lymphoma	t(8;14)(q24;q32)
	t(2;8)(p12;q24)
	t(8;22)(q24;q11)
Small non-cleaved cell lymphoma, large cell immunoblastic lymphoma	t(8;14)(q24;q32)
Follicular small cleaved cell lymphoma	t(14;18)(q32;q21)
Small cell lymphocytic lymphoma	trisomy 12
Small cell lymphocytic transformed to diffuse large cell	t(11;14)(q13;q32)
Polycythaemia vera	del(20q)

non-T adult ALL, while the t(15;17) associated with acute promyelocytic leukaemia (APL-M3) has never been seen in any other malignancy. The significance of this variability is unclear. Presumably the specificity of the t(15;17) in acute promyelocytic leukaemia could reflect either that this translocation is lethal in cells other than promyelocytes, or that it does not confer a proliferative advantage to other types of cells.

The regions around the breakpoints of the Philadelphia translocation and of the translocations associated with Burkitt's lymphoma have been cloned and shown to involve the cellular oncogenes c-*abl* and c-*myc*, respectively (see on). Cellular oncogenes may be implicated in other specific translocations where the breakpoints have not yet been cloned. For example, the oncogene c-*ets* maps to the region of chromosome 11 which is involved in the t(4;11) in ALL, while the oncogene c-*erbA1* maps to the region of chromosome 17 that is involved in the t(15;17) in APL–M3. However, it is not yet known whether these oncogenes are directly affected by the rearrangements.

11.4.2 *Chronic granulocytic leukaemia*

Bone marrow cells of approximately 90 per cent of patients with chronic granulocytic leukaemic (CGL) contain the Philadelphia (Ph[1]) chromosome, which is derived from a reciprocal translocation between chromosomes 9 and 22, t(9;22)(q34;q11) (Fig. 11.2). The presence or absence of the Ph[1] chromosome in CGL has been shown to be clinically relevant, as Ph[1]–positive CGL patients have a longer median survival time (42 months) compared with Ph[1]–negative CGL patients (15

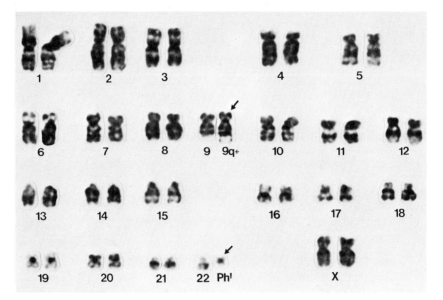

Fig. 11.2 G-banded karyotype showing the Philadelphia chromosome.

months). The question whether Ph¹–negative CGL is, in fact, the same disease as Ph¹–positive CGL is still undecided.

Leukaemic cells of approximately 80 per cent of CGL patients entering the terminal acute phase of the disease (blast crisis) show further chromosome abnormalities superimposed on the t(9;22). A change in karyotype in CGL is a grave prognostic sign, with death usually occurring within a few months. These secondary changes are non-random with at least one of three particular changes, +Ph¹, +8, +iso(17q) usually occurring, suggesting that genes on these chromosomes confer a proliferative advantage to the cells carrying them. These genes remain to be identified.

The Philadelphia translocation is one of the two specific chromosome rearrangements occurring in tumours which have thus far been shown to involve cellular oncogenes directly. The oncogene c-abl on chromosome 9 becomes transferred to the Ph¹ chromosome as a result of the translocation (Fig. 11.3). Although the breakpoint on chromosome 9 is located upstream of the c-abl gene, it appears to be variable and occur over a relatively large distance in different patients. In contrast, the breakpoint on chromosome 22 in different patients appears to be restricted to a small region (5.8 kb) of DNA. The genes on chromosome 22 adjacent to the translocation breakpoint have not been identified, but are known not to be the immunoglobulin λ light chain genes, which map below the breakpoint on chromosome 22. The oncogene c-sis is transferred from chromosome 22 to chromosome 9 as a result of the translocation, but is located some distance away from the breakpoint and appears not to be affected by the translocation. The most interesting aspect of this translocation is that an abnormally long transcript of the c-abl gene has been detected in CGL cells containing the Ph¹ chromo-

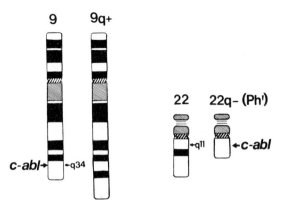

Fig. 11.3 Schematic representation of the t(9;22) in CGL.

some, but not in normal cells or in other leukaemias without the Ph[1] translocation. These results suggest that this abnormal transcript plays an important role in the development of CGL.

Five to ten per cent of CGL patients with classical features of the disease have variant translocations. These can be either of the simple type involving chromosome 22 and a chromosome other than 9, or of the complex type involving both chromosomes 9 and 22 as well as one or more other chromosomes. Recent analyses using *in situ* hybridization have shown that c-*abl* is involved in both the simple and complex variant translocations, and that in complex translocations, the c-*abl* gene consistently appears to become located contiguous to sequences from chromosome 22.

The typical Ph[1] chromosome has also been observed in some forms of AML, and is the most frequent chromosome rearrangement in adult non-B, non-T ALL. The factors determining which type of leukaemia develops from a Ph[1]–containing cell remain to be established, but presumably involve other steps in the transformation process as well as the stage of differentiation of the cell in which the Ph[1] chromosome originates.

11.4.3. *Burkitt's lymphoma*

The specific chromosome translocations associated with this B cell malignancy have been subjected to rigorous molecular analysis. An (8;14)(q24;q32) translocation is present in the malignant cells of approximately 90 per cent of patients with the disease (Fig. 11.4). One of two variant translocations, t(2;8)(p12;q24) and t(8;22)(q24;q11), is present in approximately 10 per cent of patients (Fig. 11.4). All three translocations have also been observed in B cell ALL. Chromosomes 14, 2 and 22 carry the genes for the immunoglobulin heavy (IgH), and the kappa (κ) and lambda (λ) light chains (discussed below), respectively. In the typical t(8;14) in Burkitt's lymphoma, the oncogene c-*myc* which is normally located on band q24 of chromosome 8, translocates to the IgH locus on chromosome 14. In the variant translocations, c-*myc* remains on chromosome 8 while sequences from the κ and λ light chain loci translocate to the vicinity of the c-*myc* gene. Analogous translocations between c-*myc* and immunoglobulin loci are present in rat and mouse plasmacytomas which are also derived from B cells. All three rearrangements in human tumours, and those in rat and mouse plasmacytomas, result in enhanced transcription of the translocated c-*myc* gene. A large amount of circumstantial evidence has emerged from molecular analyses of these translocations suggesting that c-*myc* activation occurs by physical separation of the gene from its normal regulatory elements.

A brief introduction to the immunoglobulin (Ig) and c-*myc* genes helps

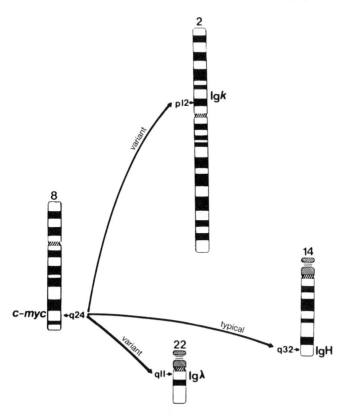

Fig. 11.4 Schematic representation of the typical and variant translocations in Burkitt's lymphoma.

in understanding the mechanisms involved in c-*myc* activation. Antibody molecules are composed of two identical light chains and two identical heavy chains (see Chapter 18). The light chains each have a variable region and one constant region domain, whereas the heavy chains each have a variable region and three or four constant region domains. The Ig loci have a large number of variable (V) region genes located upstream from the constant (C) region genes (Fig. 11.5). These loci have a very unusual property: during B lymphocyte differentiation they undergo recombinations that are crucial for the generation of antibody diversity (see Chapter 15). The first step is a rearrangement that joins one of the V-region segments with a C-region segment, separated by the small D (diversity) and J (joining) segments in the case of the heavy chains or by a J segment in the case of the light chains. The promoter of the V-segment that has been moved is thus brought under the influence of an enhancer

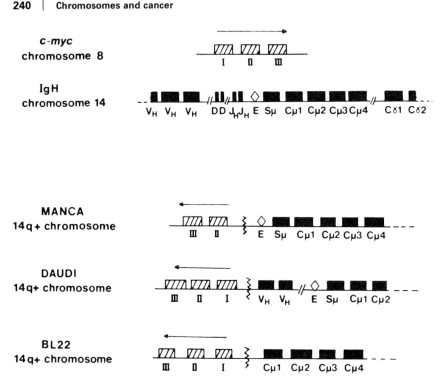

Fig. 11.5 Schematic representation of c-*myc* and IgH genes, and the arrangement of these genes at the translocation breakpoints in three cell lines derived from Burkitt's lymphoma with the typical t(8; 14) (see text). Boxed regions: exons (coding regions). Arrows indicate direction of transcription of c-*myc*.

sequence immediately upstream of the C-segment, which leads to the production of a complete Ig transcript. The enhancer is, by definition, tissue specific and can enhance transcription of genes on either side of it. Enhancer sequences have so far been found in Ig heavy chain genes and κ light chain genes, but not yet in λ light chain genes. In the case of the heavy chain loci, further rearrangements occur later that involve a switch in the C gene expressed with a given V segment. In any one B cell, these recombinations occur at only one allele of each Ig locus, resulting in the production of only one type of light chain and one type of heavy chain.

Although the normal function of the c-*myc* protein is not known, other than that it is found in the nucleus bound to double-stranded DNA, the detailed structure of the gene has been determined. The c-*myc* gene consists of three exons (i.e. coding regions) separated by two introns (non-coding) (Fig. 11.5). The first exon has a number of interesting features: it has two active promoters with transcription initiation sites from which two transcripts are synthesized; it also contains multiple termination codons which preclude its translation into protein; the sequence of this exon is highly conserved between mouse and man, suggesting some crucial role for this region.

The molecular cloning of the translocation breakpoints and analyses of c-*myc* transcription in a number of Burkitt's lymphomas has brought to light several features about the translocations.

1. The translocated c-*myc* gene becomes transcribed at significant but variable levels.

2. The breakpoints vary considerably in different tumours; they have been located upstream of the first exon of c-*myc*, as well as in the intron between exons 1 and 2; they have also been located in different positions in the Ig loci, although in most Burkitt's lymphomas with a t(8;14) they are within the μ constant region of the heavy chain locus.

3. The orientation of c-*myc* often becomes reversed so that the first or second exon becomes placed alongside Ig sequences.

4. The translocation always involves the non-functional Ig locus in which no recombination has occurred.

The variability in the locations of the translocation breakpoints makes it difficult to draw conclusions about a general mechanism for c-*myc* activation in Burkitt's lymphomas. In one case, transcriptional activation has been shown to be due to the Ig enhancer element (see Fig. 11.5, Manca). In other cases, however, the enhancer is either too far away to influence c-*myc* expression (Daudi, Fig. 11.5) or else it has been transferred to chromosome 8 (BL22, Fig. 11.5). It has also been proposed that sequences within the first exon of c-*myc* are involved in regulating expression and that removal of this exon in some tumours may be responsible for activation of the oncogene. Extensive mutation of the first exon has also been found in one case, but not in others. The fact that the first exon is absent from the viral *myc* oncogene lends further support for its regulatory role in normal cells.

While explanations for the mechanisms of c-*myc* activation in B cell tumours are for the most part speculative at this stage, the general principle remains remarkably clear: that c-*myc* becomes activated as a result of its relocation into the immediate vicinity of the Ig loci. Our understanding of the role played by the *myc* protein is also limited, although we have evidence for its involvement in other types of tumours (e.g. see section 11.6 below). Preliminary experiments have suggested that the *myc* protein may immortalize cells, with the activity of other oncogenes being necessary for full transformation. It remains to be determined whether the regulation of oncogenes by tissue specific sequences proves to be a more general phenomenon in tumorigenesis.

It is interesting that chromosome band 14q32, on which the IgH genes are located, is also involved in recurring chromosome translocations in other B cell malignancies (Table 11.2). Sequences designated *bcl*-1 and *bcl*-2 (B cell lymphoma/leukaemia) are translocated from their normal locations on chromosomes 11 and 18, respectively, into the IgH region. Neither *bcl*-1 or *bcl*-2 is homologous to any known retroviral oncogene, but if a similar mechanism operates here as in Burkitt's lymphoma, these sequences may be activated as a result of their juxtaposition with IgH genes.

11.4.4 *Acute myeloid leukaemias*

The most frequent numerical aberrations observed in AML are trisomy 8 (13 per cent of all cases), monosomy 7 (9 per cent) and monosomy 5 (6 per cent). Recurring structural chromosome rearrangements have now been identified in different subtypes of AML, which represent different lineages of myeloid cell differentiation. The rearrangements described below are thus of particular interest since they may lead us to tissue and stage specific genes that participate in malignant transformation of these cells.

An (8;21)(q22;q22) translocation is present in 10–15 per cent of patients with AML–M2, and in a small number of patients with AML-M4, but not in other malignancies. A (15;17)(q22;q12–21) translocation associated with APL-M3 may be present in virtually all cases of this disease, but has never been seen in any other malignancy except in one patient with a rare promyelocytic acute phase of chronic granulocytic leukaemia.

Structural rearrangements of chromosome band 16q22 have recently been demonstrated in AML-M4 with abnormal eosinophils, using high resolution banding. These rearrangements are either an inversion, inv(16)(p13;q22), or a deletion, del(16)(q22).

A translocation t(6;9)(p23;q34) has been observed in AML-M1, –M2, and –M4 in which there is an increased basophil count. The basophils appear morphologically normal. The breakpoint in chromosome 9 is in the same band as the cellular oncogene c-*abl*.

Structural rearrangements, translocations or deletions involving the long arm of chromosome 11, particularly bands 11q23–24 but also 11q13–14, have been observed in acute monoblastic leukaemia. In one study, six of eight children and five of sixteen adults with poorly differentiated or monoblastic leukaemia, M5a, had abnormalities of 11q, while only one of three children and none of seven adults with well differentiated or monocytic leukaemia (M5b) had these abnormalities. It is of interest that the breakpoints on 11q can vary and that where the abnormality is a translocation, the other chromosome is variable, although the most common translocation is t(9;11)(p22;q23).

11.4.5. *Secondary acute myeloid leukaemia*

An association can be seen between carcinogenic agents and karyotypes in the resulting secondary tumours. It is now established that leukaemia can arise after radiation or chemotherapy for a previous malignancy, and these secondary tumours have been shown to have characteristic chromosome aberrations. In one study, 61 of 63 patients with secondary AML had chromosome rearrangements, and of these, 55 patients had deletions of the long arm of either or both chromosomes 5 and 7, as shown in Table 11.3. Regions 5q22–23 and 7q33–36 are commonly

Table 11.3 Deletions of 5q and 7q in secondary AML

Number of patients	Chromosome aberrations
6	monosomy 5
8	deletion of 5q
22	monosomy 7
2	deletion of 7q
17	abnormalities of both 5 and 7

deleted, although the extent of the deletion varies. In an earlier study, patients with AML who had been previously exposed to insecticides or petroleum products were found to have deletions of 5q and 7q in their leukaemic cells.

11.4.6 *Acute lymphocytic leukaemia*

Good chromosome preparations are more difficult to prepare from ALL than AML patients, for reasons that are still unknown. Improved cytogenetic techniques have been developed and, at the 3rd International Workshop on Chromosomes in Leukaemia in 1980, two thirds of 330 ALL patients were shown to have clonal chromosome aberrations. Of the 213 aneuploid cases, 35 per cent were pseudodiploid, 25 per cent were hyperdiploid, and 7 per cent were hypodiploid. Numerical aberrations were non-random, with chromosomes 6, 8, 18, and 21 being preferentially gained, and chromosomes 7 and 20 preferentially lost. The structural abnormalities which occurred most frequently were t(9;22) in 17.9 per cent of patients with structural abnormalities, t(4;11) in 8.2 per cent, t(8;14) in 7.3 per cent, a 14q+ chromosome in 6.9 per cent, and a 6q– chromosome in 6.0 per cent of patients. The t(9;22) is identical to the Ph[1] translocation in CGL and is the most frequent rearrangement in adult ALL. Half the patients with the t(4;11)(q21;q23) were children, most of whom were less than one year old.

Karyotype is an important correlate of survival in ALL. Patients with leukaemias showing modal chromosome numbers greater than 50 respond best to treatment, with children in this group frequently being cured. Patients without apparent chromosome abnormalities in their leukaemias also do well, while those with the t(4;11) or t(8;14) respond particularly poorly and have the shortest survival times.

11.5 Solid tumours

11.5.1 General survey

The identification of consistent chromosome aberrations in solid tumours has lagged far behind studies on leukaemias and lymphomas, largely because of the difficulty in obtaining sufficient numbers of dividing cells, and also because there are greatly increased chromosome numbers in many tumours. The use of enzymes for disaggregating tumour tissue, the addition of growth factors or feeder layers to short term cultures, and the use of improved cytogenetic techniques have recently demonstrated consistent chromosome aberrations in solid tumours (Table 11.4). Figure 11.6 shows an example of a karyotype from a cell line derived from solid tumour.

Activated oncogenes of the c-*ras* family have been identified in 10–15 per cent of solid tumours and derived cell lines (see Chapter 10). Altered activity of cellular oncogenes in solid tumours has also been associated with the presence of homogeneously staining regions in chromosomes, and small acentric chromosomes called double minutes (described below in Section 11.6).

11.5.2 Recessively acting genes

Wilms' tumour and retinoblastoma occur in both dominantly inherited and spontaneous (sporadic) forms. Specific deletions involving chromo-

Table 11.4 Consistent chromosome aberrations in solid tumours

Malignancy	Chromosomal aberration
Neuroblastoma	del(1)(p31;p36)
Small cell lung carcinoma	del(3)(p14;p23)
Melanoma	del(6)(q15;q23) and t(6q)
Mixed parotid gland tumour	t(3;8)(p25;q21)
Ewing's sarcoma	t(11;22)(q24;q12)
Meningioma	monosomy 22
Wilms' tumour	del(11)(p13)
Retinoblastoma	del(13)(q14)

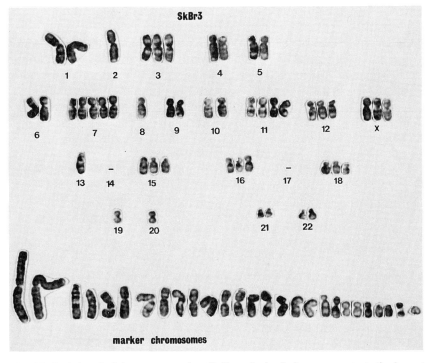

SkBr3

marker chromosomes

Fig. 11.6 G-banded karyotype of cell line derived from a metastatic breast carcinoma. Note the large number of marker (rearranged) chromosomes.

some bands 11p13 and 13q12, respectively, have been observed in a small proportion of both the inherited and the sporadic forms of these diseases. Genetic events (often submicroscopic) which result in hemi– or homozygosity (defined below) of genes within these bands on the homologous chromosomes have now been demonstrated in Wilms' tumours and retinoblastomas, implying the involvement of recessively acting genes in the genesis of these tumours. Although the identity of these genes is not known, it is postulated that if one of these chromosomes (which may be inherited) carries an inactivated or deleted allele, a second mutational event at the homologous allele that renders the first allele hemi– or homozygous, causes malignant transformation.

The methods used in these studies utilize DNA probes from chromosomes 11 or 13 which detect naturally occurring polymorphisms in the positions of sites cut with various restriction enzymes (restriction fragment length polymorphisms). In normal cells a number of restriction enzyme sites on homologous chromosomes will differ. The observation made in both Wilms' tumour and retinoblastoma is that where normal tissue is heterozygous, the tumour tissue is homozygous in about 55 per cent of patients. Mechanisms which can be detected using these techniques are (i) loss of a whole chromosome so that only one homologue remains (hemizygosity), (ii) loss of one chromosome and duplication of the other (homozygosity), (iii) mitotic recombination (crossing over between homologous chromosomes during mitosis of somatic cells), and (iv) translocations resulting in inactivation or deletion of part of the chromosome. These mechanisms are shown schematically in Figure 11.7, together with different mechanisms which may occur in the other 45 per cent of patients with Wilms' tumour and retinoblastoma.

These findings emphasize the use that can be made of sites of consistent chromosome rearrangements, even though they may not be detected in every tumour of a particular category. It remains to be

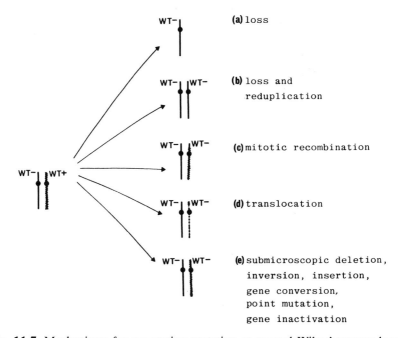

Fig. 11.7 Mechanisms for generating mutation at normal Wilms' tumour locus (WT+) in a cell already containing one inactive or deleted (WT−) allele. (a) Loss of one chromosome resulting in hemizygosity. (b) Loss of one chromosome and duplication of the other resulting in homozygosity. (c) Mitotic recombination (crossing over) between homologous chromosomes during mitosis of somatic cells, resulting in homozygosity at the WT locus. (d) Chromosome translocation resulting in inactivation or deletion of the WT locus. (e) Submicroscopic events leading to inactivation of the WT locus. (After Cavanee *et al.*, 1983. *Nature* 305, 779–84.)

established how widespread such somatic mutational events are in other types of tumours.

11.6 Gene amplification

Gene amplification was observed in Chinese hamster and mouse cell lines which became resistant after treatment with high levels of folic acid antagonists such as methotrexate. These cell lines produced elevated amounts of the enzyme dihydrofolate reductase (DHFR), due to a large increase in the number of DHFR genes (see Chapter 17). The amplified DHFR genes were found to be present either within homogeneously staining regions (HSRs) on single chromosomes, or alternatively within small acentric (centromere lacking) chromosomes called double minutes (DMs). HSRs and DMs are now known to be common features of human solid tumours, but they are only rarely seen in leukaemias or lymphomas. Because they are never seen within the same cell (although tumour cell lines may have both HSR- and DM-containing cells), HSRs and DMs are believed to represent alternate states of gene amplification.

An increase in copy number of cellular oncogenes has also been demonstrated in tumours, often in association with HSRs or DMs (Fig. 11.8). For example, the oncogene c-*myc* is amplified 16–32 fold in the acute promyelocytic leukaemia cell line HL60, and shown to be carried on DMs in this line. A related gene, called N-*myc*, has been shown to be amplified up to 900 times in human neuroblastoma cell lines carrying HSRs or DMs. N-*myc* normally maps to chromosome 2, but in three different neuroblastoma cell lines, amplified N-*myc* sequences are located on HSRs on chromosomes 4, 9, and 13. Thus, the chromosomal site of amplification is variable, suggesting that DMs carrying amplified sequences integrate into different sites in the genome to form HSRs.

11.7 Conclusions

The results presented above demonstrate that non-random chromosome defects are closely associated with a variety of human malignancies. Similar associations have also been identified in animal tumours. The defects consist of gains and losses of part or all of certain chromosomes, and of structural abnormalities, most often translocations. These non-random chromosome defects are believed to confer a proliferative advantage to cells carrying them, and to be involved in pathogenesis of tumours. Results from molecular analyses of these chromosome defects are now starting to accumulate. The findings of elevated expression and the production of abnormal transcripts of particular oncogenes have to be evaluated in relation to tumorigenicity, in the first instance by

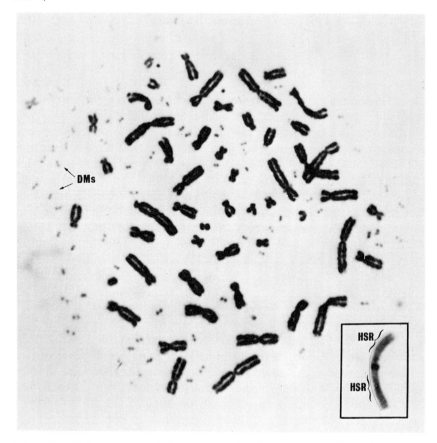

Fig. 11.8 Metaphase spread from neuroendocrine tumour cell line with multiple double minutes. Inset shows chromosome with homogeneously staining region.

identifying the normal products and functions of these genes. In the cases where reduction to hemi– or homozygosity has been observed in tumours, the recessively acting genes themselves have still to be identified.

Malignant transformation is a multistage process involving genetic alterations at several sites in the genome. While consistent chromosome aberrations provide clear indications of the locations of some of these alterations, other alterations such as the activation of cellular oncogenes by point mutation are not visible microscopically. Sequential karyotypic evolution has often been observed in experimental tumours and in human tumours where it has been possible to do serial sampling. These secondary changes, which often appear more random than the primary changes, may affect the behaviour of cells carrying them and thus be selected for by leading the cells towards increased independence from host control. In tumours which have multiple aberrations, as is often the case in the solid tumours, it is difficult to distinguish the primary and secondary changes. It is therefore important to develop techniques for karyotyping 'premalignant' lesions. For example, the hereditary disease familial polyposis coli manifests initially as multiple polyps in the colon, some of which inevitably develop into carcinoma of the colon (see Chapters 5, and 7). By analysing these benign polyps for chromosome aberrations and for activated oncogenes, it might be possible to identify genes directly involved in the genesis of colon carcinoma. Very few studies of this sort have been done so far, mainly because of difficulties in obtaining sufficient numbers of dividing cells from these benign tumours. Since carcinomas represent about 80 per cent of all human tumours, it is clear that studies should be focussed in this area to complement the extensive progress made on leukaemias and lymphomas.

The recent findings must now be used in a constructive way to decide on future avenues of research. For example, restriction fragment length polymorphisms should be used to investigate chromosome regions other than bands 11p13 and 13q12 for evidence of homozygosity. Obvious candidates for such studies are monosomy 22 in meningioma, deletions of chromosome 20 in polycythaemia vera, and the deletions of chromosomes 5 and 7 in secondary AML.

The actual mechanisms for generating consistent chromosome rearrangements are unknown. Random chromosome breakage and rejoining may occur continuously at a low frequency, with only those conferring a proliferative advantage being ultimately observed. Alternatively, certain chromosome regions may be particularly vulnerable to breakage and rearrangement. There is some evidence that spontaneous chromosome rearrangements observed in peripheral blood lymphocytes increase in frequency as a person ages, and could contribute to the age-related incidence of cancer.

Very little is known about the processes involved in the delicate balance between cell proliferation and differentiation. If we are to understand how these processes can be subverted to release cells from their normal growth controls, we need to complement our understanding of the genetic changes in tumours with studies in this area. These new approaches to understanding malignant transformation hopefully will enable major advances towards the prevention and treatment of cancer.

Further reading

Mitelman, F., and Levan, G. (1981). Clustering of aberrations to specific chromosomes in human neoplasms. IV. A survey of 1871 cases. *Hereditas* **95**, 79–139.

Rowley, J. D. (ed.) (1984). Consistent chromosomal aberrations and oncogenes in human tumours. *Cancer surveys* **3**, 360–570.

Sandberg, A. A. (1980). *The chromosomes in human cancer and leukaemia.* Elsevier, North Holland, New York.

The Third International Workshop on Chromosomes in Leukemia, 1980 (1981). *Cancer Genetics and Cytogenetics* **4**, 95–142.

For acute lymphoblastic leukaemia.

The Fourth International Workshop on Chromosomes in Leukemia, 1982 (1984). *Cancer Genetics and Cytogenetics* **11**, 251–360.

Yunis, J. J. (1983). The chromosomal basis of human neoplasia. *Science* **221**, 227–36.

For recent work on oncogenes and on Wilms' tumour and retinoblastoma, see the journals *Nature* and *Science* from 1983 onwards.

12

The role of growth factors in cancer

M. D. WATERFIELD

An understanding of the mechanisms responsible for the control of normal proliferation and differentiation of the various cell types which make up the human body will undoubtedly allow a greater insight into the abnormal growth of malignant cells. Particular attention is now focused on the role of polypeptide growth factors as signal molecules which may play a central role in both normal and abnormal growth control.

The characterization of polypeptide growth factors has resulted in part from the analysis of components of nutrient media necessary to support optimum growth of cells in tissue culture. Several polypeptide growth factors have been isolated by the use of fractionated serum and tissue extracts in assays which measure proliferation or DNA synthesis of test cells. In this Chapter, details of the structure and function of these factors will be described.

12.1 Structural and functional diversity of growth factors

The polypeptide growth factors are a class of molecules which can act as mitogens for target cells *in vivo* or *in vitro*, either alone or synergistically with other factors as a result of primary interaction with specific cell surface receptors. The expression of these receptors governs, at least in part, the cellular specificity of different growth factors. It is clear that particular cells may express several distinct growth factor receptors; therefore, responses are governed by the levels of factor(s) to which a cell is exposed and by interactions between the signal pathways generated by the receptor(s) following ligand binding. The study of such interactions provides clues to the synergistic effects of mixtures of growth factors and other molecules on the proliferation of target cells.

The types of cells that synthesize specific growth factors are often ill defined and, in some cases, it seems that almost every cell tested may be able to synthesize particular factors. This observation and others suggest that factor synthesis is not confined within particular endocrine organs, as is the case with the signal molecules grouped together as hormones (see Chapters 13 and 14), and has led to the hypothesis that three different levels or systems of signalling may exist.

The first system has been termed endocrine, in which synthesis takes place in a specific tissue or organ; the hormone is stored and secreted under the control of specific releasing factors which are in turn controlled by the nervous system. Delivery of hormones is carried out by the circulation. The second system is called paracrine, and here a cell may produce a signal molecule that can interact with nearby cells expressing appropriate receptors. In this case the cell synthesizing the factor would not express receptors capable of interpreting a signal from the factor. In the third type of system, autocrine, the cell could be expected to respond to signal molecules which it generates itself if the appropriate post receptor mechanisms are activated. Clearly the use of these three systems by a diverse series of hormones and factors could generate a formidable array of regulatory controls.

The amino acid sequences of a number of structurally distinct factors have been characterized, and the advent of recombinant DNA technology has provided a new tool for the characterization and production of factors which have previously been recognized only by a biological assay. Early work on the isolation of growth factors relied on biological sources where expression was abnormally high and where there was a suitable assay technique. The pioneering work of Cohen on epidermal growth factor (EGF) is a particularly good example. A factor which influenced the growth of nerves had been isolated from the salivary gland of the snake, and Cohen sought a similar activity in the mouse salivary gland. Extracts injected into newborn mice caused their eyes to open earlier and their incisor teeth to grow faster—apparent effects on tissues of epidermal origin. The factor was purified and is now called epidermal growth factor (EGF). Ligand binding and DNA synthesis assays on cells *in vitro* now provide more convenient methods of measuring EGF levels. The salivary glands of male mice which respond to male sex hormones produce and store large amounts of EGF, perhaps because a whole family of testosterone responsive genes are unusually active. The discovery of a site of synthesis and storage was critical in the isolation of EGF.

Other factors, such as platelet derived growth factor (PDGF), a potent mitogen for cells of glial and connective tissue origin, were discovered because serum, but not plasma, supported optimum growth of these cells. (Plasma is the fluid component of blood; blood clotting, involving the platelets, removes some proteins from the plasma which is converted into serum.) In this case it was clear that the serum contained products released by platelets and thus the platelet was the obvious source for the purification of a serum growth factor.

Improved analytical methods have made it possible to analyse the amino acid sequence of minute amounts of proteins involving either complete sequence analysis of the protein or generating oligonucleotide probes predicted from partial protein sequence. Such probes have been used to isolate cDNA clones of the genes encoding the factors. One can also isolate cDNA clones by selection of biologically active mRNA species assayed by translation following microinjection into frog oocytes. The clones can then be used to synthesize the growth factor in bacteria, yeast or mammalian cells, providing large amounts of the factor for further studies. These techniques have also been used to analyse the genes which encode the factors, to discover related but previously unknown factors, and to characterize possible defects which can result in disease.

The structure and function of the receptors for some factors have been elucidated at the molecular level. Detailed primary structures of the cell surface receptors for EGF, IL2 (interleukin 2) and insulin are now known (see on) and provide models for understanding the processes of transmembrane signal transduction.

It is necessary to link the structural data with biological studies in whole animals, organ culture or tissue culture. Biological and molecular genetic studies of growth factors have assumed a particular relevance in studies of the abnormal proliferative properties of tumours and tumour derived cell lines because close links have been made with the effects on cells induced by certain oncogenes and tumour promoters (see also Chapters 7 and 10).

Several growth factors can be grouped into families based on shared structural or functional features. Other features have yet to be classified. The spectrum of tissue specificity and size of these polypeptides is presented in Table 12.1.

12.1.1 *Haemopoietic cell growth factors*

The variation in target cell specificity of growth factors is well illustrated by the group of factors which act on cells of haemopoietic origin (see Chapter 3). The protein erythropoietin, originally isolated from enormous quantities of human urine, has now been sequenced and the gene isolated. Erythropoietin is involved in the regulation of the differentiation and proliferation of normal red cells before haemoglobin synthesis begins (the BFU-E, see Chapter 3).

Four major types of colony stimulating factors (CSFs) have been well characterized as a result of pioneering work by Metcalf who studied them in mice (Table 12.1). Thus, M-CSF seems specific for the macrophage lineage, G-CSF for granulocytes, GM-CSF for macrophage and granulocyte lineages, and multi-CSF for neutrophil, eosinophil, megakaryocyte, erythroid, and mast cell lineages. The major CSFs have now been analysed both at the protein and nucleotide levels.

A major result of the studies with CSFs has been the development of the concept that different cell lineages are produced from a multipotential stem cell precursor pool through the regulation of differentiation by these, and perhaps other, factors. CSF production occurs in several different tissues such as thymus, kidney, spleen, and uterus, and a variety of mitogen treated cells. This suggests that target cell specificity is generated by receptor expression, or by turning on post-receptor functions. Alternatively, more subtle mechanisms may operate *in vivo* to control production of factors which could be synthesized by a wide variety of cells.

Particular interest has centred on the role of CSFs in various leukaemias since it may be possible to treat patients with appropriate factors to promote normal differentiation or inhibit proliferation of leukaemic cells; for example, G-CSF has a suppressive effect on myeloid leukaemia in mice. It is too early to draw conclusion about the potential of these factors *in vivo*, but the availability of large amounts of protein will make a new generation of studies possible.

The interleukins are factors that modulate lymphocytes, and are likely to be a subset of the lymphokines which mediate interactions in the immune system (see Chapter 15). One of the first events in T cell activation is probably presentation of antigen by the macrophage to a T cell with a specific receptor (Fig. 12.1). Structural details of the T cell receptor for antigen have recently been elucidated, as have the gene rearrangements associated with generation of receptor binding diversity. The interaction of antigen, macrophage and T cell results in release of interleukin 1 (IL1) which induces expression of the receptor for interleukin 2 (IL2) and eventually cells producing IL2 appear. In this system it is unclear whether paracrine of autocrine factor synthesis of IL2 occurs.

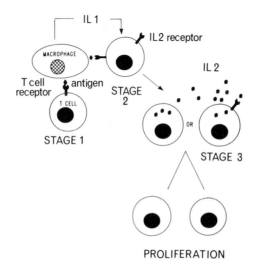

Fig. 12.1 The role of antigen, macrophage, and growth factors in the proliferative response of T cells to antigen.

This description of the factors induced by antigen stimulation is a broad summary of what is undoubtedly a much more complex series of closely regulated steps. At present, our understanding of factors which are involved in stimulating proliferation of B cells is far less clear; details of the role of the various factors and receptors are likely to be elucidated very soon.

12.1.2 *Nervous system growth factors*

The isolation of a factor with target cell specificity for cells of the nervous system was one of the pioneering events in the whole growth factor field. Levi-Montalcini, Hamburger, and Cohen in 1960 were

Table 12.1 Growth factors

Factor	Tissue specificity	Source	Size[1]
Haemopoietic			
Erythropoietin	Regulation of erythropoiesis	Urine	166 aa
IL1 (interleukin 1)	Stimulation of TCGF production	Conditioned media	156 aa
IL2 (T cell growth factor, TCGF)	Activated T cells	Conditioned media	153 aa
M-CSF	Macrophages	Conditioned media	two 14 000 M_r chains
G-CSF	Granulocytes	Conditioned media	23 000 M_r
GM-CSF	Granulocytes and macrophages	Conditioned media	118 aa
Multi-CSF (interleukin 3, IL3)	Neutrophils, eosinophils, megakaryocytes, erythroid cells, and mast cells	All tissues surveyed	166 aa
Nerve and brain			
Glial growth factor (GGF)	Astrocytes and Schwann cells	Pituitary gland	31 000 M_r
Nerve growth factor (NGF)	Neurites in sensory and sympathetic ganglia	Mouse submaxillary gland	116 aa
'Mostly mesenchymal'			
Epidermal growth factor (EGF)	Wide variety of cells from all three germ layers (not lymphoid or haemopoietic)	Mouse submaxillary gland	53 aa
Transforming growth factor type I (TGFα)		Conditioned media	48 aa
Vaccinia virus growth factor (VVGF)		Virus infected cells	77 aa
Transforming growth factor type II (TGFβ)	Action modulated by TGFα; similar to growth inhibitor of Holley	Normal kidney, platelets	two identical 14 000 M_r chains

Factor	Action	Source	Size
Insulin like growth factor I (IGF-I) and Somatomedin C	Growth hormone dependent plasma factors with sulphation activity in cartilage; insulin like effects on non-skeletal muscle; synergistic with PDGF in growth effects	Serum	70 aa
Insulin like growth factor II (IGF-II) also WSA and Somatomedin A		Serum	73 aa
Platelet derived growth factor (PDGF)	Mesenchymal and glial cells	Platelets	two homologous chains 109 and 104 aa
Fibroblast growth factor I, II, III	Adult endothelial cells and other mesenchymal derived cells, but not endodermal or ectodermal cells	Pituitary gland and brain?	16 000 M_r

[1] aa = amino acids; M_r = apparent molecular weight.

responsible for the assay and purification of nerve growth factor (NGF) from snake venom and the mouse submaxillary gland. Once again the male mouse provided a convenient source for purification. It has been suggested that NGF acts as a neurotrophic factor in the mammalian nervous system; this role for NGF remains controversial. No specific disease state has been linked to defects in NGF function; however, antisera to NGF produce a neuropathy when injected into the mouse. NGF from submaxillary glands is synthesized and exported as a pentamer of three distinct polypeptides (α_2, β, γ_2) which associate non-covalently with two atoms of zinc. The structures of the precursors of the α, β and γ subunits have been established. Interestingly, the β subunit of NGF shares structural features with insulin, relaxin, and the insulin like growth factors (see on).

Other mitogenic factors from the nervous system include fibroblast growth factors (FGFs), neuropeptides, astrocyte growth factors, and growth factors from Schwann cells. The characterization of the FGFs has been beset with problems because of difficulties in purification. The pituitary gland and brain contain a basic FGF, whereas the brain and other tissues contain acidic FGFs. These factors are potent mitogens for cells of mesodermal origin. Recent advances in the ability to grow *in vitro* and classify particular cell types from the nervous system have made it possible to characterize a glial growth factor (GGF) which may have a role in amphibian limb regeneration. GGF acts on Schwann cells and fibroblasts, and is produced in the pituitary (and perhaps other places).

Many neuropeptides act as mitogens for fibroblasts in combinations with other growth factors. The usual test cell employed is the Swiss 3T3 fibroblast. The neurohypophyseal peptides, vasopressin (nine amino acids) and bombesin (14 amino acids), have been studied in detail using these cells. Their role in development, regeneration, or proliferative disorders of the brain or peripheral nervous system is unclear. However, certain lung tumours are potent producers of various peptides including bombesin and it is possible that they have a functional autocrine role in stimulation of abnormal proliferation in these diseases.

12.1.3 *Epidermal and transforming growth factors*

Studies on EGF have provided a general model for most growth factors. EGF binds to a specific cell surface receptor present on a variety of cells; using binding assays, the binding characteristics and numbers of receptors on different cells can be measured (Fig. 12.2). The A431 cell line, derived from a human vulval carcinoma, has approximately 100 times more receptors than most 'normal' fibroblasts and other cells, and consequently is useful in EGF receptor studies and provides information on the mechanism of signal transduction. The overexpression of

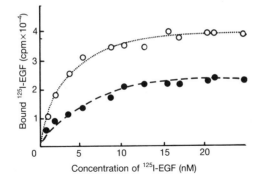

Fig. 12.2 The assay of epidermal growth factor and its receptor using A431 cell membranes or placental syncytiotrophoblastic membrane vesicles. Increasing concentrations of ^{125}I-EGF bound to A431 cell (O) or placental vesicles (●) was measured with a radioimmunoassay where bound ligand was separated from free ligand with a monoclonal antibody against the EGF receptor. The data obtained can be used to measure the number of receptors on A431 cells and on placenta.

receptors on the A431 cell is probably related to amplification of the receptor gene (see on).

Many transformed and tumour derived cell lines produce factors called transforming growth factors (TGFs) which change the phenotypic properties of normal fibroblasts such that they grow in soft agar media (a property typical of transformed cells and correlating well with the ability of these cells to form tumours in nude mice). TGF$^{\alpha}$ has now been purified from rat and human sources and their amino acid sequences determined. A search of protein and nucleic acid sequence computer data showed that EGF and TGF$^{\alpha}$ were related, and that vaccinia virus encoded an EGF related peptide (called VVGF).

The biosynthetic precursors of these three members of the EGF family, predicted from nucleic acid sequences, have several interesting features (Fig. 12.3). The putative precursors have amino terminal sequences which could function as 'signal peptides' for directing the polypeptides into intracellular membranes. A hydrophobic sequence near the carboxyl terminus could serve to lock the precursors into the plasma membrane, with their amino terminal regions containing the active peptide growth factor displayed on the exterior of the cell. It is not yet known if this in fact happens. However, the active growth factors are cleaved from larger precursors by proteolytic cleavage. In the case of the putative EGF precursor, which is 1100 amino acids long, a number of peptides, similar in size and structure to EGF, may be processed into other growth factors.

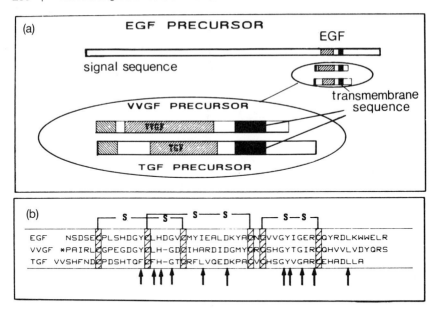

Fig. 12.3 The structure of EGF and the related factors, TGF and VVGF. (a) The predicted precursors of EGF, VVGF, and TGF are represented as linear polypeptides with the position of particular amino acid residues indicated. The amino terminal signal sequence (▨▨▨) used for membrane insertion is shown, together with the location of the processed active factors as crosshatched zones within the precursor molecules. The shaded zone ▨▨ represents the predicted transmembrane sequences. (b) The amino acid sequence of the growth factors are aligned for homology. Disulphide bonds for EGF are indicated. The arrows indicate conserved amino acids.

The amino acid sequences of the active processed growth factors (Fig. 12.3) have conserved cysteine residues, linked in disulphide bonds in mouse EGF. Several other residues are conserved and presumably these are essential for the shared properties and presumed three dimensional conformation of this group of factors. EGF, TGF$^\alpha$, and VVGF all bind to the A431 cell EGF receptor in a manner suggesting that there is a single binding site on the receptor for which these factors compete, although it is possible that a distinct TGF$^\alpha$ receptor exists.

It is not yet clear if TGF$^\alpha$ and EGF have distinct biological functions. Both factors induce early eye opening in mice and both are mitogenic for a range of test cells. VVGF might be used to subvert cellular functions of the EGF or TGF$^\alpha$ receptor, thus providing vaccinia with increased biological capabilities. The production of TGF$^\alpha$ seems to be associated with abnormal proliferation since only transformed or tumour derived cell lines are known to produce this factor.

12.1.4 *Transforming growth factor* β

The characterization of growth factor activities found in the medium of transformed cells resulted in the isolation of TGF$^\beta$, a distinct polypeptide which acted as a mitogen only in the presence of added EGF. TGF$^\beta$ (or TGF type II) has subsequently been purified from normal tissues such as kidney and platelets. Partial amino acid sequence analysis and the use of molecular cloning techniques show that the active polypeptide is a disulphide bonded homodimer.

TGF$^\beta$ induces more diverse cellular responses than does TGF$^\alpha$. TGF$^\beta$ has its own receptor distinct from EGF (and TGF$^\alpha$), and appears to be closely related, if not identical, to a growth inhibitor purified from the medium of African green monkey kidney cells. The observation that a single polypeptide may act as a growth stimulator and a growth inhibitor probably depends on the particular assay systems. TGF$^\beta$ may also alter the time course of the mitogenic response of cells to other growth factors such as EGF. TGF$^\beta$ is produced by almost all cell lines (normal or transformed) that have been examined.

12.1.5 *Insulin and the insulin like growth factors*

The hormones insulin and relaxin form part of a family of structurally related polypeptides which includes NGF and two potent growth factors known variously as somatomedins, non-suppressible insulin like activities or insulin like growth factors (IGF-I and IGF-II). The common structural features of these factors are summarized in Figure 12.4. The known three dimensional structure of insulin provides a model for predicting the structures of the other molecules which have shared regions of homologous amino acids. Insulin and relaxin are synthesized as precursors that are processed to remove the C peptide sequences, whereas this region is retained in the IGFs and NGF. This family of molecules shows how a basic structure can be modified in evolution to generate factors with distinct biological functions.

The addition of insulin to culture medium has long been used to support optimal cell growth. It acts, at least in part, through its low affinity binding to the IGF-I receptor thus mimicking, at high concentrations, the effects of IGF-I. The factor known as 'multiplication stimulating activity' (MSA) is IGF-I. The complete structures of IGF-I and IGF-II precursors have been established, and the factors can now be produced in large amounts. Many cells possess distinct receptors for insulin, IGF-I and IGF-II. IGF-I may be necessary for some (e.g. BALB/c 3T3), but not all (Swiss 3T3), cells to complete the cell cycle in response to a mitogen such as platelet derived growth factor. It is possible that many cells in culture may produce IGFs and this could explain

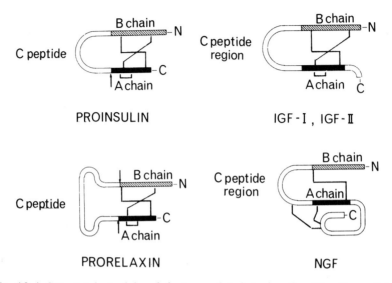

Fig. 12.4 Structural models of factors related to insulin. The C peptide is removed during precursor processing in the case of insulin and relaxin. Disulphide bonds are shown as interconnecting lines.

differences in action of both PDGF, other mitogens, and IGFs on cultured cells.

12.1.6 *Platelet derived growth factor*

The search for the factor present in serum but not plasma responsible for supporting optimal growth of fibroblasts or glial cells in culture resulted in the purification from platelets of platelet derived growth factor (PDGF). PDGF is stored within the α granules of platelets which are released during the clotting process at wound sites (or, of course, in production of serum from blood). PDGF is thought to be involved as a chemoattractant in tissue repair processes which involve migration of cells such as macrophages, smooth muscle cells, and neutrophils to the wound site, and also as a mitogen probably in a synergistic mode with TGF$^\alpha$s to promote the repair of the damaged connective tissue.

PDGF purified from outdated human platelets is a highly basic protein of molecular weight (mol. wt.) 28–32 000 daltons, which can be separated into two components, PDGF-I (mol. wt. 28–30 000) and PDGF-II (mol. wt. 30–32 000). The structural basis for the difference between these two species is unclear. Human PDGF contains two types of polypeptides named A and B held together by disulphide bonds (Fig. 12.5). The analysis of the structure of PDGF was helped considerably by the finding that the *sis* oncogene of simian sarcoma virus (SSV) encoded a polypeptide closely related to the B chain of PDGF. The B chain is 109 amino acids long whereas the A chain (only partially sequenced) is distinct but partially homologous to the B chain and is approximately the same length. It is still unclear whether active human PDGF is a hetero-dimer of A and B chains, a mixture of homodimers, or simply a homodimer of B chains. The latter hypothesis is supported by three facts: (i) porcine PDGF, purified from fresh platelets, has a single amino terminal sequence homologous to the human B chain sequence, (ii) the active transforming protein produced by SSV transformed cells also seems to be a homodimer of B chains, and (iii) expression of the cloned *sis* viral oncogene in yeast cells leads to synthesis of an active PDGF like growth factor.

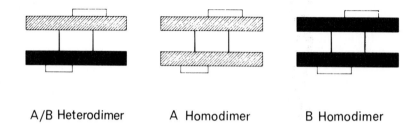

A/B Heterodimer   A Homodimer   B Homodimer

Fig. 12.5 Three possible dimeric species of PDGF composed of A (cross-hatched) or B (solid) chains.

PDGF binds to a specific cell surface receptor on cells of mesenchymal and glial origin. A high affinity receptor is not detectable in cells of epithelial origin. PDGF is the sole factor required to stimulate proliferation of Swiss 3T3 cells, and a particular glial cell line used to monitor PDGF purification. It is, however controversial as to whether PDGF alone can act as a mitogen for other mesenchymal and glial cell lines, or for cells *in vivo*. In the case of BALB/c 3T3 cells it seems that PDGF induces what has been termed the state of 'competence' and addition of IGF-I is required for the cells to complete a proliferative cycle. No doubt, cells *in vivo* are exposed to an even more complex array of factors which can act synergistically.

12.1.7 *Poorly characterized growth factors*

A number of other polypeptide growth factors could prove to be distinct factors. These include factors which act on, or are produced by, cartilage, endothelial cells, various T cells, B cells, macrophages, and a variety of neural cells.

12.2 Receptors and signal transduction

The initial interaction between a growth factor and a target cell is mediated by a high affinity receptor present on the surface of the cell. Receptors can be detected and quantified using radiolabelled ligand as described previously for EGF (Fig. 12.2). The numbers of receptors can vary from several hundred to as many as several million on certain tumour derived cell lines. Cells generally express receptors for several different growth factors and the numbers of these receptors can be independently modulated by ligand binding.

Following the interaction of ligand with receptor, a process called 'down regulation' can occur which involves loss of cell surface receptors through internalization via coated pits into the internal vesicle system of the cell. Receptor and ligand can be proteolysed inside the cell and the receptor in some cases recycled following dissociation of ligand at the acid pH of the internal vesicles. Clear experimental evidence for recycling of growth factor receptors is lacking but, for the low density lipoprotein (LDL) and transferrin receptors involved in transport functions, the receptor reappears at the cell surface after releasing its ligand into an intracellular compartment.

12.2.1 *The structure of receptors*

The molecular 'anatomy' of the receptors for the growth factors EGF, IL2, and insulin have been established. Structures have also been determined for several other cell surface receptors involved in recognition functions in the immune system (e.g. membrane bound immunoglobulin, T cell receptor, Class I and II histocompatibility antigens) or transport functions (e.g. LDL, asialoglycoprotein, transferrin, polymeric immunoglobulin A and M receptors). The range of structures predicted from evidence based on primary sequence data and immunological and biochemical studies is shown in Figure 12.6.

The receptors for EGF and insulin differ from the other predicted structures of membrane recognition molecules in that they have large cytoplasmic domains in addition to the external ligand binding domain. Thus, it is expected that the mechanisms of signal transduction for the EGF and insulin receptors are distinct from those used by the IL2 receptor, the transport receptors, and the recognition molecules of the immune system mentioned above.

12.2.2 *The structure and function of the EGF and insulin receptors*

The primary amino acid sequences of the EGF and insulin receptors predict an external ligand binding domain separated from a cytoplasmic domain by a single stretch of hydrophobic residues which, in an α helical conformation, could span the lipid bilayer of the cell. The external domain of the receptors is glycosylated at several distinct asparagine residues. The cytoplasmic domains of both receptors are homologous to the protein kinase domains of the catalytic subunit of cyclic AMP and GMP dependent protein kinases and to the *src* family of transforming proteins (see Chapter 10, and below). The receptors for EGF, PDGF, insulin, and IGF-I (but not IGF-II) all possess a ligand stimulated tyrosine kinase activity which autophosphorylates the protein and also phosphorylates a number of cytoplasmic proteins. The location of a major *in vivo* autophosphorylation site in the EGF receptor occurs in a cytoplasmic domain not found in the insulin receptor (Fig. 12.6). The tyrosine

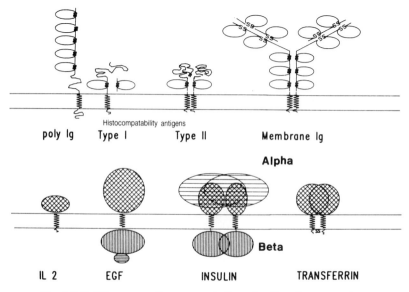

Fig. 12.6 Diagrammatic representation of cell surface receptors.

kinase activity is as yet the only known intrinsic function of the receptors. It is not clear how the signals generated by the ligands are transduced across the membrane.

Receptors for different growth factors can be 'transmodulated', i.e. they communicate. For example, PDGF or phorbol esters induce a reduction in EGF binding affinity for the EGF receptor. Protein kinase C, the phorbol ester receptor, will phosphorylate the EGF receptor on a threonine residue. The introduction of an acidic phosphate group could alter the receptor conformation. The consequence of the phosphorylation, whatever the mechanism, is a change in binding affinity for EGF.

12.2.3 *The structure of other growth factor receptors*

The IGF-I receptor, like the insulin receptor, is known to be a homo-dimer made up of two α chains (mol. wt. 95 000) and two β chains (mol. wt. 105 000). The IGF-II receptor is, however, a single chain of mol. wt. 250 000 and it is possible that this will be a novel structure unrelated to the insulin and IGF-I receptors. The PDGF receptor is known at present only as a 185 000 mol. wt. protein which has a ligand stimulated tyrosine specific protein kinase.

12.2.4 *Growth factor signal transduction*

The interaction of a growth factor such as EGF or PDGF with its receptor produces a complex cascade of morphological, physiological, and biochemical events which eventually, after a lag of eight or more hours, can result in stimulation of DNA synthesis and cell division in target cells. As yet one cannot explain how the signal cascade leads to the alterations in gene expression which are clearly necessary for stimulation of cell proliferation. The mechanisms of signal transduction have been studied using cells in culture where the spectrum of responses depends on the cell type, the effects of other compounds in the medium which can act independently or synergistically, and on the ability to study cells which behave in a synchronized fashion with respect to the cell cycle. Cells employed for these studies are usually synchronized by serum deprivation prior to challenge with mitogen in a defined medium. The responses of fibroblasts to various growth factors will be discussed as a guide to further reading about signal transduction.

Following the interaction of the growth factors EGF, PDGF, IGF-I, and insulin with their receptors, there is rapid autophosphorylation on tyrosine residues of the receptor proteins themselves. A number of cellular proteins are also phosphorylated on tyrosine residues but the functional significance of this tyrosine modification, as yet, remains elusive. With PDGF, a rapid stimulation of phospholipase activity occurs, generating arachidonate (through the action of phospholipase A2) from diacylglycerol, and inositol triphosphate (IP3) (through phospholipase c activity). Further metabolism of arachidonate can lead to synthesis of various leucotrienes and prostaglandins, several of which have potent biochemical effects. These phospholipase dependent events are not detected with EGF. The generation of IP3 is thought to mobilize calcium ions from internal pools which, as a consequence, allows the modulation of many calcium dependent processes. Rapid sodium/hydrogen exchange also occurs with compensating movements of potassium ions; this could result in alkalinization of the cell by altering the activity of an, as yet, unidentified $Na+/H+$ pump. Phosphorylation of the pump by the enzyme protein kinase C may cause the activation. Protein kinase C is activated by diacylglycerol, which is produced by phospholipase c during the generation of IP3. It is also activated by the phorbol ester promoters (e.g. TPA), thus providing a. link to explain the known effects of TPA on cell proliferation. The impact of protein kinase C activation may be multifunctional. One effect is a decrease in affinity of EGF for its receptor, induced by both PDGF and TPA, and is likely to be caused by protein kinase C phosphorylation of the receptor as mentioned earlier. These effects can now be produced *in vitro* with purified kinase and EGF receptor. Protein kinase C probably mediates many other regulatory processes. The effects of some of these may be far-reaching. For example, the protein kinase C mediated phosphorylation of ribosomal protein S6 may cause a selective alteration in protein synthesis.

It is still controversial whether internalization plays an important signalling role. In the case of EGF, some experiments suggest that a sub-population of receptors remains on the surface. It is important to consider that cells must be exposed to the growth factor for several hours, suggesting that a persistent signal is needed to induce proliferation.

The search for a mechanism which could explain the effects of growth factors on gene expression has been stimulated by the exciting observation that transient transcription of the c-*fos* protooncogene, which encodes a nuclear protein (see on), and of the actin gene occurs within minutes after PDGF or TPA (but not EGF) treatment of cells. Other mRNA species may be rapidly modulated by growth factors.

It is remarkable that we know so little about mechanisms of signal transduction. The advent of new protein purification techniques, using monoclonal antibodies and high pressure liquid chromatography together with recombinant DNA techniques, provides methods for expression of normal and mutant proteins and allow site specific muta-genesis in particular kinds of cells where the correlation of structure and function can be pursued.

12.3 Subversion of growth control by oncogenes

The retroviruses and their viral oncogenes have already been introduced in Chapters 9 and 10. The nucleotide sequences of each oncogene have been determined and hence we know the amino acid sequence of the putative transforming proteins which these oncogenes encode. Antisera to transforming proteins allow detection of these products in virally trans-formed cells, tumours from experimental animals or, in some cases, in human tumours, tumour cell derived lines and normal cells. Because the viral oncogenes are usually altered or aberrantly expressed counterparts of normal cellular genes, it is of great interest to determine the function of the normal genes so that their aberrant expression can be related to the causation or progression of cancer. In some cases, discrete differences in structure of the oncogene and its normal gene (protooncogene) are known, but in most cases the functions remain elusive. For two oncogenes, the function of the normal gene is known and establishes a link with the pathways used by growth factors to regulate normal proliferation.

12.3.1 *The* sis *oncogene encodes PDGF*

The discovery that the *sis* oncogene of SSV encoded a transforming protein closely related in amino acid sequence to PDGF was made through the use of amino acid sequence data banks. The predicted amino acid sequence of the *sis* oncogene was almost identical over a stretch of about 100 amino acids to that of the B chain of PDGF. This result was particularly provocative because it brought together two fields of research—those of oncogenes and growth factors—and suggested that the reduced requirements of certain transformed and tumour derived cell lines for serum and PDGF might be mediated by autocrine production of this factor in these cells.

Further molecular genetic and protein chemistry studies have established that the v-*sis* sequences are derived from the normal gene which encodes PDGF—the c-*sis* gene (Fig. 12.7). The normal c-*sis* gene, located on human chromosome 22, is transcribed in human placentas and in various tumour derived cell lines of connective tissue origin as a

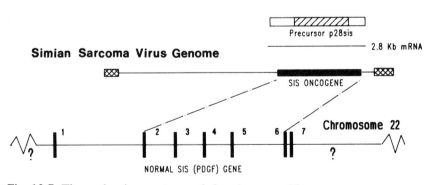

Fig. 12.7 The molecular anatomy of the *sis* genes. The structures are represented as lines which indicate nucleic acid or protein sequences. The solid bars or boxes are coding sequences of the genes. The crosshatched areas are the virus LTRs (long terminal repeats) and the shaded regions are the biologically active peptides.

4.2 kb mRNA. In some tumour cell lines, notably HTLV transformed lymphocytes, an additional transcript of 2.7 kb has been detected. Removal of amino and carboxyl terminal sequences from the polypeptide precursor gives the 109 amino acid B chain of human PDGF.

The v-*sis* sequences have been acquired by SSV from part of exon 2, exons 3,4,5, and part of exon 6. Exon one, however, is important in addition to exons 2–7 for transformation of NIH/3T3 cells. This exon probably encodes a sequence important for correct processing of the precursor polypeptide which is provided by SSV in the oncogene. The coding sequences of v-*sis* and the region of c-*sis* defined so far could only encode the B chain of human PDGF. As mentioned above, it is possible that the A chain sequences found in human PDGF from outdated platelets are artificially linked to the B chain by disulphide interchange. Because v-*sis* sequences expressed in an appropriate construct in yeast cells make active PDGF, it seems likely that SSV transformed cells make an active homodimer.

SSV transformed cells secrete a PDGF like molecule which can act as a mitogen for fibroblasts. The synthesis of a secreted factor by SSV seems to be achieved by the use of the SSV envelope gene signal sequence. The mitogenic activity of the partially purified factor is markedly inhibited by antisera raised against purified human PDGF. SSV transformed cells may secrete other mitogens as well. Antisera to PDGF partially block proliferation of SSV transformed cells, suggesting that an autocrine pathway may be used. The results described above demonstrate that the normal gene can be converted to an oncogene by abnormal expression of a truncated normal protein, and therefore PDGF production at the wrong time or place may result in altered proliferation and transformation.

The normal site of synthesis of PDGF found in platelets is thought to be the megakaryocyte. This cell is the progenitor of platelets; it becomes multinucleate, incapable of further proliferation, and is thought to shatter to form the platelets that circulate in the blood. The platelets themselves do not have the capability for protein synthesis. Important points may be inferred from these observations. For example, it is the platelet rather than a PDGF synthesizing cell which delivers the mitogen PDGF to a site of tissue damage. Furthermore, the megakaryotype 'self destructs' as part of the process of platelet formation, thus ensuring limits on the continued proliferation of the cell which synthesizes the mitogen. A possible reason for this mechanism may be that regulating the PDGF gene in a cell at a wound site may be less controllable than delivering a 'defined dose' in platelets. However, studies show that, when blood vessel damage is mimicked by stripping the lining of a vessel with a catheter, the *sis* gene is turned on in the endothelial cell. These cells lack PDGF receptors and thus PDGF release may serve to stimulate the smooth muscle and other connective tissue cells which surround the damaged vessel. Also, PDGF is produced during the early proliferation of the placenta. These results imply that the *sis* gene can be turned on at the sites of tissue damage and during development. Clearly the role of PDGF in normal growth, development, and tissue repair is not yet fully understood.

Transcriptions of *sis* has been measured in a small number of tumours and tumour cell lines. It seems to be transcribed selectively in tumours of mesenchymal and glial origin. A larger number of tumour cell lines and, most importantly, primary human tumours, need to be examined.

An hypothesis developed from these observations is that the *sis* gene, when turned on for whatever reason (mutation of the *sis* gene control region, expression of a protein which alters *sis* gene transcription, etc.) in a cell capable of responding by proliferation may result in uncontrolled growth through an autocrine mechanism. Since control of proliferation may be exerted at several levels, it is probable that *sis* expression is just one of several subversive steps that result in a tumour.

12.3.2 *The* erbB *oncogene encodes a defective EGF receptor*

The origin of the acquired cellular sequences of the *erbB* oncogene of avian erythroblastosis virus (AEV) was revealed by a computer search of a protein sequence data bank. Using the amino acid sequence of 20 distinct tryptic peptides derived from the human EGF receptor obtained in my laboratory, it was found that seven of those peptides were almost identical to regions of the protein encoded by the v-*erbB* oncogene. Based on the predicted domain structure of the EGF receptor, v-*erbB* would encode a truncated EGF receptor lacking the external EGF binding domain of the receptor (Fig. 12.8). Truncated receptor may possibly deliver a continuous proliferation signal in transformed cells. The v-*erbB* sequences encode only 65 amino acids of this external domain; this finding is substantiated by studies showing that AEV transformed erythroblasts fail to bind EGF.

The v-*erbB* transforming protein has the putative transmembrane domain and most of the cytoplasmic domain of the EGF receptor. This cytoplasmic domain is homologous over a stretch of 250 amino acids to the tyrosine protein kinase domain of the *src* family of oncogenes (see Chapter 10) and to the kinase domain of the insulin receptor.

The ability to express a truncated EGF receptor must contribute in some way to the proliferative disease caused by AEV. Since the only known intrinsic function of the EGF receptor is a tyrosine protein kinase activity, this enzyme activity has been sought in AEV transformed cells. We have recently demonstrated that, using antisera raised against synthetic peptides from the kinase domain of the EGF receptor, the

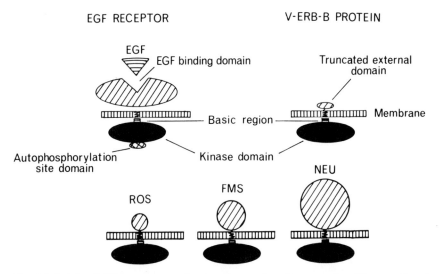

Fig. 12.8 The EGF receptor and related transforming proteins. The predicted structures of the polypeptides are represented as domains on the outside and inside of the lipid membrane. The structures of *ros* and *fms* are based on sequence homologous with the EGF receptor and *neu* is largely hypothetical since only preliminary data are available.

immunoprecipitated v-*erbB* protein phosphorylates exogenous substrates and also phosphorylates a protein of the same molecular weight as v-*erbB* on tyrosine residues. It remains to be seen whether purified v-*erbB* is a constitutively activated kinase, and it must be proved that the activity is not due to a contaminating kinase. As yet, we do not know the function of the tyrosine kinase activity of any of the oncogene proteins or of the EGF receptor. With insulin receptor, tyrosine phosphorylation activates and makes the kinase ligand independent. The consequences of this activation are a mystery.

12.3.3 *Transformation by* erbB *related oncogenes*

The v-*erbB* oncogene is a member of the multigene tyrosine kinase family of oncogenes, and these share regions of amino acid sequences homologous to the catalytic subunits of the cAMP and cGMP protein kinases and, of course, to the cytoplasmic domains of the EGF and insulin receptors. The region of amino acid sequence homology contains particular conserved residues which are thought, by analogy with known three dimensional structures, to form part of the nucleotide binding site. A comparison of the amino acid sequences of these kinases shows a clear division into two sub-families based on particular amino acid substitutions.

The individual transforming proteins are, in many cases, synthesized as fusion proteins retaining portions of the progenitor virus encoded proteins such as the *gag* or envelope proteins (see Chapter 10). In addition, the transforming proteins may have amino and/or carboxyl terminal extensions of the kinase domain which could contribute functional specificity to the protein. The structure of the normal protein encoded by the protooncogene has been established for some but not all of these oncogenes. In all cases, mutation involving truncation and/or addition of novel sequences is found.

It might be anticipated that the genes for other growth factor receptors may have been acquired by other members of this family of oncogenes. The recent determination of the human insulin receptor sequence has failed to demonstrate a clear relationship with any viral oncogene; although the *ros* oncogene (from an avian sarcoma virus) encodes a protein more closely related to the insulin receptor kinase domain than other members of the family, but has probably been acquired from a different gene. Additionally, the *fms* oncogene (from a feline sarcoma virus) appears highly related, if not identical, to the receptor for M-*CSF* discussed earlier. With *fms* and *ros* transforming proteins, it is possible to define a hydrophobic sequence similar in length to that which is thought to cross a lipid bilayer (see Fig. 12.8). Recent studies show that v-*fms* is a carboxyl terminally truncated version of c-*fms*, lacking part of the internal domain which might transduce the ligand signal. c-*ros* may have similar features. The predicted sequences of the other transforming proteins of this family of oncogenes do not reveal a transmembrane protein domain structure.

A new oncogene called *neu* has been found in neuroblastomas from newborn rats after treatment of pregnant rats with a chemical carcinogen. Preliminary evidence suggests that *neu* may encode a defective receptor.

12.3.4 *Altered* EGF *receptor expression in tumours*

The observation that expression of a truncated growth factor receptor encoded by a retroviral oncogene may play a pivotal role in transformation and induction of tumours suggests that similar but non-viral mechanisms could be involved in the formation or progression of human tumours. Several abnormalities in the structure and function of the EGF receptor in tumour derived cell lines and primary tumours have been observed. It has been known for several years that the A431 (vulval carcinoma) cell line expresses as many as 100 times more EGF receptors than most 'normal' cells. Preliminary examination of other squamous tumour cell lines, primary squamous tumours, and a number of brain tumours of glial origin have suggested that overexpression of EGF receptors may be a common feature. In a significant number of glial and squamous tumours the EGF receptor gene is amplified and in some cases rearranged. A surprising finding was that A431 cells expressed a major aberrant transcript which encoded a truncated external domain rather than the truncated internal domain expressed by v-*erbB*.

In other tumours, high levels of receptors are detected without gene amplification, suggesting that abnormal expression can be mediated by alterations in control of transcription. Whatever the mechanism, the net effect is the production of high levels of receptor in certain tumours. It is difficult to show experimentally that such receptor defects cause or alter the progression of tumours.

12.3.5 *Receptor links to* fos *and* myc *oncogenes*

The transforming proteins encoded by oncogenes are intimately involved with alterations in control of cell proliferation, and therefore a number of laboratories have investigated the temporal expression of various c-*onc* gene products in response to mitogens.

The addition of PDGF to fibroblasts, and concanavalin A or lipopoly-saccharide to lymphocytes, has been shown to induce c-*myc* RNA within 1–2 hours. Similar studies in fibroblasts have shown a rapid transient stimulation of c-*fos* transcription within 5 minutes (with a return to normal levels within 45 minutes) after exposure to PDGF, FGF or TPA. Similar responses have been deleted in a rat neuronal tumour cell line following exposure to NGF. The effect on transcription can be observed in the presence of cycloheximide, indicating that protein synthesis is not required to mediate transduction of this effect. Such rapid transient effects on transcription are not limited to c-*fos* since transcription of the actin gene is also stimulated within 15 minutes; indeed, it is possible that a large subset of genes may respond to mitogen stimulation with a burst of transcriptional activity. It is particularly interesting that EGF does not stimulate transcription of c-*fos*. However, a note of caution must be introduced here since the growth state of the cells (cell density, etc.) may have influenced these experiments. If validated, these results further establish the distinction between the signal pathways mediated by these factors as discussed previously.

12.3.6 *Does* ras *subvert a receptor signal?*

Each member of the *ras* multigene family (see Chapters 9, and 10) differs from its normal counterpart by a single amino acid substitution in a poly-peptide of mol. wt. 21 000 which is associated with the inner surface of the plasma membrane. The *ras* gene product (normal or mutant) binds GTP and is a member of a family known as G proteins (GTP binding proteins). Additionally, the product is capable of GTP hydrolysis (a GTPase).

Partially characterized G proteins seem to mediate transduction of signals from specific cell surface receptors into changes in intracellular cyclic nucleotide levels. The G proteins are found in a complex of three subunits α, β, and γ. Activated receptors stimulate binding of GTP to the α subunit which then interacts with an effector molecule such as adenlyate cyclase. Hydrolysis of GTP by the α subunit terminates signal transduction.

The finding that certain mutant *ras* proteins have diminished GTPase activity suggests that, if continuously activated, it might mimic a continuous receptor signal. The result would be an increase in cAMP which in turn regulates pathways linked to cAMP dependent protein phosphorylation.

The precise role of the *ras* protein has yet to be established, but the evidence suggests that the mutation of *ras* at a single amino acid causes defects in a major second messenger system linked to an enormous family of receptors. Virtually all classical hormones and drugs require guanine nucleotides for stimulation of adenyl cyclase, suggesting mediation of signal transduction by G proteins. In Swiss 3T3 cells, an increase in cytoplasmic cAMP is mitogenic and various agents that do not directly raise cAMP levels can act synergistically with agents that do. Within the cell, it seems that a number of distinct but interconnected signal pathways exist which are linked to various types of receptors (Fig. 12.9). Subversion of the earliest steps in transduction could induce a plethora of disturbances in what are normally carefully regulated pathways.

12.3.7 *Links to the effects of tumour promoters*

Recent studies of the effects of phorbol esters on the physiology and biochemistry of platelet activation have provided new insight into the control of cell proliferation and the interpretation of multistage processes in causation of cancer. Nishizuka and colleagues showed that phorbol esters (such as TPA) mimic effects mediated by the ubiquitous enzyme, protein kinase C, which was subsequently shown to be the major receptor for TPA. As mentioned earlier, protein kinase C can be activated by diacylglycerol liberated as a result of phospholipase c activity generated by, for example, PDGF. In fact, the treatment of cells with a diacylglycerol analogue increased proliferation. Mounting evidence suggests a major role for protein kinase C as a mediator of signal transduction for various receptors, and the identification of this enzyme as the tumour promoter receptor gives a major focal point for studying the promotion stage in the generation of tumours in response to carcinogens (see Chapter 7).

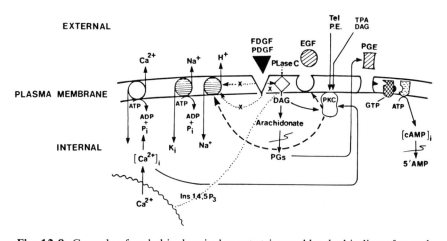

Fig. 12.9 Cascade of early biochemical events triggered by the binding of growth factors to specific receptors. Binding of growth factors (e.g. PDGF) stimulates phospholipase (PLase) C activity leading to the generation of diacylglycerol (DAG) and inositol and (Ins) $1,4,5,P_3$. The mechanism by which receptor occupancy leads to the activation of this enzyme remains unknown. DAG and Ca^{2+} activate protein kinase C (PKC) activity. Protein kinase C can also be directly activated by phorbol esters (PE) such as TPA, teleocidin (Tel), or by DAG. This phosphotransferase system is implicated in the transmodulation of EGF receptor and in enhancing the activity of the Na^+/H^+ antiport system (broken lines). It is also likely that monovalent cation fluxes are stimulated by other mechanisms not yet identified (X). PDGF also causes rapid mobilization of Ca^{2+}, a process that could be mediated by Ins 1,4,5, P_3. The increase in cytosolic Ca^{2+} may co-operate with DAG in activating PKC. A feature that distinguishes PDGF and FGF from many other mitogens is that these factors elicit a massive release of arachidonic acid from the cell. The source of this arachidonic acid remains unclear, but at least is partly derived from DAG. Arachidonic acid is converted into many metabolites including stable E-type prostaglandins (PG) which, in turn, exit the cell and stimulate adenylate cyclase activity via their own receptor. (Courtesy of E. Rozengurt.)

12.4 Abnormal growth control in cancer—a summary

It is evident that enormous progress is being made in our understanding of the structure and function of growth factors and their receptors. One central theme has emerged through the interaction of several different fields of research—that subversion of normal growth signals at the level of membrane signal transduction can be responsible for loss of control of cell proliferation. In two related but distinct ways the effects of growth factor can be mimicked by oncogenes. In one case, by the abnormal production of PDGF, and in the other by expression of a truncated EGF receptor. Growth factor production is a part of the transformed pheno-type of many tumour cells but direct links to oncogenes have not been established. Amongst the oncogenes of the *src* family, it appears that *ros* and *fms* (and perhaps *neu*) could encode truncated cell surface mole-cules like *erbB*; perhaps these are defective receptors for as yet unknown growth factors. The other members of this family may interact at the cell membrane to transduce or modulate various signals relevant to control of proliferation. Evidence is accumulating that the *ras* protein is also intimately involved with transmembrane signalling—this time with recep-tors linked to a multitude of different ligands, many of which are known to act synergistically with growth factors in influencing cell proliferation. Further links to membrane associated events are provided by protein kinase C which may function as a second messenger in signal transduc-tion and can be subverted by tumour promoters. Lastly, the oncogenes *myc* and *fos* respond to signal pathways of growth factors and might encode DNA binding proteins that could clearly modulate gene expres-sion.

Thus a picture is emerging of subversion at key points in transduction of normal growth–factor generated regulatory pathways. Experimental studies of human tumours, which support the observations summarized above, are in progress and, together with the accumulated knowledge of cancer research, may provide clues to novel therapeutic strategies.

Further reading

Cuatracasas, P., and Greaves, M. F. (eds.) (1976–78). *Receptors and recognition, Series A.* Chapman and Hall, London.

Guroff, G. (ed.) (1983–85). *Growth and maturation factors* Vols. **1, 2,** and **3.** Wiley Interscience, Chichester.

Hunter, T. (1984). The proteins of oncogenes. *Scientific American* **251,** 60–9.

—— and Cooper, J. A. (1985). Protein tyrosine kinases. *Annual Reviews of Bio-chemistry* **54,** 897–930.

Li, C. H. (ed.) (1984). *Hormonal proteins and peptides.* **Vol 12,** Growth factors. Academic Press, NY, London.

Rozengurt, E. (1983). Growth factors, cell proliferation and cancer: an overview. *Molecular Biology and Medicine* **1,** 169–81.

Waterfield, M. D. (1985). Subversion of growth factor signal transduction by oncogenes in the molecular biology of tumour cells. *Progress in Cancer Research and Therapy* **32,** 71–85.

13

Hormones and cancer

W. I. P. MAINWARING

13.1 Introduction

Cancer is not a modern disease. Skin cancers were lucidly described in the Ebers papyrus, dating about 1770 BC, and because of its external location and ready observation, breast cancer was well known to Hippocrates and his acolytes. This was the phase of medicine based on his humoral theory of disease, and breast cancer was attributed to an 'excess of overheated black bile'. During the latter part of the 18th century the Scottish surgeon, John Hunter, established that removal of the gonads led to a dramatic shrinkage in the size of the accessory sexual glands in both sexes in animals. This glandular atrophy was particularly noticeable in the case of the prostate in males and the uterus in females.

These observations provided the basis for investigations into the part played by hormones in human cancer. Indeed, Hunter subsequently devised a remarkably sound system for the classification of human breast cancers and did a vast amount of work on their pathology; many of his specimens are still in the Hunterian Museum in London. Research began in earnest in 1889 when Schinzinger proposed a relationship between ovarian function and breast cancer. In clinical terms, the years 1894–96 were the watershed between speculation and reality. In this period, Beatson described the palliation of breast cancer in some patients after ovariectomy, and Rann and White advocated castration for the arrest of prostate cancer. Research in this area then gathered real pace with the purification and characterization of the principal steroid and polypeptide hormones in the years 1905–35. The synthesis of very active analogues and hormone antagonists has also had a profound effect on research progress, opening up genuine possibilities for the successful treatment of cancer by hormonal means. For example, in 1941 Huggins and Hodges introduced the non-steroidal oestrogen, diethylstilboestrol, for the treatment of prostate cancer, a therapy still widely used today.

The incidence of cancers is markedly different in the two sexes and this may be largely explained by the different hormonal status of men and women. Breast cancer, for example, can occur in both sexes but is 100 times more prevalent in women. This difference is attributable to the different types of hormones secreted after birth and most strikingly after puberty. On the other hand, prostate cancer does not occur in women because during embryonic life the structural progenitors (or anlagen) for this organ disappear and persist only in the male. Similar arguments explain the absence of uterine and cervical cancer in men.

A deeper understanding of the mechanism of action of hormones in molecular terms has also provided an impetus to our knowledge of how hormones are implicated in cancer. The cornerstone of current thinking on hormone action is the target cell concept in which specific organs respond to only a restricted number of hormones. It is widely accepted that this distinctive pattern of response reflects the types of receptors present in different cells; a target cell contains the appropriate receptors whereas a non-target cell does not. Certain aspects of earlier studies on receptors have recently been challenged but the essential foundations of the target cell concept remain both persuasive and tenable. Indisputably, certain cells respond more dramatically to hormonal stimuli than others and this is particularly true for prostate, uterus and breast. It is hardly coincidental that these are the major sites for the development of hormone sensitive tumours. While many target organs respond to the same hormone, not all of them become malignant. For example, the production of keratin by hair follicles requires a combination of hormones but tumours in these cells are rare. In the kidney the secretion of renin is under stringent hormonal control but tumours of renin secreting cells are very rare. Current evidence suggests that a target cell is at risk of malignant change only if the appropriate hormones prompt it to divide, as in the case of prostate, breast and uterus.

It is not clear how the distinctive distribution of receptors occurs, but certainly it is laid down during differentiation in the embryo, foetus and neonate. There is some evidence that certain hormones promote the synthesis of their own receptors; this may be true for the receptors for sex hormones in the urogenital tract just before and during puberty.

Since the malignant process is typified by dedifferentiation, carcinogenesis may result in profound changes in the concentrations of receptors. Indeed the assay of receptors has proved useful in monitoring both the appearance and successful treatment of certain forms of cancer.

The course of many types of cancer is profoundly influenced by hormonal imbalance. During neoplasia, several relevant intracellular changes may occur. A cell normally secreting a hormone may produce more or less as a consequence of neoplasia. On the other hand, a cell which normally cannot synthesize a hormone may acquire this ability as the result of malignant change.

Cancer endocrinology is concerned with the role of hormones in cancer induction and their effects on tumour growth. Some tumours, particularly those which arise from hormone responsive organs, may require hormones for their continued growth. Accordingly, alterations in the concentrations of these hormones can be exploited as a method of treatment.

13.2 Basic endocrinology

13.2.1 *Types of hormones*

As defined by Starling, a hormone (from Greek, to arouse) is a compound secreted into the vascular system by one organ to enhance the activity of other organs distant from the site of synthesis. While still true in many respects, this definition needs qualification with respect to many recently described situations (see also Chapter 14). First, testosterone has a direct effect on certain organs, such as muscle and testis, but in many others it must undergo obligatory metabolism to elicit a biological response; in cancer, its necessary conversion to 5α-dihydrotestosterone in accessory sexual organs, such as the prostate, is particularly important. Second, cholesterol is not a hormone but may be converted to the important steroid like hormone, $1\alpha,25$-dihydroxycholecalciferol (formerly termed vitamin D_3), by a sequence of reactions occurring in the skin, liver, and finally kidney. Third, many hormones have direct effects on their organs of synthesis, as in the case of sex hormones. Fourth, many hormones work via second messengers, as originally proposed by Sutherland with cyclic AMP as the 'middleman'; it is now clear that cyclic GMP, Ca^{2+} ions, phosphoinositol, and even polyamines can serve as second messengers. Last, hormones do not invariably activate the biochemical processes in their target cells; glucocorticoids, for example, kill T lymphocytes, granulocytes and macrophages, and tumours derived from them.

Many hormone–like growth factors have been extracted and purified from serum in recent years; these are discussed in Chapter 12. This Chapter will be concerned with those hormones secreted by the ovary, testis, adrenal cortex, and anterior pituitary. In chemical nature, these important hormones are either steroid or polypeptide hormones. In addition, the thyroid hormone, thyroxine, must be taken into account.

The secretion of all these hormones is regulated by precisely co-ordinated activity of the hypothalamus, pituitary, and the secretory (endocrine) glands themselves (Fig. 13.1). The hypothalamus is part of the central nervous system and controls the release of tropic hormones from the pituitary gland at the base of the brain. The pituitary has two parts, anterior and posterior, each of which produces different hormones. The regulatory system is a closed loop, requiring releasing hormones and stimulatory hormones or tropins; both of these classes of hormones are polypeptides. The crucial interaction is between complex nerve centres in the hypothalamus and the anterior pituitary which contains specialized cells responsible for the production of a distinctive tropin.

In response to appropriate external and internal stimuli, the hypothalamus secretes releasing hormones into a system of veins which drain directly into the anterior pituitary and stimulate the selective synthesis of tropins. There are different releasing hormones for thyrotropin (TRH), corticotropin (CRH) and one for the two gonadotropins (GnRH), lutropin and follitropin. The gonadotropins stimulate the production of the female sex hormones (oestrogen and progesterone) from the ovary or male sex hormones (androgens) from the testis. The tropins are secreted into the general circulation where they stimulate the synthesis of hormones from target cells. Thyrotropin stimulates thyroxine secretion from the thyroid. Corticotropin promotes the synthesis of the gluco-corticoids, cortisol and cortisone, from the adrenal cortex, together with a small but significant amount of testosterone. There are two mechanisms to prevent excessive hormonal stimulation. First, the steroid hormones and thyroxine are distributed strongly bound to specific transport proteins in serum; indeed, 0.5 per cent or less of free biologically active hormone may be available to the cells of the body. Second, there are powerful enzymes for steroid breakdown (catabolism) in the liver in both

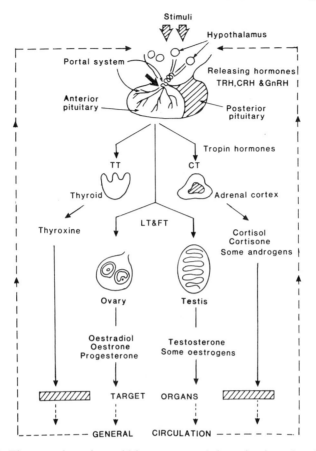

Fig. 13.1 The secretion of steroid hormones and thyroxine is under the control of the hypothalamic pituitary axis. Specific tropins are secreted by the anterior pituitary, including thyrotropin (TT), corticotropin (CT), and the gonadotropins, lutropin (LT) and follitropin (FT). The secretion of the tropins is triggered by specific releasing hormones, TRH for TT, CRH for CT and GnRH for both LT and FT. An excess of hormones in the blood switches off the secretion of releasing hormones by the hypothalamus by closed negative feedback loops.

sexes. Should these latter control mechanisms fail, there is a dramatic rise in the concentration of free active hormone in serum with potentially dangerous consequences.

As well as the polypeptides already described, the anterior pituitary secretes two other polypeptide hormones, somatotropin and prolactin, in response to a variety of stimuli. Somatotropin promotes the growth of many cells and clearly may be important in the cancer process. Prolactin, as its name suggests, was originally identified by its powerful role in inducing lactation. Further research has shown, however, that prolactin has diverse functions and is certainly implicated in the carcinogenic process in many organs, notably breast and prostate.

As an aside, two other points should be made. The mineralocorticoid steroid hormone, aldosterone, is regulated by a novel means and although its level in serum may rise enormously in Conn's syndrome (tumour in the zona glomerulosa of the adrenal cortex), it plays no significant part in the process of carcinogenesis. The hypothalamus also secretes two polypeptide hormones, oxytocin and vasopressin, along with carrier proteins known as the neurophysins, into the posterior pituitary; again, there is no proven involvement of either hormone in neoplasia.

All classes of steroid hormone have diverse effects on a wide range of target cells but, as stated before, their most important feature as far as cancer is concerned is whether they can stimulate cell division. The oestrogens and androgens are powerful mitogens and promote growth and mitosis in many target organs, such as breast, uterus, and prostate; these are potentially dangerous hormones as can be demonstrated experimentally. By contrast, glucocorticoids and progestins are protective agents and generally inhibit cell multiplication; there are certain exceptions and these will be discussed later.

13.2.2 *Mechanisms of hormone action*

13.2.2.1 *Steroid hormones and thyroxine.* Most of the responses to steroid hormones are mediated by specific and seemingly mobile receptor proteins; a few responses related to gluconeogenesis and secretion may be promoted by other means. Steroids enter all cells from the blood by passive diffusion but there is some evidence that certain tumours may possess mechanisms for the facilitated or active transport of steroid hormones. If specific receptors are present, a high affinity hormone receptor complex is formed which, after a conformational change or 'activation', is translocated to the nucleus to occupy large numbers of so called acceptor sites, composed of DNA and non-histone nuclear proteins (Fig. 13.2). Most responses are evoked by the selective acceleration of gene transcription, i.e. specific changes in gene expression. We do not really understand why different cells respond in such contrasting ways to the same hormonal stimulus or why only certain target cells can be driven into mitosis. The extreme specificity of response to steroid hormones depends largely on whether receptors are present or not, and on the binding of steroid which is a very selective process indeed. The concentration of the hormones themselves is an additional factor. Under normal circumstances, for example, oestrogen receptors bind physiological concentrations of androgens very weakly, if at all. In both sexes, however, certain tumours in the adrenal cortex

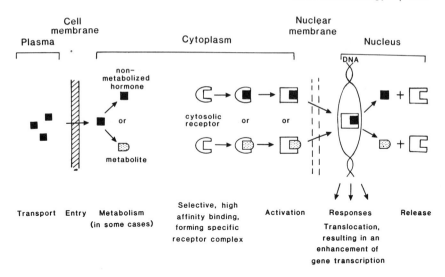

Fig. 13.2 A scheme of the mode of action of steroid hormones and thyroxine. Metabolism of the secreted hormone within its target cells is important only in the case of the androgen, testosterone. Cytosolic receptors for thyroxine have not been identified, yet the hormone still accumulates within the nucleus of its target cells. Based on Mainwaring (1980) In: *Cellular receptors* pp. 91–125 (eds. D. Shulster and A. Levitski). John Wiley and Sons, Chichester.

produce such massive amounts of androgens (virilizing hyperplasia) that the oestrogen as well as androgen receptors are fully occupied, and elicit certain oestrogenic as well as androgenic responses, even in males.

The thyroid gland produces iodine containing hormones, thyroxine (tetraiodothyroxine) and triiodothyroxine. These have a profound effect on cell metabolism and growth of many cells, including some tumours. A deficiency in infants leads to mental and physical stunting (cretinism). Iodine deficiency causes an overgrowth of the thyroid cells leading to the formation of tumour like nodules (goitres) but these rarely if ever become malignant.

Soluble cytosolic receptors have not been identified for thyroxine, but the hormone is bound to a nuclear receptor in the chromatin of its target cells. Its precise role in tumour cell growth is still to be defined.

13.2.2.2 *Polypeptide hormones and growth factors.* Both these classes of compound have specific receptors as integral components of the outer surface of the plasma membrane. The receptors have a close structural and functional association with enzyme systems and ion gates capable of generating a wide range of second messengers. Occupation of the specific receptor sites enhances the synthesis of second messengers, and since the subsequent steps are operational cascades, the hormonal signal is amplified and a few molecules of hormone can evoke a very pronounced effect. Some internalization of polypeptide hormones has been detected in the Golgi apparatus and lysosomes of target cells; this may represent a mechanism for their degradation but may be a more subtle reflection of a wider influence on cellular function. There are defences against excessive hormonal stimulation. Excess polypeptides are degraded by proteases in the walls of arteries and capillaries. A long biological life for cyclic nucleotides is prevented by the ubiquitous presence of phosphodiesterases. Finally, there is evidence that protracted exposure of specific receptors to their appropriate hormone leads to a very significant decrease in the number of receptors (down regulation); this phenomenon is being exploited in novel approaches to the hormonal therapy of certain tumours. It follows from this general discussion that tumours may arise from hormone producing or hormone responsive cells (see on).

13.3 Hormones and carcinogenesis

The first hint that hormones were potential carcinogens came in 1932 when Lacassagne induced mammary tumours in male mice with the oestrogen, oestrone benzoate. Using a similar approach, Kirkman induced kidney tumours with oestrogens but only in hamsters and not other rodents. This unexpected finding showed that hormones may influence organs not usually thought to be hormone sensitive. The synthesis of the non-steroidal oestrogen, diethylstilboestrol, by Dodds in 1935, provided researchers with an extremely powerful research weapon. Of all the classes of steroid hormones, the sex hormones, and oestrogens in particular, are the most potent carcinogens. Work in this area is not without its controversies. There are often conflicting results when the effects of hormones are compared in different species. Of greater importance, data obtained from experimental animals often conflict with findings in the human. Taking an overall view, hormones can be carcinogenic under certain circumstances or can provide the means for the arrest of tumours. Our knowledge in this area is based on studies on animals, in man, and on cells in tissue culture.

13.3.1 *Animal studies*

The literature on this topic is now vast and will only be covered briefly. In experimental animals prolonged exposure to oestrogens and their analogues, such as stilboestrol, results in cancer formation in many organs, but most commonly in reproductive organs, kidney, liver, and anterior pituitary, but there is a considerable variation between species. It has also been reported that protracted treatment of dogs with potent androgens may lead to prostate tumours. Concomitant administration of carcinogenic hydrocarbons, such as dimethylbenzanthracene, often enhances the tumour incidence achieved by hormones alone; in addition, hydrocarbons may help to induce tumours in organs normally insensitive to hormones. So far, tumours have not been consistently induced in experimental animals even by chronic treatment with polypeptide hormones including prolactin and somatotropin.

Two examples illustrate interspecies differences. Tumours of the uterine cervix can be induced in mice by extremely low doses of oestrogens; under similar, dose corrected conditions, all other species are refractory. Mammary tumours are common in some mouse strains and are often associated with a mammary tumour virus. Repeated pregnancies tend to increase the incidence of these tumours. In human breast cancer there is no evidence of a virus and pregnancy tends to protect (see Chapter 4). Prostate tumours are very rare in most animals although common in man. Such anomalies create problems when trying to assess the potential danger of hormones in humans.

This problem has been approached by Dunning in 1963. From a spontaneous rat prostate tumour, she developed a whole range of transplantable, androgen sensitive and androgen insensitive tumours; these tumours are stable and can be grown in tissue culture.

While studies on experimental animals have taught us much about hormones and cancer, they have not shed any light on certain pressing human problems. Taking the prostate, for example, experimental studies have failed to explain why cancer is so prevalent in the human prostate, yet rare in adjacent accessory sexual glands which are subject to a similar if not identical hormonal milieu. Further, animal studies have failed to explain why the male dog is the only species to share a high incidence of prostatic cancer. Prostate cancer in humans is a disease of old age, and there have been some reports on a spontaneous prostate tumour arising in aged AxC rats. The incidence of prostate tumours was raised to 70 per cent if the animals were exposed to exogenous androgens. While of considerable interest, these studies may tell us little about the human disease, because ageing men are unlikely to be exposed to exogenous androgens and the endogenous production of testosterone tends to decline during ageing. Answers to such questions could provide invaluable insights into the aetiology of the human disease.

The use of animals for testing potentially dangerous hormones has prompted many controversies. Perhaps the most notorious centres on synthetic progestins related to 17-hydroxyprogesterone. When tested in beagle dogs, but not other animals, these compounds were found to induce mammary tumours. Despite lengthy debate, these synthetic progestins were banned from inclusion in contraceptive pills on the evidence obtained from one experimental species only.

13.3.2 *Studies in man*

Evidence that hormones are carcinogenic in man comes largely from clinical observations and epidemiological studies. Many relevant observations, still largely unexplained, have been made. For example, prostate cancer has never been recorded in eunuchs or castrati, and there is a high incidence of breast cancer in socially enclosed female communities, such as nunneries.

13.3.2.1 *The hormones and cancer in women.* There is a rapidly growing body of evidence that prolonged exposure to sex hormones, especially oestrogens, results in a high incidence of several forms of human cancer. Women are more usually affected since they tend to take more hormone preparations largely for obstetric and gynaecological reasons. Nonetheless, androgen containing formulations markedly increases the risk of hepatoma in men and transvestites with oestrogen implants have a higher incidence of breast cancer than normal men. The contraceptive pill (see Chapter 4) contains a combination of oestrogen and progesterone; the critical point in terms of potential danger is the relative proportions of the two hormones. While essential for contraceptive function, the oestrogen is the potentially threatening component, whereas the progesterone is protective or 'anti-oestrogenic'. Early preparations containing a high oestrogen to progesterone ratio have all now been banned because they markedly increased the risk of endometrial (uterine) cancer. Contraceptive preparations containing a very low oestrogen to progesterone ratio are currently considered safe and indeed may well provide protection against cancer of the ovary, breast and endometrium. There has been one cautionary report, yet to be substantiated, of a high incidence of breast cancer in young women who have been taking oral contraceptives since just after the menarche. Fortunately, such dangers to health may be obviated in the future by the wider use of contraceptive implants containing only a synthetic progestin, levonorgestrol. These subdermal implants are effective, long lasting, and have a reduced risk of cancer.

Formulations containing oestrogens alone, so called 'happy pills', became fashionable for helping certain women through the undesirable psychological and physical aspects of the menopause. Many such preparations have now been withdrawn for, although achieving the proposed objectives, patients also ran a higher risk of endometrial cancer and possibly breast cancer as well. Such postmenopausal treatments are ethically acceptable only if progestins are also included in the regimen.

A most distressing illustration of the dangers of hormones is provided in reports of vaginal cancer in young women whose mothers took stilboestrol during early pregnancy to prevent threatened abortion.

Extensive epidemiological studies have established the major risk factors for breast cancer (see Chapter 4). These include early menarche, late menopause, having close relatives with the disease, infertility, obesity, geographic location and having the first pregnancy late in life. The current strategy is to try to explain these findings in terms of hormonal imbalance, but no unequivocal conclusions can yet be drawn. Nonetheless, breast cancer is generally considered to result from over-exposure to oestrogens and underexposure to progesterone. The risk associated with obesity can be partly explained by the ability of adipose cells to synthesize oestrogens, but impaired activity of detoxification mechanisms in the liver and elsewhere may also be implicated. The beneficial effect of having a child early in life could be due to the high concentrations of progesterone like hormones in pregnancy protecting the breast cells against oestrogens in the long term. The risks of early menarche and late menopause can be combined in that a high number of menstrual cycles may be dangerous in terms of the repeated surges of oestrogens ultimately providing the stimulus for malignancy. No convincing correlation has yet been drawn between endocrine imbalance, family history, and domestic locality.

All of these epidemiological considerations apply equally forcibly to endometrial cancer. One possible clue, as with prostate cancer in men, is provided by studies on Japanese migrants to Western cultures. Breast and endometrial cancer increase in these women, possibly a result of changing diet. Western foods tend to be richer in fat and this may cause subtle but significant changes in the hormonal milieu and even hormonal imbalance. This is considered in more detail in Chapter 4.

13.3.2.2 *Hormones and cancer in men: prostate cancer.* The high incidence of prostate cancer in the human male remains an enigma and, as in so many cancers, we have no real idea why the incidence rises so sharply in old age. Certainly, the precise involvement of androgens remains to be elucidated. The only real clue so far is that the malignant prostate has a marked ability to form and retain elevated concentrations of 5-α-dihydrosterone; this androgen is a far more powerful mitogen than testosterone itself. The disease is associated with westernized, industrialized societies and remains relatively uncommon in Mongoloid races. In several studies, it has been shown that when Chinese and Japanese emigrated to California and Hawaii, their risk of developing prostatic cancer rose significantly. The formerly low incidence of prostate cancer in Japan itself is now gradually increasing, whereas formerly common cancers, especially of stomach, are gradually decreasing. While not a complete explanation, there is plausible evidence suggesting that the newly acquired risk is attributable to the adoption of social customs and particularly the diet more typical of the West.

In contrast to breast cancer, epidemiological studies on prostate cancer are much less extensive. In the United States, this cancer is higher in blacks than Caucasians and lower in Jewish immigrants. Throughout Europe, no relationship has been established between the high incidence of prostate cancer and socioeconomic status, marital status, fertility, social habits, hair distribution, and physical size. There are hints of a possible connection with recurrent prostatitis, repeated infections, and venereal disease. A remarkable connection has been drawn in several reports between prostate cancer and 'sustained sexual interest' and 'sex drive'. Needless to say, these terms are difficult to qualitate, let alone quantitate. Investigators have used various parameters to measure sexual activity, and it remains possible that increased activity in some form is associated with prostate cancer.

Although a considerable literature has been amassed on the epidemiology of many human cancers, it is surprising that measurements of oestrogens and androgens in blood, urine, sebum, and even saliva, have so far failed to show that abnormalities in the concentrations of sex hormones are associated with the disease states. It should be stressed, however, that measurements in the past have been as total hormone concentrations. In biological terms, it is the concentration of free, unbound hormone which is important. In keeping with this change in analysis, elevated concentrations of free oestradiol are present in the plasma of women with breast and endometrial cancer as compared to normal, age matched controls. Similar measurements in other cancers could be vital in the future for diagnostic and prognostic purposes.

13.3.3 *The actions of hormones on tumour cells in culture*

Some stable lines of tumour cells have been established and these provide an invaluable approach for studying the direct effects of hormones on tumour cells. Such studies are expanding rapidly, because cells in culture, rather than in intact animals, have the advantages of easy manipulation, high biochemical activities, and ethical acceptance. A major problem is that only a small proportion of tumours can be established in culture. Three experimental systems will be briefly reviewed.

13.3.3.1 *Human breast cancer cells.* Because of the understandable concern about the present scale of the breast cancer problem, a great deal of effort has been directed to the establishment of such tumour cells in culture. The driving force behind these enterprises is the ability to screen the effects of hormones and other drugs on the tumour cells directly. The MCF-7 line of breast tumour cells has been investigated in detail.

The growth rate of these cells is enhanced by low concentrations of oestrogens and prevented by antioestrogens, such as nafoxidene and tamoxifen. Such studies have helped to clarify many aspects of the hormonal management of breast cancer and certainly provided hints for the improvement of clinical treatment. First, the cells can be maintained in the complete absence of oestrogens, so that hormones exert their influence by accelerating or modulating an existing, basal rate of cell proliferation. Second, antioestrogens inhibit basal proliferation in the absence of oestrogens. It is now clear that antioestrogens, such as tamoxifen, bind extensively to the oestrogen receptor and are efficiently translocated to nuclear chromatin, but the antioestrogen receptor protein complex is biologically inactive. Third, oestrogens also enhance the density to which the cells will grow. In particular, the cells can proliferate in the presence of powerful oestrogens without attaching to an artificial substrate, such as agar or collagen, which mimics the underlying stroma and mesenchyme present in the intact breast. It has been postulated that oestrogens change the social behaviour of these tumours cells in such a way that inhibitory influences on their growth, such as contact inhibition, are largely offset. Finally, the tumour cells grow best in culture medium containing serum, but this can be replaced by an artificial medium containing transferrin, insulin, cortisol, thyroxine, prolactin, and epidermal growth factor.

These observations have considerable relevance in the clinical context. It would seem that the responses are mediated by the classical receptor machinery and so treatment with anti-oestrogens can be predicted to be successful only if the tumour contains receptors, and is therefore r^+ rather than r^-. On current evidence, it would seem that oestrogen deprivation alone will only slow tumour growth to a basal rate, but certainly not stop it completely. Nonetheless, the importance of antioestrogens in the palliation of breast cancer is experimentally and now clinically proven. Clearly, growth of the breast tumour cells requires a variety of polypeptide and steroid hormones, and these are yet to be investigated *in vitro*. Antagonism of these hormones may therefore be useful in the management of breast cancer and such possibilities are currently the centre of active clinical trials.

As a final point, very high doses of steroids and related compounds, such as stilboestrol, inhibit the growth of MCF-7 cells. This restraint on

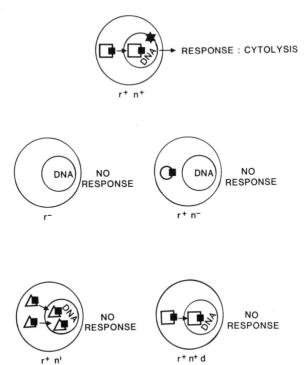

Fig. 13.3 In normal lymphocytes and many lymphomas, a receptor complex containing glucocorticoids, such as prednisolone, translocates to the nucleus and, by activating gene expression from DNA, produces proteins (★) which promote cytolysis. Such cells are r^+n^+. Many lines of lymphomas resist the cytocidal effects of glucocorticoids. Some are r^-; others contain structurally different receptors, which cannot translocate to the nucleus and are r^+n^-; other modified receptors may translocate in great numbers yet not evoke a response and are r^+n^i; and finally, there are resistant lines, r^+n^+d, in which only the crucial change in gene expression is impaired.

cellular proliferation cannot be mediated by the oestrogen receptor machinery and the molecular basis for such cytocidal effects remains to be clarified.

13.3.3.2 *Prostate cells in culture.* Various sublines of the Dunning prostate tumour have been used to confirm the hormonal effects found in the MCF-7 cell line. The prostate cells grow best in the presence of powerful mitogens, such as 5-α-dihydrotestosterone, mibolerone and certain 5-androstanediols, but are inhibited by antiandrogens, including the non-steroidal compound, flutamide. Autonomous sublines contain few if any androgen and prolactin receptors, and antiandrogens occupy the receptor sites of androgen sensitive sublines but the resultant complex is without biological activity. Although a number of cell lines derived from human prostate tumours are available, few respond to hormones in the same way as the cells do *in vivo*.

A promising approach to endocrine studies both in the breast and prostate is the use of organ cultures in which small pieces of tissue, with epithelium and stroma in their normal relationship, can be maintained. These techniques have given useful information but are still to be exploited fully.

13.3.3.3 *Rat lymphomas cells.* Powerful glucocorticoids are used in transplantation surgery to suppress the immune system and there is now some evidence that these steroids not only kill some lymphoid cells but may also act as a trigger for the development of some leukaemias and lymphomas.

Studies on rat lymphomas cell lines have provided explanations for the cytocidal effects of glucocorticoids, and also led to a better understanding of the mechanism of action of steroid hormones in general. This work has been expedited by the availability of powerful analogues of cortisol. Many of these analogues, such as dexamethasone, fluoprednisolone, and triamcinolone acetonide, contain substituent fluorine atoms at positions 6 or 9 of the steroid ring system. The halogen substitutions greatly potentiate the biological activity of these synthetic glucocorticoids because they do not bind to the transport protein, corticosteroid binding globulin, in serum and also resist catabolism within glucocortocoid target cells.

The anti-inflammatory action of glucocorticoids, namely the killing of B lymphocytes and tumours derived from them, was first described by Daughaday in 1943. Subsequent research has shown that cell death is mediated by glucocorticoid receptors in the lymphocytes and lymphomas, followed by synthesis *de novo* of many species of mRNA encoding proteins responsible for the lethal process. The hormone induced cytolysis is clearly a complex process; certainly the uptake of life maintaining glucose is completely suppressed, together with the intracellular accumulation of toxic fatty acids and powerful DNAases.

Certain sublines of lymphomas have been found to be resistant to glucocorticoids and their study has been of fundamental importance. Resistance can be explained by several types of change in the receptor system for binding glucocorticoids (Fig. 13.3). The majority of resistant lines are termed r^-, meaning that they have either lost the ability to synthesize the receptor protein or produce a modified and biologically inactive receptor. Other resistant lines contain the normal complement of receptors but translocation of the receptor complex to the nucleus is either lost (r^+, n^-) or even increased (r^+, n^i). A final class of resistant cells has a normal receptor system but complete resistance to glucocorticoids; these cells have been described as deathless (r^+, n^+, d).

The identification of the r^-, n^i, and r^+, n^+, d sublines raises some very interesting questions. Clearly the occupation of surface receptor and nuclear acceptor sites is not the full explanation for hormonal responses in molecular terms. Other biochemical events after receptor occupation and translocation are clearly involved. We know now that higher eukaryotes contain genes that may be the ultimate regulators of the biochemistry of cells in terms of their viability, sensitivity to mitogens, and response to hormones. Along these lines, it could be argued that these deathless mutants have structural defects in such genes. Such possibilities could be vital to future research. In the final analysis, however, these seemingly encouraging results on cultured tumour cells must be viewed with caution, tinged even with disappointment, when applied to the human equivalents of these cancers.

13.3.4 *A comparison of hormones and chemical carcinogens*

Because of their potential danger in ecological and industrial terms, a great deal of effort has been directed towards elucidating the general mechanism of action of chemical carcinogens. With a few exceptions, chemical carcinogens exist as precarcinogens which must be activated, usually in the target organ, before their carcinogenicity can be maximally expressed (see Chapter 7). Such activation is also necessary with many naturally occurring carcinogens, including the aflatoxins, quercitin and cycasin. In the latter activation is carried out by intestinal microorganisms. Before examining the carcinogenic properties of hormones in detail, it is useful to compare their mechanism of action with that of carcinogens (Table 13.1). It is clear that the mechanisms are very different except that both hormones and chemical carcinogens need dividing cells as targets for the malignant process to develop.

13.4 The mode of action of hormones in carcinogenesis

As described in Chapters 1 and 7, the original concept of Berenblum, that carcinogenesis consists of a first phase of initiation followed by various phases of promotion, is now widely accepted. With a few notable exceptions, hormones act as promoters or cocarcinogens. There are only a few instances where they may be considered as genuine initiators, like the chemical carcinogens. Generally, hormones enhance the rate of initiation and development of tumours induced by all of the proven classes of initiators, such as chemical carcinogens, viruses, and ionizing radiations. A crucial point which argues against hormones being initiators is that

Table 13.1 A comparison of the mechanism of action of hormones and chemical carcinogens

Property	Hormones	Chemical carcinogens
Mutagenicity	Not mutagenic	Mutagenic
Site of action	mRNA and proteins	DNA
Latent period	Long	Short
Nature of tumours	Benign or locally invasive	Highly malignant and metastatic
Activation	Not necessary	Necessary
Species- and sex-dependency	Very marked	Barely relevant
Nature of exposure repeated	Prolonged	Single exposure may suffice
Expression of carcinogenicity	*In vivo* only	*In vivo* and *in vitro*
Regression after ceasing exposure	Regression	No regression
Need for cell division	Needed	Needed

they are not mutagenic, whereas almost all genuine initiators are powerful mutagens.

Perhaps one case where hormones may act as genuine initiators is the vaginal cancer in young women whose mothers took stilboestrol during pregnancy. At various stages in development, human embryos are acutely sensitive to damage by a wide range of exogenous agents. In this case, traces of stilboestrol could pass the protective barrier of the placenta and initiate carcinogenesis in oestrogen target organs, such as the vagina. The cancer may only develop after birth under the promoting influence of oestrogens after purberty.

In acting primarily as cocarcinogens, hormones could exert their influence in any of three ways, namely in classical promotion, in accelerating tumour growth, or in sensitizing target cells to initiating agents. Hormones may also have a significant role in tumour progression (see on).

13.4.1 *Cocarcinogenesis*

13.4.1.1 *Promotion*. There are many examples in experimental systems where hormones act as promoters and greatly increase the incidence of tumour development by initiators. Particularly good examples, although by different mechanisms, include the promoting influence of glucocorticoids thyroxine and somatotropin on the induction of skin tumours in mice by methylcholanthrene and croton oil, and the activation of mouse mammary tumour virus by glucocorticoids.

Another good example is that of mammary tumours induced in rats by dimethylbenzanthracene. This chemical is a potent inducer of breast tumours in the rat if it is administered at precisely 50 days of age; if administered at other times, its carcinogenicity to breast epithelium is markedly decreased (Table 13.2). Seemingly, the hormonal milieu and the developmental state of the cells at this time are optimal for tumour induction. Removal of the ovaries at any time reduces the induction of tumours and this may be reversed by administration of oestrogens. In hypophysectomized rats, oestrogens are ineffective as promoters and it seems their influence is expressed via the hypothalamic pituitary axis by the accelerated secretion of prolactin. This may be an authentic example of prolactin sensitive tumour induction. Progesterone has a complex influence in this experimental system. When administered prior to the initiating carcinogen, tumour incidence decreases but, when given after the initiator, tumour incidence increases. This paradox remains to be clarified. Certainly, it would be dangerous to extrapolate these findings to breast cancer in women. As emphasized before, data from animal work are not always consistent with clinical findings, and in this particular case, the very nature of the tumours may be fundamentally different.

Table 13.2 The influence of hormones on the induction of mammary tumours by dimethylbenzanthracene

Additional treatment	Number of tumours	Day of appearance of tumours
None	Many	90–94
Ovariectomy, 30–35 days	Few	106–110
Ovariectomy, 65–70 days	Few	106–110
Progesterone, 30–35 days	Few	106–110
Progesterone, 60–70 days	Very many	79–83

Dimethylbenzanthracene was given through a stomach tube to female Sprague-Dawley rats of 50 days of age, either alone, with administration of progesterone or to ovariectomized animals. The days when palpable tumours were observed is given along with the relative numbers.

The involvement of oestrogens in the development and course of endometrial cancer is much clearer, although it is difficult to draw an absolute distinction between initiation and promotion. Certainly, oestrogens promote the disease, after earlier phases of hyperplasia and pre-neoplasia, and these are all countered by progesterone or synthetic progestins. While this is a striking example of tumour promotion in the human, it is surprising that oestrogens rarely induce endometrial cancer in experimental animals. The difference could be of some importance, because it could imply that induction of tumours by the sex hormones is not simply to evoke changes in cell proliferation and mitosis; other factors are almost certainly involved.

We know very little about the relationship between other hormones and carcinogenesis. Although it has been suggested that there is a close relationship between the androgens and tumour growth in the prostate, firm evidence that it plays any role in tumour induction is lacking.

13.4.1.2 *Tumour growth.* There are many striking examples in the literature of the profound influence of the sex hormones on tumour growth. This was very evident in work on Shionogi mouse breast tumour cells, an unusual androgen responsive tumour, but most strikingly demonstrated in recent research on the transplantable Dunning prostate tumours in the Copenhagen rat. Growth of the androgen sensitive tumour lines is effectively suppressed by castration or a variety of antiandrogens, including cyproterone acetate and flutamide; powerful oestrogens, such as stilboestrol, also strongly inhibit growth of these tumours.

In considering tumour growth, two aspects are particularly important. Tumour cells may divide more slowly than many normal cells, but are distinguished by their inexorable rather than their rapid growth. Second, an increase in tumour size occurs only when cell multiplication exceeds cell death; in the prostate and breast, it has been estimated that between 25 per cent and 45 per cent of new cells soon die. From these considerations, hormones could exert an influence on tumour size by maintaining exponential growth or slowing cell death. There is little sound evidence on the latter point. Clinically, it is not possible to distinguish between promotion and tumour growth; nonetheless, there is no reason *a priori* why results from hormone sensitive, experimental tumours are not germane to the human disease.

Although hormones may affect tumour growth by direct action on the cells, indirect mechanisms may also play a part. The influence of hormones on the growth of common human tumours, such as prostate and breast, is complex. These tumours are composed of epithelium, stroma, and blood vessels. In the normal breast, oestrogens promote the proliferation of the endothelial cells in the capillaries and this may provide an indirect way in which these hormones modulate tumour growth by increasing the supply of nutrients. In the prostate, there has been a belief for many years that a close structural and functional interaction between the stromal and epithelial elements is mandatory for the coordinated normal growth of the organ. Prolonged exposure to androgens, especially 5 α-dihydrotestosterone, could upset this delicate stromal–epithelial interaction. Future research in this area has been given a strong boost by the successful maintenance of separated stromal and epithelial elements of both dog and rat prostate in culture; this breakthrough should provide new insights into the mechanism controlling prostate growth and the part played by the androgens in the process.

13.4.1.3 *Sensitization.* Dividing cells are prime targets for carcinogens. Both classes of sex hormone are powerful mitogens and promote division, and even hyperplasia, in certain of their target organs, including prostate, breast, and cervix. These hormones, therefore, increase the potential number of cells that will be at risk on exposure to initiating agents. This process may simply be termed sensitization. Using the rat prostate as the model system, new insights have recently been gained into mechanisms by which androgens enhance DNA replication. After the rapid saturation of nuclear acceptor sites by receptor 5 α -dihydro-testosterone complex and an accompanying phosphorylation of certain nuclear proteins, the subsequent responses evoked by androgens proceed in a precise biphasic manner (Fig. 13.4*a*). The first (Group I) responses are not implicated in DNA replication whereas the later (Group II) responses involve the synthesis de novo of the biochemical machinery for DNA unwinding proteins. After reaching a zenith just prior to and during the S phase, the synthesis of these components then ceases (Fig. 13.4*b*) despite continued androgenic stimulation. These changes are attributable to a temporal distinction in the expression of the structural genes representative of Group I and Group II components. Importantly, the occupation of the nuclear acceptor sites by 5 α -dihydrotestosterone is also biphasic, the two phases coinciding precisely with the synthesis of Group I and Group II components (Fig. 13.4*c*). It is to be hoped that

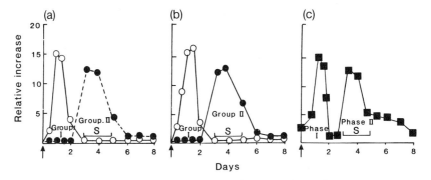

Fig. 13.4 Changes evoked in the prostate of castrated rats by testosterone are biphasic. Group I responses occur early and are not associated with DNA replic-ation; Group II occur later, during synthetic (S) phase of the cell cycle when DNA synthesis is in progress. The changes are presented relative to measurements in castrated animals prior to implantation with testosterone, marked by arrows. (a) Changes in the activities of aldolase (Group I, ○) and thymidylate synthetase (Group II, ●). (b) Changes in the amounts of the specific mRNAs for aldolase (○) and thymidylate synthetase (●). (c) Changes in the concentration of androgen receptors in the nucleus (■).

these results can be confirmed by careful studies on oestrogen target cells, as in rat uterus, but they do provide a pointer to the molecular basis of stringent control being lost and the transformed prostate cells permanently retaining the machinery necessary for continuous replication of DNA. These important results are currently being applied to the androgen sensitive and insensitive Dunning tumours.

Hormones may influence DNA synthesis in ways other than by gene expression. They may induce the synthesis of growth promoting factors in their target cells or in other cells of the body, but there is scant evidence on these points.

13.4.2 *Tumour progression*

Progression in tumours has been unequivocally demonstrated in many experimental systems and is supported by clinical observations. In general, hormone sensitive tumours progress to an autonomous hormone insensitive state, but whether this is due to changes in the cells or to selection of resistant cells already present in the tumour is not known. A good example is seen in the BR6 mouse which develops multiple mammary cancers very frequently. The tumours appear and grow rapidly during pregnancy and may regress after birth, but grow again at precisely the same site during the next pregnancy (Fig. 13.5). The tumours each behave independently. Some regress completely after pregnancy, others show incomplete regression and others become completely autonomous, i.e. they are no longer dependent on pregnancy associated hormones for their growth. It should be stressed that progression is not invariably from

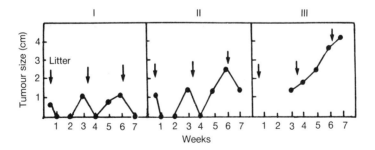

Fig. 13.5 Three mammary tumours with different properties in a single BR6 mouse. The tumours arise during pregnancy, and may disappear (responsive tumours) or persist (unresponsive tumours), after delivery of the litters, marked by arrows (data from Foulds, 1969. *Neoplastic development.* Academic Press, London).
I   Left groin—pregnancy–responsive—complete regression.
II Right axilla—pregnancy–responsive—incomplete regression.
III Right neck—pregnancy–unresponsive.

normal hormone responsive to hormone unresponsive; there may be a direct transition from the normal to a hormone unresponsive stage. Since the information given in Figure 13.5 was taken from one mouse, it is clear that the hormonal responsiveness of a given tumour is intrinsic and not determined by the environment.

An observation of fundamental importance is that during progression of the Dunning prostate tumour, there are major changes in the complement of chromosomes, i.e. during progression to autonomy gene changes are involved. It seems very likely that similar changes occur in other tumours but the precise gene changes involved have still to be discovered.

13.5 Types and nature of hormone sensitive and hormone producing tumours

From the earlier discussion it is clear that endocrine associated tumours fall into two groups, hormone sensitive from target organs, and hormone producing from endocrine glands (but see also Chapter 14).

13.5.1 *Hormone sensitive tumours*

Tumours arising from target organs should be described as hormone sensitive rather than hormone dependent. This is not simply a semantic distinction. Hormone dependence implies that certain tumours could only persist during hormonal stimulation and would atrophy if the source of hormone was removed. Both clinically and experimentally this is rarely the case. All tumours are heterogeneous with respect to cell types, and it follows that certain cells may be amenable, and even acutely sensitive, to hormonal manipulation whereas others certainly are not. However, by prudent handling of the hormonal environment of certain tumours, the disease may be checked in many cases and, in the most encouraging situations, even cured. These human tumours are best described as hormone sensitive. When considering hormone sensitive tumours, it may well be that the future will hold some remarkable surprises. Traditional endocrinology has been set on its head over the last decade by the discovery of a bewildering array of polypeptide hormones, from coded neurotransmitters to growth regulators (see Chapters 12 and 14). Few investigators would have anticipated the identification of the naturally occurring analgesics, the endorphins, or predicted that hormones classically associated with the gastrointestinal tract, such as gastrin, glucagon and cholecystokinin, could also be synthesized within the central nervous system. Our traditional tenets of endocrinology are probably very insecure and many growth factors and hormones of great relevance to human cancer, are just being isolated and characterized.

13.5.1.1 *Steroid sensitive tumours.* Tumours in the accessory sexual glands are among the most common forms of cancer in men and women and these tumours are rightly described as hormone sensitive. The aetiology of these diseases is clearly complex and changing. At the turn of the century, for example, carcinoma of the uterus was the most common hormone sensitive tumour in women; since then the incidence of this tumour has decreased and has been superceded by the pronounced and increasing incidence of breast cancer. This change is baffling but could reflect hormonal changes resulting from improved hygiene, better contraception, and better medical care in general. This particular tumour highlights a major problem for modern investigators; it is clearly imperative to find a plausible explanation for such important changes, but early medical records are often wanting and experimental animal models are few. The only animal equivalent for uterine cancer is the rabbit, and even here the disease is endocrinologically and pathologically distinct from the human disease.

Breast cancer is a major threat to the health of the female population in all westernized societies. Benign tumours, fibroadenomas, are rare before puberty but represent the commonest form of breast tumour in the age span 25–30 years. Carcinoma of the breast is age associated, and becomes more common from about 30 years of age (see Chapter 4). There is a clear endocrinological basis for the disease and, as described later, this provides the rationale for clinical manipulation and arrest of the disease in many women. Growth abnormalities in the breast can also result in papillomas, which range from well to poorly differentiated tumours. A rarer condition is Paget's disease, which is defined as a primary malignancy of the nipple but is often associated with a tumour of the breast. Tumours in other organs of the female reproductive tract, e.g. the vulva and vagina, are relatively rare, but may be induced by oestrogens under certain circumstances (see on). In both cases, a hormonal imbalance, and particularly an excess of oestrogens, is involved.

In Western societies, cancer of the prostate is the fourth most common male cancer. It usually appears in men of 60 years or older and increases in frequency with age. The tumours vary enormously from highly invasive poorly differentiated tumours to relatively slow growing and well differentiated forms. Cancers in other male accessory organs, such as epididymis and seminal vesicle, are rare. In all cases, there is a hormonal aetiology for the disease. Cancer of the penis and scrotum is also very rare; a hormonal basis for these tumours is possible but not proven.

Circumcision certainly is accepted as the prime defence against cancer of the penis; for reasons unknown, this cancer is particularly frequent in the stallion. No other animal shares this risk.

13.5.1.2 *Polypeptide sensitive tumours.* It is now clear that the cells of the body are continually exposed to a wide battery of polypeptide hormones. Although many cells respond to somatotropin and virtually all cells respond to insulin by increasing uptake of glucose and amino acids, very few tumours seem to be sensitive to these polypeptide hormones. There is growing evidence for the involvement of prolactin in the induction and progression of certain tumours. The first indication of the involvement of prolactin in carcinogenesis came from studies on the growth of several lines of transplantable mammary tumours in the AxC rat. This hormone may also play a significant role in the growth of cancers in the breast and prostate; in the latter case, prolactin may enhance the uptake of androgens from the peripheral circulation. There are indirect indications but little definite information that polypeptide hormones of the pituitary may modulate the growth of certain tumours. The effects of other polypeptides are considered in Chapters 12, and 14.

13.5.1.3 *Hormone producing tumours.* All organs producing steroid hormones (ovary, testis, adrenal) are potential sites for malignancy. Tumours, as well as producing effects by their size and position, may cause symptoms by interfering with the normal production of hormones by the organ, by overproduction of normal hormones, or by the production of hormones not normally produced.

Ovarian tumours most commonly occur in the age range 40–60 years. Benign conditions are also quite common. Ovarian cancers are of many different types. The most common tumours arise from the surface epithelium and have a wide range of structure; the second group are of germ cell origin, and a third rare group arises from sex cord stromal cells (these cells normally surround germ cells and are responsible for the production of ovarian steroid hormones). Tumours from these latter cells are likely to be hormone producing and may produce oestrogens or androgens.

Testicular tumours, although not common, are increasing in frequency and are the most frequent form of cancer in young men. As outlined in Chapter 4 there is strong evidence that hormonal changes *in utero* may be a factor in their development. As in the ovary, tumours may arise from the germ cells or *much* less often, from specialized androgen producing interstitial cells or oestrogen producing Sertoli cells. Some germ cell derived tumours, for reasons unknown, may produce a hormone, human chorionic gonadotropin (HCG), normally produced by the human placenta.

The adrenal gland has two parts, an inner medulla and an outer cortex, each having a different embryological origin. The medulla can be considered as a neuroendocrine organ and its tumours are discussed in Chapter 14. The cortex produces steroid hormones, mainly gluco– and mineralo–corticoids but it may also produce oestrogens and androgens. Tumours in the adrenal cortex have been widely investigated and have very interesting properties. Small, benign adenomas are quite common, but carcinomas are rare. The tumours show no age dependency and can occur from infancy to senility, with women tending to be more prone to the disease than men. The tumours are often well differentiated, with an almost normal glandular appearance, but in many cases they may grow to a remarkable size. The disease is usually fatal because of metastasis to vital organs, rather than a lethal deterioration in the synthesis of life supporting glucocorticoids and mineralocorticoids.

The physiological outcome of cancer in steroid producing organs can often be profound. Tumours may lead to overproduction or impairment of steroid secretion, either of hormones normally produced or of other steroids. In either event, the clinical consequences can be dramatic, often dangerous and even socially distressing. For example, certain adrenal tumours in women result in virilization due to excessive secretion of androgens, with consequent psychological and physical disturbances such as abundant growth of bodily hair and voice changes.

Tumours in organs producing polypeptide hormones can also have dire consequences. In many pituitary tumours, the secretion of tropins is anomalous, with dramatic interference, for example, in sexual activity and fertility. Similarly, tumours of the pancreas can either curtail or overproduce the secretion of insulin and glucagon, with dangerous and even fatal consequences (see Chapter 14). Tumours of other endocrine organs, e.g. thyroid, can produce similar effects.

Human cancers can cause unexpected clinical difficulties. Some tumour cells may acquire the ability to synthesize hormones; for example, certain types of lung cancer actively secrete the normal pituitary hormone, adrenocorticotropin. This is generally referred to as ectopic hormone secretion. Similarly, in women tumours of placental origin (hydatidiform mole and choriocarcinoma) may secrete vast quantities of gonadotropins. The progression or cure of many cancers can be monitored by the cessation of abnormal hormone secretion.

13.6 Treatment of hormone sensitive human cancers

From the overview of general endocrinology presented earlier (see Fig. 13.1), there are many opportunities for curtailing the supply of hormones to tumours. Some of the approaches are far more radical than others and in recent years ingenious and less stressful approaches have been actively explored. Means have also been found to reduce the harmful effects of many drugs and hormones on normal cells.

13.6.1 *Hormonal manipulation*

Endocrine treatment for prostate cancer has been used for more than 40 years. Huggins and Hodges argued that since the normal gland required androgens for its growth, antiandrogenic treatment might inhibit the growth of prostatic tumour cells. This can be done either by removing the main source of androgen—the testes—or by antagonizing androgens with oestrogen administration, usually by giving stilboestrol orally. In many cases this proved to be effective. About 80 per cent of all cases respond at first but eventually most relapse. It was thought that this may have been due to the production of androgens by the adrenals, perhaps stimulated by pituitary hormones produced in increased amounts as a result of castration or oestrogen treatment. Removal of the adrenals or pituitary was then used but these operations are life threatening themselves and the results were not satisfactory. Most tumours eventually become hormone independent and continue to grow. The use and dosage of stilboestrol remains a very controversial issue. Certainly, it is accepted that only low doses should be used, to reduce the risk of breast enlargement, electrolyte and cardiovascular disturbances, as well as psychological problems. Obviously better forms of treatment are required.

Great thought has been given to the targeting principle in the therapy of tumours (see Chapter 18). The ideal is to deliver the drug selectively to the tumour itself, eliminating deleterious side effects. For example, thyroid cancers can be selectively and effectively killed by low doses of radioactive ^{125}I because of the remarkable penchant of the organ for concentrating this halogen. In the prostate, the perceptive suggestion was to use phosphorylated forms of stilboestrol and oestradiol-1β. Until the phosphate groups are removed, the drugs have little if any biological activity; however, the prostate has a remarkably high activity of phosphatases, thus ensuring that the prostatic tumour will tend to concentrate the active drug component specifically, but the clinical results are still uncertain. Another approach of great promise is the development of drugs which selectively inhibit the enzyme, 5 α-reductase, responsible for forming the powerful mitogen, 5 α-dihydrotestosterone, within the prostate tumour itself. Active inhibitors, such as a wide range of 4-azasteroids, are currently on clinical trial; the preliminary findings look encouraging. Prostate cancer produces extremely painful metastases in the bones and relief from this has recently come from a rather surprising quarter. Ketoconazole was originally developed as an antifungal agent and it is now the principal means for relieving bone pain. While the drug is clearly an inhibitor of cytochrome P450 systems, the reason for its action on relief from bone pain remains unknown.

Two areas of recent and very extensive research on prostate cancer have been very disappointing. A lot of effort has been applied to the development of antiandrogens which block the function of the androgen receptors. Many such compounds have been synthesized, including the steroid, cyproterone acetate and the non-steroidal compound, flutamide. Clinically, neither have proved useful in curing prostate cancer, although they have been effective in individual cases. Indeed, the usefulness of cyproterone acetate has been limited virtually to its legal acceptance as the means for chemical castration of persistent sexual offenders throughout Western Europe. A real problem that remains is how hormone sensitive an individual prostatic tumour really is. It seems that measurement of androgen receptors is not the way forward. Persuasive evidence is beginning to emerge that the activity of 5α-reductase is a far better indicator of the hormone sensitivity of a given tumour; after all, it is beyond doubt that this enzyme complex is induced and stringently regulated by androgens.

The most revolutionary proposal for the successful arrest of prostate cancer by hormonal means has come from research in Canada; suppression of androgen secretion in patients with prostatic cancer, by a drug combination of antiandrogens, such as flutamide or anandron, plus a powerful range of synthetic analogues of gonadotropin releasing hormone. The antiandrogens block the peripheral effects of any androgens while the GnRH analogues suppress the hypothalamic pituitary axis and also reduce the gonadotropin receptors in the testis by down regulation, thus effectively suppressing the secretion of androgens. Early results on this approach seemed to be promising but later work has not supported the original enthusiasm. Nonetheless, new approaches for the hormonal manipulation of prostate cancer are needed, because radical surgical removal of the prostate is now seen as a difficult and unsatisfactory procedure; metastases of the disease cannot be treated by surgical means.

Many of the considerations on prostate cancer are relevant to breast cancer in women. Methods are being sought to replace radical surgery on the breast or on the endocrine glands. Such practices as hypophysectomy and radical mastectomy of the breast tumour are much rarer now than in the past (see Chapter 16). As in the prostate, the normal breast, and many of its tumours, respond to the relevant sex hormones, mainly oestrogens and progestins.

Two aspects of the research and management of breast cancer have been most encouraging. First, it is now accepted that measurements on the concentrations of oestrogen and progesterone receptors is valuable in the successful management of individual patients. The measurement of progesterone receptors is based on sound evidence that they are oestrogen induced proteins. If the tumour is receptor positive, r^+, then hormonal manipulation is advised; if r^-, then chemotherapy should be used. Second, there are several antioestrogens available now and tamoxifen in particular has been of striking benefit in the treatment of many women; about 30 per cent of all patients had an objective response and a further 20 per cent showed some clinical improvement. The results are better in postmenopausal women. For premenopausal women, ablation of the ovary, either by surgery or X–rays, remains the first choice for reduction of oestrogen levels.

Synthetic progestins, of long biological life and which may be taken orally, are finding wide and successful use in the treatment of endometrial cancer. Antioestrogens may also have an important role to play here in the future.

Synthetic glucocorticoids, especially prednisone, prednisolone, and their fluorinated counterparts, have also been invaluable for the treatment of many types of lymphoma and leukaemia, as well as Hodgkin's disease. Such approaches are only of value if the malignancy is r^+, containing receptors for glucocorticoids; this is not always the case. Even if cells are r^+, hormones alone will not eradicate the disease and additional chemotherapy is required (see Chapter 17). Novel glucocorticoids which are more specific in their action on r^+ cells are currently under study. For example, triamcinolone acetonide 21-oic acid methyl ester is a potent glucocorticoid without the side effects of any of its structural congeners; in particular, it neither suppresses the secretion of natural glucocorticoids from the adrenal glands nor promotes involution of the thymus. A major problem in treatment of hormone responsive tumours is the growth of hormone independent tumour cells.

13.6.2 *Chemotherapy*

We have not yet explored all the possibilities for the successful treatment of breast and prostate cancer by hormonal means. Surprises and new opportunities may be in store. For example, there is a growing and impressive body of evidence that aminoglutethimide may be very valuable in the treatment of most hormone sensitive tumours; this drug, like ketoconazole, is an inhibitor of enzyme complexes containing cytochrome P450 and thus provides a clinical means of suppressing steroid hormone synthesis. In both these tumours, the administration of pharmacological doses of steroid hormones, including glucocorticoids, has often been found to be beneficial. There is no plausible explanation of these observations in molecular terms. As mentioned earlier, the final arrest of hormone sensitive human tumours will depend on a combination of hormonal manipulation and chemotherapy.

Further reading

Henderson, B. E., Ross, R. K., Pike, M. C., and Casagrande, J. T. (1982). Endogenous hormones as a major factor in human cancer. *Cancer Research* **42**, 3232–39.

Lupulesco, A. (1982). *Hormones and carcinogenesis.* Praeger Press. A book containing sound and detailed information. Highly recommended.

14

The neuroendocrine system and its tumours

J. M. POLAK and S. R. BLOOM

The classical view of endocrinology, meaning the study of hormone producing glands and their disorders, has been challenged seriously following the discovery that many body tissues contain the so called 'diffuse neuroendocrine system' (see on). The cells of this system produce 'regulatory peptides', capable of acting not only at a distance, as chemical messengers or hormones, but also locally as paracrine substances or as neurotransmitters/neuromodulators (see Fig. 14.1). The reason for this multiplicity of actions is that regulatory peptides are produced by two different classes of tissue cells. Active peptides can be produced by endocrine cells or by neural elements. The former release the peptide either into the blood stream (circulating hormones) or locally, in a paracrine manner, whereas the latter release the peptide from the nerve terminal after neuronal depolarization to act as neurotransmitters/neuromodulators.

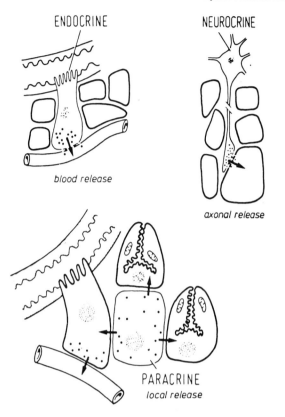

Fig. 14.1 Diagrammatic representation of the tripartite mode of action of the component cells of the diffuse neuroendocrine system.

Peptide producing endocrine cells are dispersed throughout the body, often intermingled within non-endocrine tissue. These cells were first recognized by Feyrter who called them 'clear cells' due to their weak histological staining, or cells of the 'diffuse endocrine system', in view of their dispersed, intermingled localization and possible regulatory function. The special histochemical properties of these cells led Pearse to apply the term 'APUD' (amine precursor uptake and decarboxylation) to them whereas the similar morphological characteristics these cells share with neurons (i.e. dense core secretory granules) led Fujita to propose the term 'paraneurons'. The recognition that neural tissue, often anatomically closely associated with endocrine cells, is also capable of producing and secreting active peptides led to the expansion of the 'diffuse endocrine system' to 'diffuse neuroendocrine system'.

Regulatory peptides are being discovered at an exponential rate, due to advances in chemical extraction procedures and, in particular, to molecular biology. The latter approach has been instrumental also in the determination of the chemical structure of the pre-pro-molecules from which smaller active peptides are generated (Fig. 14.2).

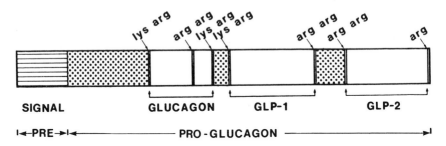

Fig. 14.2 Schematic representation of the pre-pro-glucagon molecule indicating the positions of peptides of the glucagon family.

It is beyond the scope of this short review to describe in detail the characteristics of each individual peptide. The reader is, however, referred to a number of extensive review articles and to Table 14.1.

14.1 Morphological features of peptide containing endocrine cells and nerves

Peptide containing endocrine cells are found scattered throughout the body and those cells located in hollow organs frequently possess microvilli extruded into the lumen. The latter can be visualized better at the electron microscope level. Endocrine cells have intracytoplasmic secretory granules, the morphology of which, including their electron density and their limiting membrane and size, permits separation into various cell types. Secretory granules tend to be located at the basal pole of cells, close to the basement membrane and to the organ blood supply. Endocrine cells frequently display a cytoplasmic elongation along the basement membrane. The arrangement of these features suggests functional properties: receptor functions are attributed to microvilli; peptide product is stored in secretory granules and a cytoplasmic extension indicates a possible local or paracrine role for some of the peptide containing endocrine cells.

Numerous neurotransmitters have been identified now in the nervous system and these include not only the classical neurotransmitters, acetylcholine and noradrenaline, but also amino acid neurotransmitters and, in

Table 14.1 Neuroendocrine regulatory peptides

Peptide	Distribution	Endocrine cells (C) Nerves (N)	Main known actions
Insulin	Pancreatic islets (β cells)	C	Blood sugar
Glucagon	Pancreatic islets (α cells)	C	Blood sugar
Enteroglucagon	Intestine	C	Trophic to gut
Secretin	Small intestine	C	Pancreatic bicarbonate secretion
Gastric inhibitory polypeptide (glucose dependent insulino-tropic peptide) (GIP)	Small intestine	C	Insulin secretion, gastric acid secretion
Vasoactive intestinal polypeptide (VIP)	Central and peripheral nervous system	N	Muscle relaxation, vasodila-tation, secretion
Peptide with histidine	Central and peripheral nervous system	N	Muscle relaxation, secretion
Growth hormone-releasing	Hypothalamus	N	Growth hormone production
Gastrin	Pyloric stomach and small intestine	C	Gastric acid secretion
Cholecystokinin (CCK)	Small intestine	C	Gall bladder contraction, pancreatic enzyme secretion
CCK-8	Central and peripheral nervous system	N	Excitatory
Gastrin-releasing peptide (GRP) (see also Neuromedin C)	Lung, central and peripheral nervous system	C, N	Trophic, release of other regulatory peptides
(Bombesin)	Amphibian skin and gastro-intestinal tract	C	
Neuromedin B, Neuromedin C (=GRP main form)	Spinal cord (porcine)	N	
Growth hormone-releasing factor (GRF)	Hypothalamus	N	Growth hormone production
Substance P	Central and peripheral nervous system	N	Sensory: vasodilatation, muscle contraction

Table 14.1 —*continued*

Peptide	Distribution	Endocrine cells (C) Nerves (N)	Main known actions
Neurokinin A (= Substance K, Neuromedin L); Neurokinin B (Neuromedin K)	Spinal cord (porcine)	N	
Pancreatic polypeptide	Pancreatic islets	C	Pancreatic enzyme secretion, gall bladder contraction
Peptide with C– and N–terminal tyrosine (PYY)	Intestinal system	C	
Neural peptide with tyrosine (NPY)	Central and peripheral intestinal tract	N	Vasoconstriction
Motilin	Small intestine	C	Gut motility
Somatostatin	Stomach, intestine, pancreatic islets, thyroid gland, central and peripheral nervous system	C, N	Release and action of many peptides; may be antitrophic
Neurotensin	Intestine, adrenal medulla, central nervous system	C	Vasodilation, gastric acid secretion
Parathyroid hormone	Parathyroid gland	C	Blood calcium
Calcitonin	Thyroid gland	C	Blood calcium
Calcitonin gene-related peptide (CGRP)	Central and peripheral nervous system	N	Vasodilatation; sensory
Adrenocorticotrophic hormone (ACTH)	Anterior and intermediate lobes of pituitary gland; central nervous system	C, N	Production of adrenal corticosteroids
Corticotrophin-like intermediate lobe peptide (CLIP)	Intermediate lobe of pituitary gland	C	
Melanocyte-stimulating hormone (MSH) (α, β, γ)	(Anterior) and intermediate lobes of pituitary gland, central nervous system	C, N	Skin pigmentation

Hormone	Source	Classification	Action
Endorphin (α and β)	Anterior and intermediate lobes of pituitary gland, central nervous system	C, N	—Opioid
β-lipotrophin	Anterior and intermediate lobes of pituitary gland, central nervous system	C, N	
Dynorphin	(Anterior) and intermediate lobes of pituitary gland, central nervous system	C, N	Opioid
Enkephalin (met- and leu-)	Central and peripheral nervous system, adrenal medulla	N, C	Opioid
Vasopressin	Central nervous system (neurosecretory)	N	Antidiuretic
Oxytocin	Central nervous system (neurosecretory)	N	Contraction of uterus and let down of milk
Thyroid hormone releasing hormone (TRH)	Hypothalamus	N	Release of TSH
Luteinizing hormone releasing hormone (LHRH)	Hypothalamus	N	Release of gonadotrophins
Corticotrophin releasing factor (CRF)	Hypothalamus	N	ACTH production
Growth hormone	Anterior pituitary gland	C	Growth
Prolactin	Anterior pituitary gland	C	Milk production
Placental lactogen	Placenta	C	Lactogenic, trophic, lipolytic
Thyroid stimulating hormone (TSH)	Anterior pituitary gland	C	Thyroid hormone production
Follicle stimulating hormone (FSH)	Anterior pituitary gland	C	Ovarian follicle formation, spermatogenesis
Luteinizing hormone (LH)	Anterior pituitary gland	C	Ovulation, gonadal hormone production
Chorionic gonadotrophin	Placenta	C	Luteotrophic
Various recently discovered peptides	Heart (atrium)	?C	Sodium excretion, diuresis, blood pressure

particular, peptide neurotransmitters. All can be identified in cell bodies, nerve fibres, and terminals by the use of specific antibodies.

14.2 Techniques for the visualization of the 'diffuse neuroendocrine system'

14.2.1 *Light microscopy*

14.2.1.1 *General markers.* Secretory granules in the cytoplasm of endo-crine cells have the ability to take up silver salts and precipitate them into a silver deposit with (argyrophilia) or without (argentaffinia) addition of a reducing agent. For amine containing endocrine cells, argentaffin (Masson) silver impregnation is used and, for other endocrine cells, a number of argyrophilic methods have been proposed. Among these, one of the most commonly used is the silver impregnation method of Grimelius. These techniques work well also in neuroendocrine tumour tissue.

Neuron specific enolase (NSE) is an isoenzyme of the glycolytic enzyme enolase. Antibodies to NSE are known to immunostain endo-crine cells and their related nerves. They are also useful for the demonstration of neuroendocrine differentiation in tumours. Neuron specific enolase is a cytosolic non-granular enzyme and thus antibodies to it will be useful for demonstrating poorly granulated neuroendocrine tissue (e.g. small cell carcinoma of the lung, Merkel cell tumours of the skin, see on).

Chromogranin is a protein(s) originally extracted from the adrenal medulla. Polyclonal sera and monoclonal antibodies have now been raised against chromagranin and shown to be excellent markers for secretory granules in normal and tumour endocrine cells.

The occurrence of intermediate filaments, e.g. vimentin, keratin, and neurofilaments, has been investigated extensively, particularly in neuro-endocrine tumours. Expression of these intermediate filaments is not a general phenomenon and occurs only in some tumours (e.g. small cell carcinoma of the lung, Merkel cell tumour).

14.2.1.2 *Peptide markers.* Immunocytochemistry, using region specific antibodies to regulatory peptides and their pre-pro-forms, has been used extensively for the visualization of the specific components of the diffuse neuroendocrine system (both cells and nerves) and of their tumours.

14.2.2 *Electron microscopy*

Electron microscopy has been fundamental in determining the neuro-endocrine differentiation of normal and tumour tissue. By electron microscopy, the presence of dense core secretory granules is easily

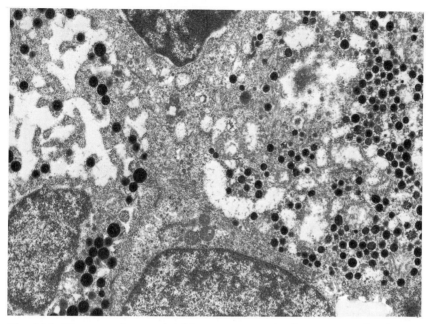

Fig. 14.3 Electron micrograph of human pancreatic glucagonoma showing two distinct secretory granule populations in neighbouring tumour cells. Glutaraldehyde fixation, uranyl acetate and lead citrate counterstains. ($\times 8600$)

distinguishable (Fig. 14.3). Secretory granules are not destroyed by poor fixation, and thus can be distinguished in tissue fixed for routine pathology. In conventional osmium staining for electron microscopy, the limiting membrane of the granule is easily distinguishable and analysis of the size, electron density, halo, and characteristics of this membrane can thus be seen. These features are indicative, especially in normal tissue, of the production by a given cell of a particular peptide.

14.2.3 *Hybridization histochemistry*

Advances in molecular biology now permit the construction of probes (nucleotide sequences) for a given peptide. The use of cDNA probes, complementary to messenger RNA directing the synthesis of a given peptide, and its use in the technique of 'hybridization histochemistry' allows morphologists to visualize the biosynthetic events prior to peptide package in granules. A number of different methods for 'hybridization histochemistry' have been proposed. These probes are labelled with radioisotope or biotin and the end product is visualized by autoradiography or by methods permitting the visualization of biotin labels.

14.2.4 *Receptor visualization*

Peptide binding sites can be visualized by autoradiography or by immunogold staining procedures. The techniques of *in vitro* auto-radiography using tissue sections and emulsion coated coverslips or sensitive film have been developed for the visualization of peptide bind-ing sites. Densitometric image analysis of these preparations is now being used for quantitation.

14.3 Neuroendocrine tumours

14.3.1 *Nomenclature*

Various terms have been used to describe tumours arising from the diffuse endocrine system, e.g. carcinoma, APUDoma; there is no general consensus on nomenclature.

 The advent of modern technology, such as immunocytochemistry and radioimmunoassay, allows further characterization of these tumours in terms of their function. Neuroendocrine tumours frequently produce more than one regulatory peptide (mixed endocrine tumours), but often one circulating peptide is responsible for the associated clinical syn-drome. In such cases the tumour is frequently referred to by the name of this active secretory product, e.g. gastrinoma and insulinoma. In view of these difficulties, we propose three levels of nomenclature. First, 'neuro-endocrine tumours' is to be used as a generic term to describe all tumours thought to be derived from the diffuse neuroendocrine system and showing the general histological, histochemical, and immunohisto-chemical features of such cells. Second, terms may refer to particular histological patterns at specific sites, e.g. islet cell tumour of pancreas or oat cell carcinoma of lung. Third, an indication of the major peptide secretions of the tumour is included. In this system each level is com-plementary to the others and a full description of a tumour should include mention of all three.

14.3.2 *General features of endocrine tumours*

14.3.2.1 *Clinical features.* It is difficult to assess the true incidence of endocrine tumours but well recognized, functioning tumours are clearly uncommon, with the exception of small cell carcinoma of the lung.

 Clinical features of some functioning tumours may be obscured by the presence in the circulation of more than one regulatory peptide with counteracting effects. In addition to hormonal effects, nonspecific mani-festations, depending on site, size, and invasion, may be present. Clinical suspicion is usually roused when more common diseases have been excluded. This sometimes delays diagnosis, with adverse effects on the prognosis. High levels of secretion of a regulatory peptide may provide a useful assay; however, it must be remembered that circulating levels of active peptides can be elevated in diseases other than tumours. Many pre-operative, non-invasive techniques are also widely used, including a series of stimulation and suppression tests for the particular hormone. Further, a series of localization techniques are used (see Chapter 16).

14.3.2.2 *Biochemistry.* Highly sensitive specific radioimmunoassays for the measurement of regulatory peptides in blood and tissue are readily available and allow early diagnosis of functioning tumours. Thus, very small tumours may be diagnosed clinically and biochemically, but localization of the precise site of the tumour may still be a problem.

14.3.2.3 *Histology.* Peptide producing endocrine cells are frequently unevenly distributed within a tumour. It is therefore very important to sample a large number of specimens taken randomly throughout the tumour mass. The growth pattern of endocrine tumours is quite characteristic. Tumours are composed of uniform cells with few mitoses arranged in irregular masses, ribbons or glandular structures. A glassy, amorphous degeneration of the tumour stroma (amyloid) is common and sometimes extensive. A more functional criterion of malignancy has recently been proposed. This is the production and release of alpha human chorionic gonadotropin (HCG) by many malignant endocrine tumours. This criterion is especially relevant for pancreatic endocrine tumours.

14.3.2.4 *Electron microscopy.* Using electron microscopy, tumours have been found to contain variable numbers of secretory granules, but often peptide producing tumour cells store less peptide than their normal counterparts. It is generally accepted that a poorly granulated tumour reflects high secretory activity, and this frequently correlates with the presence of abundant ribosomes, rough endoplasmic reticulum and prominent Golgi apparatus. Poorly granulated tumours are usually associated with significantly elevated levels of circulating hormone. This suggests that one of the metabolic defects in endocrine tumour cells resides in the control of hormone secretion.

14.3.3 *Ectopic hormone production*

By definition, ectopic hormones are produced by a tumour arising in an organ which does not secrete the substance normally. For example, Cushing's syndrome, caused by the overproduction of adrenal hormones, may develop as a result of the production of adrenal corticotrophic hormone (ACTH), a pituitary hormone which stimulates the adrenal glands, e.g. by neuroendocrine tumours of the pancreas or of the lung. Synthesis and sometimes secretion of a number of peptides by endocrine and non-endocrine tumours may be much more common than is realized. Proof of ectopic hormone production is difficult and requires clinical and biochemical methods as well as morphological techniques and cell culture. Symptoms of ectopic hormone secretion as tumour markers are important. Ectopic hormone production may occur in tandem with normal hormone secretion. The pathogenesis of ectopic hormone production has not been elucidated yet. It has been postulated that some or all tumour cells have abnormal regulation of DNA transcription, mRNA processing, or even, perhaps, defective post-translational modification of pre-pro-hormone.

14.3.4 *Multi hormonal tumours*

Multiple hormone production may be caused by single or multiple endocrine neoplasia (MEN). The production of more than one hormone by a single endocrine tumour was thought to be uncommon. This was due mainly to the fact that the effects of one secreted hormone were clinically predominant and thus obscured the presence of other less active peptides. It is now recognized that some patients have symptoms attributable to the simultaneous secretion of more than one hormone and may show a transition of effects from one to another, sometimes due to treatment (chemotherapy). In most instances the appropriate hormones have been shown to be produced by separate cell types both at the light and electron microscopical levels.

14.4 Individual tumours

14.4.1 *Tumours of the pancreas and gut*

14.4.1.1 *Insulinomas.* β-cells in the pancreatic islets secrete insulin, and insulinomas are one of the many causes of hypoglycaemia (low blood sugar). They constitute 70–75 per cent of all pancreatic endocrine tumours and are about equally common in both sexes. All patients with insulinomas should also be checked for other endocrine disturbances since β or non-β cell adenomas can be associated with other inherited endocrine neoplasms of the multiple endocrine neoplasia (MEN) syndrome. Clinical features are almost always present, even with small tumours. Hypoglycaemia is manifested by headaches, blurred vision, sweating, hunger, and palpitations. Symptoms are usually intermittent and thus a patient can be misdiagnosed as having psychiatric, cardiac or neurological disease. The highest incidence of insulinomas is found between the ages 30–60 years. Virtually all insulinomas are localized in the pancreas. About 90 per cent of them are solitary and most (84–96 per cent) are benign.

Insulinomas, like most other endocrine tumours, produce different molecular forms of insulin, C peptide, and pro-insulin in variable proportions.

14.4.1.2 *Tumours associated with the Zollinger–Ellison syndrome (gastrinomas).* Gastrinomas represent 20–25 per cent of pancreatic endocrine tumours. They occur most often between 30 and 50 years of age and there is a slight male preponderance. The clinical features, as originally described by Zollinger and Ellison, are intractable gastric, duodenal and jejunal ulceration, bleeding, and very high gastric acid secretion. These features are rarely found nowadays since the tumours are usually diagnosed at an earlier stage due to the increasing awareness of the condition and availability of assays. Plasma gastrin levels are usually very high, but calcium stimulation of gastrin levels, a commonly employed diagnostic test, permits the distinction between a gastrinoma and other hypergastrinaemic conditions associated with recurrent peptic ulcers. Eighty-five per cent of gastrinomas are found in the pancreas. Extra pancreatic gastrinomas are found, for instance, in the duodenum (13 per cent) and in other areas (1 per cent), including the stomach, upper jejunum, and bile ducts. This distribution in the frequency of anatomical sites for gastrinomas does not fit with the distribution of gastrin-containing (G) cells in normal tissue; in particular, gastrin containing cells are not found in the adult human pancreas but have been described in the foetal pancreas.

At least 60 per cent of gastrinomas are malignant. The tumours frequently metastasize, especially to the liver. Histologically these tumours have the typical appearance of neuroendocrine tumours, e.g. immunoreactivity for neuron specific enolase, chromogranin, and various segments of gastrin and pre-pro-gastrin. Tumours producing gastrin frequently secrete other regulatory peptides, in particular pancreatic polypeptide.

14.4.1.3 *Diarrhoeagenic (WDHA) tumour syndrome, VIPomas or PHMoma syndrome.* Certain patients with non-β islet cell tumours and severe diarrhoea did not meet the criteria for the diagnosis of gastrinoma. The absence of gastric acid hypersecretion in such patients was also reported. Since the discovery that vasoactive intestinal polypeptide (VIP) is produced frequently and in large concentrations by such tumours, the word VIPoma was coined. VIPomas represent 3–5 per cent of all pancreatic endocrine tumours. The syndrome is characterized by watery diarrhoea. Approximately two thirds of patients complain of abdominal colic and some have intermittent high faecal fat output. There is often a significant weight loss. At operation, a high amount of alkaline secretion from the pancreas is found. Some patients may also suffer from occasional flushing attacks. Fifty to seventy-five per cent of tumours are malignant. The tumours are often quite large (2–7 cm). VIP is known to be produced both by endocrine and neural tumours, and histologically tumours show either classical features of islet cell tumours of the pancreas or features of ganglioneuroblastomas.

14.4.1.4 *Glucagonomas.* The typical clinical picture shows the following symptoms: a migratory skin rash localized to the lower abdomen, perineum and legs, an abnormal glucose tolerance test, anaemia, a sore red tongue, angular stomatitis, severe weight loss, depression, tendency to develop overwhelming infection, and venous thrombosis (in about one third of patients).

The awareness of the characteristic skin rash as a cutaneous marker of internal malignancy and the availability of plasma analysis for glucagon opened the way for a large number of case reports, and it now seems that glucagonomas are more frequent than was previously thought. Administration of zinc induces a fast remission of the skin rash. This led to the postulate that the skin condition may be due partly to zinc deficiency. The disease occurs most often between 40–70 years of age and appears to be slightly more common in women than in men. More than 60 per cent of glucagonomas causing the symptoms are malignant. The mixed nature of glucagonomas, also quite a common feature, is further validated by peptide immunocytochemistry. Pancreatic polypeptide producing cells are found frequently, but also insulin, somatostatin and gastrin producing cells may be found. Glucagon producing pancreatic adenomas constitute part of the MEN Type I syndrome.

14.4.1.5 *Tumours producing pancreatic polypeptide (PP): PPomas.* Oversecretion of PP is one of the most frequent associations noted with well defined functioning neuroendocrine tumours. Tumours most frequently containing PP cells include VIPomas, glucagonomas, and insulinomas. Gastrinomas show a lesser frequency of PP production. PP is rarely present in other classes of neuroendocrine tumours (ileal or lung carcinoids (see on) may occasionally also produce PP). Therefore, PP positive immunostaining in a metastasis of an endocrine tumour of unknown origin points to the possibility of the primary tumour being present in the pancreas.

14.4.1.6 *Somatostatinomas.* The association of somatostatin production by endocrine tumours, with a defined clinical syndrome, remains in dispute. Most somatostatinomas are solitary and localized in the pancreas; fewer tumours have been described in the gut. Somatostatin containing tumours are frequently malignant and their growth pattern is similar to that described for other neuroendocrine tumours.

14.4.1.7 *Growth hormone releasing factor (GRF) producing tumours, or GRFomas or acromegalic tumours.* Tumours of the pancreas associated with acromegaly have frequently been described in the literature, and GRF has now been found to be produced by pancreatic endocrine neoplasms.

14.4.1.8 *Carcinoids and serotonin producing tumours.* As the term carcinoid has been associated at various times with a morphological appearance, a clinical syndrome and a biochemical feature (the production of serotonin), its usage has often been confusing. In this section, it is used to describe endocrine tumours of the gut whether or not they are associated with the clinical features of serotonin production. The typical carcinoid syndrome consists of episodes of flushing, hypertension, diarrhoea, cough, wheezing, and localized capillary dilatation. Fibrosis, oedema, pellagra-like lesions of the skin, peptic ulcer, and abdominal fibrosis can also be present. The symptoms described above are particularly prominent once the tumour has metastasized to the liver, allowing the tumour products to enter the circulation. Seventy-five per cent of serotonin producing tumours arise from the gastrointestinal tract. Unlike other endocrine neoplasms, the size of the tumour may be considered as a prognostic factor. When a tumour measures more than 2 cm in diameter it is considered malignant and it is likely that metastases are already present. Frequently carcinoids are multiple and sometimes associated with other malignant neoplasms. Serotonin can be demonstrated by use of specific antibodies, which are now widely available, and is particularly prominent in midgut carcinoids but is usually absent from foregut and hindgut tumours. Apart from serotonin, carcinoid tumours of the bowel have been reported to produce other regulatory peptides. Gastric carcinoids are a separate entity. These have been shown to occur in association with mucosal atrophy (atrophic gastritis) and pernicious anaemia or may occur in patients in which acid secretion has been blocked completely by newly discovered drugs for ulcer treatment. These gastric tumours have been reputed to produce histamine.

14.4.1.9 *Pituitary gland tumours.* In man the pituitary is divided into two lobes, with the anterior lobe being known as the adenohypophysis and the posterior, or neural, lobe as the neurohypophysis (Chapter 13). The former produces at least six hormones having major effects on metabolic processes and on other endocrine glands. Hormone production is stimulated or inhibited by hypothalamic factors arriving at the anterior pituitary via the hypothalamic-hypophyseal portal circulation and by feedback from the hormonal secretions of the target organs. The neurohypophysis is an extension of the brain containing a variety of peptides and amines, in addition to the main neurosecretory hormones, vasopressin and oxytocin.

Tumours of the pituitary gland are relatively frequent. Prolactin secreting tumours are by far the most common and are followed by growth hormone secreting tumours and then ACTH secreting tumours. Gonadotropin and thyrotropin secreting tumours are infrequent although recent reports subclassify the so called 'chromophobe' adenomas as gonadotrophin producing tumours. Mixed tumours, secreting more than one hormone, are a common finding. The cell of origin of all these tumours has been disputed but the frequent occurrence of 'mixed' pituitary adenomas might be thought to favour the existence of precursor cells which give rise to all tumour cell types.

Prolactin secreting adenomas cause infertility and impairment of testicular function, milk secretion, and amenorrhoea. Tumours of this type are frequently poorly granulated. Thus, attempts to immunostain prolactin in an actively secreting, poorly granulated tumour may be unrewarding or the peptide may be present in the Golgi area.

Pituitary tumours associated with Cushing's syndrome have been shown to react with antibodies to various portions of peptides of the ACTH and related hormones. Tumour secreting peptides of the ACTH family are thus a very variable entity.

14.4.1.10 *Thyroid tumours.* Two classes of neuroendocrine tumour of the thyroid, medullary carcinoma, are now recognized: the sporadic, and the familial types. The medullary carcinoma is one of the few malignant tumours with an inheritance of an autosomal dominant type with high penetrance. Twenty per cent of all cases of medullary carcinomas are thought to be genetically determined and these usually present with phaeochromocytomas (tumours of the adrenal medulla) and other tumours as part of the multiple endocrine neoplasia (MEN Type II) syndrome. The tumour arises from special calcitonin producing cells (C cells) in the thyroid and C cell hyperplasia precedes and accompanies inherited medullary carcinoma. The defect is probably at the level of C cell hyperplasia and the development of the malignancy is possibly a secondary defect. It is, therefore, exceedingly important to screen relatives of a patient with inherited medullary carcinoma for the possibility of C cell hyperplasia, by measurement of plasma calcitonin. Furthermore, it is necessary to analyse the entire thyroid of sporadic medullary carcinomas for the possible presence of C cell hyperplasia, and organize subsequent screening of relatives.

Medullary carcinomas present all the classical features of neuroendocrine neoplasms and a wide variety of histological types has been described. Calcitonin and its flanking peptide PDN-21 or katacalcin are the peptides most frequently found in medullary carcinomas. Calcitonin gene related peptide (CGRP) is also found often in medullary carcinomas. Other peptides or substances have also been shown to be produced by medullary carcinomas, and these include ACTH, neurotensin, bombesin, somatostatin, serotonin, prostaglandins, and substance P. The production of multiple hormones or other peptides may explain the bizarre clinical features often encountered in medullary carcinomas, including protracted diarrhoea.

14.4.1.11 *Tumours of the adrenal medulla and paraganglia.* Phaeochromocytoma is the most frequently found tumour of the adrenal medulla, but ganglioneuromatous differentiation can also be found. A phaeochromocytoma is clinically recognized in the following circumstances: as a familial case, episodic hypertensive episodes, persistent hypertension with increased urine excretion of vanillyl mandelic acid, noradrenalin or adrenalin.

The size of the tumour ranges from a microscopic lesion to over 2 kg in weight, but most are about 5–6 cm diameter and weigh an average of 9 g. Histologically, the appearance of phaeochromocytomas is quite bizarre, with very many irregular cells of variable size, structure, and arrangement. Many multinucleated, gigantic cells can be found which, at the ultrastructural level, contain numerous distinctive electron dense secretory granules. Until recently, the normal adrenal and derivative tumours were regarded as producing catecholamines, but lately regulatory peptides have been found increasingly to be produced by both the normal and tumour tissue. These include peptides of the enkephalin/dynorphin family, neurotensin and, very recently, a novel peptide known to produce marked vasoconstriction, neuropeptide Y.

Phaeochromocytomas may be a component of the familial MEN II syndrome together with medullary carcinoma of the thyroid, parathyroid hyperplasia or adenoma. Phaeochromocytomas are usually benign tumours but malignancy can occur when tumours are found bilaterally. They occur in adults between the ages of 25–55 years.

Tumours of paraganglia are called extra-adrenal phaeochromocytomas in Europe, and paragangliomas in America. These can occur all along the sympathetic chain and in the para-aortic bodies. Paraganglia form a widely disseminated system of small sensory and perhaps local neurosecretory organs that develop in foetal life, persist in infancy and thereafter become smaller and more difficult to find in certain parts of the body such as the fibrous tissue behind the peritoneum along the aorta. Several lie close to other major blood vessels, in or near nerves or ganglia, or are located in organs such as the lung or duodenum. The urinary bladder also contains paraganglia and phaeochromocytomas of the urinary bladder have been reported.

14.4.2 *Respiratory tract tumours*

The respiratory tract is also a common site for neuroendocrine tumours. This is logical as the 'diffuse neuroendocrine system' is well represented in the normal respiratory tract. In fact, one of the active peptides frequently produced by small cell carcinomas is bombesin/GRP which is also present in normal mucosal endocrine cells. Within neuroendocrine tumours of the lung, the carcinoid seems to represent the benign end of a continuous spectrum which ends in the small cell carcinoma, the malignant counterpart of neuroendocrine tumours. The lung is a fairly frequent site of carcinoids, in fact 12 per cent of all carcinoids arise in the lung. However, carcinoids represent only 1 per cent of all lung tumours. The highest incidence of bronchial carcinoids occurs in the 31–40 years age group, with a slight preponderance in females (62 per cent). The tumour usually arises in the main bronchi but may be located in the lung periphery. Multicentric growth has been described and carcinoids may be part of a plurigiandular syndrome. Carcinoid tumours are generally well demarcated and may either just protrude into the bronchial lumen ('iceberg' tumour) or may be predominantly endo-bronchial in their growth pattern. Microscopically, carcinoids of the lung do not differ from other carcinoids or neuroendocrine tumours, although broncial carcinoids grow slowly and have a low malignant potential. Ultrastructurally, carcinoid tumours of the lung are frequently well granulated. Immunocytochemistry reveals a variety of products being produced by carcinoid tumours, in particular serotonin, bombesin, PP, and occasionally ACTH, with or without overt clinical syndromes. Small cell carcinoma of the lung is the malignant counterpart of lung endocrine tumours. It is one of the most frequent neuroendocrine tumour types and comprises 20 per cent of all bronchial carcinomas. Small cell carcinomas are divided into two main types depending on cell size: (i) oat cell type, consisting of small oat shaped cells with a finely granular chromatin pattern, no nucleolus and very sparse cytoplasm, and (ii) intermediate cell type, composed of slightly larger cells with characteristics similar to the oat cell type but with more abundant cytoplasm. There does not seem to be a correlation between the histologial sub type and patient survival. The best neuroendocrine marker for the characterization of small cell carcinomas is the non-granular marker neuron specific enolase. Small cell carcinomas of the lung have long been associated with hormonal abnormalities, particularly Cushing's syndrome and inappropriate anti-diuretic hormone secretion. Extensive data are now available indicating that bombesin released from tumour cells of the small cell carcinoma acts in an autocrine (paracrine) manner. The tumour cells release their product into the vicinity and in turn activate tumour cell receptors to enhance growth.

Small cell carcinomas of the lung are aggressive neoplasms, having the poorest prognosis of all lung tumours with an overall five year survival rate of only 2 per cent. The tumour is generally extremely sensitive to combined chemotherapy and radiotherapy, whereas other lung tumours are more amenable to surgery.

14.5 Conclusions

Studies of the 'diffuse neuroendocrine system' are a new facet of endocrinology and expand the classical view of glandular endocrinology. Regulatory peptides are still being discovered and their role in the control of body functions is being firmly established. Advances in molecular biology make possible determination of the structure of peptide precursors and the use of region specific antibodies to the various portions of the molecule are opening up new investigative areas of peptide neuroendocrinology. The application of other modern techniques now allows not only investigation of the stored peptide but of all intracellular steps leading to this peptide synthesis, including visualization of the mRNA. It is predictable that more functional studies will be forthcoming, analysing the quantities of messenger in relation to peptide biosynthesis. The site of action of regulatory peptide receptors can now be analysed and therapeutic agents are being developed to interact with particular regulatory peptides specifically, either at the site of their production or release or at their receptor level, and therefore new avenues for the treatment of this very interesting group of tumours are becoming available.

Further reading

Bloom, S. R., and Polak, J. M. (1981). *Gut hormones* (2nd Edition). Churchill Livingstone, Edinburgh.

Polak, J. M., and Bloom, S. R. (1985). *Endocrine tumours.* Churchill Livingstone, Edinburgh.

—— and —— (1985). Pathology of peptide-producing neuroendocrine tumours. *British Journal of Hospital Medicine* **53**, 153–7.

—— and —— (1983). Regulatory peptides: key factors in the control of bodily functions. *British Medical Journal* **286**, 1461–6.

—— and Van Noorden, S. (1983). *Immunocytochemistry: practical applications in pathology and biology.* Wright, Bristol.

—— and Varndell, I. M. (1984). *Immunolabelling for electron microscopy.* Elsevier, Amsterdam.

Varndell, I. M., Polak, J. M., Sikri, K. L., Minth, C. D., Bloom, S. R., and Dixon, J. E. (1984). Visualization of messenger RNA directing peptide synthesis by *in situ* hybridization using a novel single-stranded cDNA probe: potential for the investigation of gene expression and endocrine cell activity. *Histochemistry* **81**, 597–601.

15

Immunology of cancer

PETER BEVERLEY

15.1 Introduction to the immune system

Animals or men born without a properly functioning immune system suffer from multiple infections and usually die at an early age. Thus the primary function of the immune system is to defend the animal against pathogenic microorganisms, but the system will also react against other foreign substances. It was proposed, as long ago as the turn of the century by Paul Ehrlich, that the immune system might also prevent, or at least retard, the growth of many tumours. In this Chapter I shall examine this hypothesis but to do this it is necessary to explain first how the immune system works.

15.2 Organization of the immune system

Many of the cells of the immune system (white cells or leucocytes) are found throughout the body because they circulate in the blood stream and also migrate into tissues, particularly at sites of inflammation. Lymphoid cells are also found in specialized lymphoid organs, the bone marrow, thymus, spleen and lymph nodes (Fig. 15.1). The lymph nodes are widely distributed throughout the body. The tonsils and adenoids are specialized lymph node organs in the pharynx; the lymph nodes in the intestine are known as Peyer's patches. All the cells of the immune system originate from self-replacing stem cells in the bone marrow, as do red blood cells and platelets (see Fig. 3.1, Chapter 3). In this Chapter we

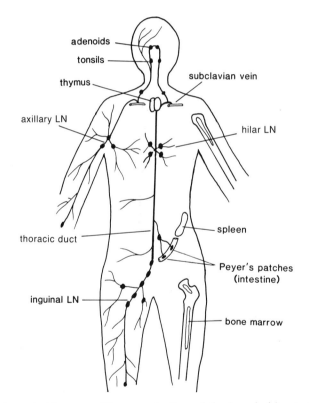

Fig. 15.1 Lymphoid organs. The organization of the lymphoid organs is shown schematically. Afferent lymphatics drain the tissues and enter regional lymph nodes (LN). Efferent lymphatics from the lymph nodes drain into the thoracic duct which enters the venous system. The spleen, thymus, and bone marrow connect to other lymphoid organs mainly via the blood circulation (not shown in the figure).

shall be mainly concerned with the function of lymphocytes because these cells are responsible for specific immunity. In contrast granulocytes mediate non-specific protection, particularly against bacterial pathogens. Granulocytes and macrophages are attracted to sites where invading microorganisms are present and are able to ingest (phagocytose) and often kill the microorganisms. They lack the two major properties of lymphocytes: specificity and memory. Granulocytes are also shortlived (hours) whereas lymphocytes are long lived (months or years). There are two main classes of lymphocytes. Bone marrow derived (B) lymphocytes mature in the marrow and then migrate directly to the spleen and lymph nodes. They are then ready to react to foreign substances (antigens). Thymus derived (T) lymphocytes migrate from the bone marrow to the thymus where they mature before migrating to the peripheral lymphoid organs (spleen and lymph nodes). These two types of lymphocyte, although morphologically very similar, can be readily distinguished by their differing cell surface phenotypes; that is, the array of glycoproteins carried in the lipid bilayer of the cell surface membrane. T and B lymphocytes also have very different functions although they interact during most immune responses.

15.2.1 B lymphocytes and antibody

The principal function of B lymphocytes is to synthesize and secrete antibodies. When these cells are stimulated by encountering a foreign antigen, they first go through several cycles of cell division and then differentiate into specialized antibody secreting cells called plasma cells. Antibodies are globular glycoproteins (hence immunoglobulins) found in the blood plasma. The general structure of an immunoglobulin molecule is shown in Figure 15.2. It consists of two heavy (H) and two light (L) chains. The H and L chains are each divided into two portions, the N-terminal portion (approximately 110 amino acids) being termed the variable part and the remaining portion (approximately 330 or 110 amino acids for H and L chains respectively) being termed the constant part. The variable part of a heavy and light chain form an antigen binding site while the constant part of the heavy chain determines the biological function of the molecule. Differences in the amino acid sequence of the constant part of the H chain determine the class of the immunoglobulin molecule. There are five major immunoglobulin (Ig) classes, IgA, D, E, G, and M, with H chains designated by the Greek letters α, δ, e, γ, and μ (Table 15.1). The two light chain types which also differ in their constant parts are called κ and λ. Each class has different properties which are summarized in Table 15.1. IgM and IgD are found on the membrane of resting B lymphocytes and act as receptors for antigen. When B cells are stimulated they first secrete IgM. Secreted IgM is a pentamer of subunits

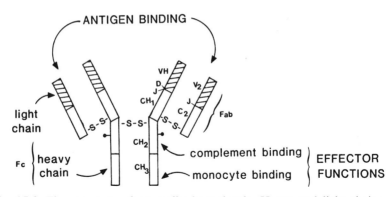

Fig. 15.2 The structure of an antibody molecule. Heavy and light chains are linked by disulphide bonds (S–S). A further disulphide bond joins the two heavy chains. There are further intrachain disulphide bonds in each variable (V) and constant (C) domain of the protein. The symbol —• denotes the site of carbohydrate attachment. The antigen binding fragment (Fab) and crystallizable fragment (Fc) of the molecule are indicated.

Table 15.1 Properties of human immunoglobulins

Property	IgG	IgM	IgA	IgD	IgE
Mol. wt.	150 000	900 000	400 000	180 000	190 000
Concentration in serum (mg/ml)	10	1	2	0.03	<0.001
Relative amount in secretions	Low	Low	High	Very low	Low
Crosses placenta	Yes	No	No	No	No
Complement fixation	Yes	Yes	No	No	No
Transport across epithelia	No	No	Yes	No	Yes
Allergic reactions	No	No	No	No	Yes
Fc binds to cells	Yes	Yes	Yes	No	Yes

joined by an extra polypeptide, the J chain. Later most B cells switch to secreting IgG, A or E. IgG is the main class present in the blood and is a monomer of the basic four chain immunoglobulin molecule. In man there are four subclasses of IgG termed IgG1, IgG2, IgG3, and IgG4 which have closely related H chains. In the mouse and rat there are corresponding IgG subclasses called IgG1, IgG2a, IgG2b, and IgG3. IgA and IgE are minor components of serum and have specialized functions relating to protection of mucous membranes and allergic reactions respectively.

It is a remarkable property of the immune system that it can produce specific antibodies (able to bind with high affinity) to almost any antigen encountered. This is possible because each B lymphocyte synthesizes and secretes a different immunoglobulin molecule. The molecules differ mainly in the variable part and this variability is achieved by several mechanisms. These include selection from a large pool of variable (V) genes, random joining of V genes to regions coding for diversity (D) and joining (J) segments, random combination of heavy and light chains, and somatic mutation. This allows for the production of millions of different antigen binding sites. Each combining site has a unique structure (idiotype) and by immunizing an animal with homogeneous Ig it is possible to raise anti-antibodies (anti-idiotypes) which react only with the immunizing Ig and not other Ig molecules (see Chapter 18).

Generally when an animal encounters an antigen, for example a virus, many B cells are stimulated. Each B cell carries on its surface membrane immunoglobulin molecules with different antigen binding sites. These act as the receptors for antigen and the secreted immunoglobulin of each cell has the same antigen binding site (specificity) as the membrane bound immunoglobulin. Each B cell will divide to produce a clone of daughter cells all producing immunoglobulin with the same specificity, but since many B cells bind the antigen the serum of the immunized animal will contain a mixture of the antibodies produced by many clones. A second contact with the same antigen elicits a greater and more rapid antibody response (immunological memory).

15.2.2 *Monoclonal antibodies*

Antisera made by animals in response to an antigen are the product of many different clones (polyclonal) of B lymphocytes and individual antibodies react with many different sites (epitopes) on the antigen. If the antigen is complex, as are bacterial or mammalian cells, it may be very difficult to determine exactly which molecules of the cell the antibodies are directed toward. For many years the complexity of antigens hampered efforts to produce antibodies which would distinguish between tumour and normal cells although, in principle, the exquisite specificity of antibodies made this an attractive approach to understanding the changes of malignant transformation. In 1975 Kohler and Milstein provided a solution to this problem when they published a method for immortalizing single antibody secreting B lymphocytes by fusing them to a plasma cell tumour (myeloma) to produce a hybrid cell (hybridoma).

All the progeny of such a hybridoma cell produce identical (monoclonal) antibody molecules (for futher details see Chapters 3, and 18). The ability to produce unlimited quantities of homogeneous antibody of any desired specificity has had a major impact in many areas of biology including tumour immunology.

15.2.3 T lymphocyte function

Until recently the functions of T cells were far less well understood than those of B cells. T lymphocytes do not secrete a single major protein product such as immunoglobulin but carry out their functions either by direct contact with other cells or by producing lymphokines (secreted proteins that have powerful biological effects on other cells and are active at very low concentrations). A further difficulty in understanding T cell function was that no T cell receptor for antigen was identified until 1983, and even now it is unclear exactly how T cells 'see' antigen because they seem unable to bind soluble antigen molecules. Antigen is always 'seen' in association with 'self'; the phenomenon of genetic restriction. The nature of this phenomenon can be made clearer by describing one of the earliest experiments to demonstrate it. If an animal (or man) is immunized with a virus, for example influenza A, immune T cells from the animal are able to kill influenza A infected cells but not uninfected target cells or cells infected with a different virus such as influenza B. The immune T cells are therefore specific for influenza A virus. The experiment, however, has a second part. The infected target cells must come from the same animal (or inbred strain) as the immune T cells or they cannot be killed. Thus the T cells do not recognize virus only; they appear to 'see' virus + self. Further genetic experiments showed that the self components required were membrane glycoproteins coded in a region of the genome called the major histocompatibility complex (MHC) (see also Chapter 5). This name derives from older experiments which showed that the same gene products are responsible for the rejection of organ grafts, a reaction also known to be initiated by T lymphocytes. Thus in both the response to foreign pathogens and to tissue grafts T lymphocytes recognize and respond to MHC antigens although in one case foreign MHC and in the other self MHC + antigen. Exactly how T cells 'see' self + antigen is still not clear but this genetic restriction creates a problem for the experimenter wishing to study T cell immunity to tumours since in order to observe a reaction to a tumour cell, the T lymphocytes and tumour cells must be MHC identical.

While the nature of the antigenic complex seen by T cells is still ill defined, studies using T cell clones, monoclonal antibodies, and molecular cloning techniques have at last revealed the structure of the T cell receptor for antigen. This is a molecule of 90 000 daltons consisting of two chains with similarity to immunoglobulin light chains. Early evidence suggests that the mechanisms for generating diversity of T cell receptors are similar to those for B cell immunoglobulin (described briefly in Chapter 11). In contrast to B lymphocytes, however, T cells do not appear to secrete their surface receptor in measurable amounts and carry out their multiple functions by other means. Table 15.2 lists some of the activities of T cells. Some of these can be carried out by T cells alone. Typical of this type of reaction are graft rejection or protection against virus infection mediated by the 'cytotoxic' (cell killing) T cells described above. Many other functions involve other cell types as well as the responding T cells. Very often these responses are immunoregulatory; that is, the T cells control the responses of other cell types. Thus helper T cells stimulate B lymphocytes to secrete antibody and suppressor T cells can switch off antibody production. This latter response is important in terminating a response to a foreign pathogen but may also prevent inappropriate immune responses to self antigens (autoimmunity).

Many immunoregulatory functions are mediated by lymphokines. They have powerful effects on the growth and differentiation of their target cells and act as local hormones within the immune system. They are similar in many respects to the growth factors discussed in Chapter 12. Table 15.3 lists some of the better characterized lymphokines as well as the monokine interleukin 1 which plays a role in the initial activation of T cells. One of the best characterized lymphokines is interleukin 2 (IL2) which is produced by activated T cells and can stimulate both the producing cell (autocrine stimulation) and other T cells to divide. Only T cells which have been first stimulated by contact with antigen express receptors for IL2. The growth promoting effects of IL2 are very powerful

Table 15.2 T lymphocyte functions

In vivo
  Delayed type hypersensitivity
  Graft rejection
  Graft versus host response
  Protection against viral and fungal infections

In vitro
  Help for antibody responses
  Mixed lymphocyte responses—proliferation
                           —cytotoxicity
  Proliferation in response to non-specific mitogens
  Proliferation in response to specific antigens
  Cytotoxicity against specific antigens (in association with MHC antigens)
  Suppression of antibody, proliferative or cytotoxic responses

---

Table 15.3 Functions and properties of lymphokines

Lymphokine	Effect	Molecular weight and properties
Macrophage migration inhibition factor (MIF)	Inhibition of macrophage migration *in vitro*	Heterogeneous 12–70 000
Macrophage activation factors (MAF)	Activates macrophages to become bactericidal or tumoricidal	Similar to MIF
Chemotactic factor(s)	Attraction of monocytes and granulocytes	12–38 000
Colony stimulating factor(s)	Promote growth and maturation of progenitor cells	23 000
Lymphotoxin(s)	Cytostasis or cytolysis of target cells *in vitro*	Heterogeneous 20–140 000
Tumour necrosis factor	Necrosis of tumour *in vivo*	17 000 and multimers; non-glycosylated
Interleukin 1	Activation of T cells; pyrogenic response	Heterogeneous 2–50 000
Interleukin 2	Growth of T lymphocytes	13 500
B cell growth factor(s)	Growth of B lymphocytes	15 000
Interferon α	Inhibition of viral replication	15 000
Interferon γ	Increase in MHC expression	38 000

and it is used to grow antigen activated T cells *in vitro*. So potent a growth stimulus is IL2 that it is possible to grow a large number of cells from a single T cell. This is known as an IL2 dependent T cell clone. Such clones are being used to analyse the specificity and functions of T cells and are the T cell equivalent of monoclonal antibodies.

In contrast to IL2 and B cell growth factor (BCGF) which promote cell division, other interleukins promote differentiation into effector cells. B cell differentiation factor (BCDF), for example, stimulates B cells to stop dividing and secrete antibodies. In other cases the main functions of lymphokines are not yet clear. The interferons are examples of this category. Interferons have effects on many different cell types which include stimulation of cytotoxic activity, anti-proliferative effects, and the induction of increased expression of MHC molecules at the cell surface. Because lymphokines have such powerful regulatory effects it is possible that derangements in their production or receptors might play a role in disease processes, particularly malignancy. As yet there is little evidence for this but abnormal expression of IL2 receptors has been documented in some T cell tumours, so that this is a field which requires further study.

15.3 The immune system and cancer

15.3.1 *Immune surveillance*

As the importance of the immune system in protection against infection became apparent, it was suggested that immunity to tumours might also be important. In 1909 Paul Ehrlich postulated that we might all die of tumours if the immune system did not remove 'aberrant germs' (nascent tumours). This idea led to many attempts to demonstrate immunity to tumours in which tumours were transplanted from one animal to another. The transplants were rejected and this was taken as evidence of immunity to the tumour. Only later was it recognized that these experiments demonstrated not tumour immunity but transplantation immunity directed against MHC antigens.

Only when genetically homogeneous inbred animals (mice) became available was it possible to carry out experiments on tumour immunity and it was then shown that if a growing tumour was excised from a mouse and the animal was challenged with a graft of the same tumour, the graft was rejected. The animal was thus immune to the tumour cells but not to a graft of a different tumour. At about the same time as these early experiments on tumour specific immunity, Thomas and later Burnet restated Ehrlich's hypothesis of protection against 'aberrant germs' as the theory of immune surveillance against tumours. They proposed that tumours arise frequently and that the majority were eliminated by the immune system well before becoming clinically apparent. This hypothesis stimulated a great deal of experimental work in both man and experimental animals because the theory made clear predictions which could be tested. In particular it suggested that tumours should differ antigenically from normal cells and that they would arise more frequently in circumstances when the immune response of the host is compromised. A corollary of this view was that it might be possible to use immunological means to detect tumours and perhaps to stimulate the immune system to destroy tumour cells (immunotherapy). In the remainder of this Chapter I shall examine the evidence for and against immune surveillance, discuss the nature of tumour antigens and consider the possibility of using immunological methods for detection of tumours and of harnessing the immune system for tumour destruction.

15.3.2 *Evidence for and against immune surveillance*

Burnet summarized his view of immune surveillance as follows. (i) Most malignant cells have antigenic qualities distinct from those of the cell type from which they derive; (ii) such antigenic differences can be recognized by T cells and provoke an immune response. If this view is correct it follows that; (iii) the incidence of malignant disease should be greatest in periods of relative immunological inefficiency, particularly in the perinatal period and old age; (iv) immunosuppression whether genetic or induced by drugs, radiation, infection or other causes should increase the incidence of cancer; (v) spontaneous regression of tumours may occur and evidence of an immune response should be apparent in these cases, and (vi) large scale histological examination of common sites of cancer should reveal a higher proportion of tumours than become clinically apparent. Burnet also suggested ways in which the theory of surveillance might be tested experimentally. Thus immunosuppressive agents that facilitate the transfer of tumours or damage to the T cell immune response produced by surgical removal of the thymus might lead to increased tumour incidence.

At first sight a variety of clinical and experimental data do seem to be in accordance with the surveillance theory. In man some tumours show a higher incidence in the first few years of life than in early adulthood and the incidence, but of different tumour types, then rises progressively with increasing age (see Chapter 1). There is also compelling evidence in man that the incidence of tumours is greatly increased in immunosuppressed individuals. This is true both in rare patients with inherited immunodeficiency and in the large number of kidney grafted patients who are treated with immunosuppressive drugs in order to prevent rejection of the grafted kidney. In these individuals the incidence of tumours may be as high as 1 per cent. However, a closer examination does not support the surveillance hypothesis.

The age incidence of tumours is as well explained by many other theories of cancer causation as by immunosurveillance. Tumours are caused by genetic changes in their cells of origin. These changes might be expected to occur either as errors during periods of rapid cell division (early life) or when external causes (carcinogens) have had time to take effect, as in later life.

The more persuasive data derived from immunosuppressed individuals are similarly less convincing when reexamined. While there is indisputably a large increase in tumour incidence the overwhelming majority of these tumours are tumours of the lymphoid system, whereas in normal individuals the common tumours are of epithelial origin (see Chapter 1).

The frequency of the most common tumours such as those of the lung, stomach, intestine, and breast is not increased, while those of the skin, lip, and cervix show some increase. These data are not in accord with a straightforward surveillance theory which would predict an overall increase in tumour frequency of the most common tumours. A very large study of over 15 000 nude mice, which lack a functional thymus and are therefore congenitally T cell immunodeficient, also contradicted the surveillance hypothesis since no tumours were seen. How then can the increased incidence of lymphoid tumours in immunosuppressed individuals be explained, and what role, if any, does the immune system play in protection against tumours?

Another experimental study of immunosuppression, as well as a closer examination of the nature of the tumours arising in transplant patients, provide some clues. When a large group of mice were treated from birth with anti-lymphocyte serum raised in rabbits, their T cell immunity was sufficiently depressed so that skin grafts from another mouse strain were retained indefinitely. Like the nude mice, these mice did not develop spontaneous tumours but when they inadvertently became infected with polyoma virus (see Chapter 9) a number developed multiple tumours of a type characteristically caused by this virus. Similarly the lymphoid tumours seen in transplant recipients are commonly of B lymphocyte origin and have been shown to contain both DNA and proteins characteristic of the Epstein Barr virus (EBV). This member of the herpesvirus family is implicated in the cause of Burkitt's lymphoma, a B cell tumour seen in parts of Africa, and nasopharyngeal carcinoma (see Chapter 9). The virus can also immortalize normal human B lymphocytes *in vitro*. It is certain therefore that this virus is responsible for at least one step in the transformation of B lymphocytes into malignant lymphomas which occurs in immunosuppressed individuals. These findings suggest, therefore, that the important role of the immune system in tumour protection may be in preventing the spread of potentially oncogenic viruses. This role is in accordance with the modern view of T lymphocyte function which suggests that they recognize antigen in association with self MHC and are particularly important in combating intracellular parasites such as viruses.

In the case of EBV this view agrees with experimental and clinical data. EBV is an ubiquitous infectious agent in human populations. More than 90 per cent of adults have evidence of past infection in the form of antibody to the virus in their serum. Infection may be symptomless but in young adults EBV causes infectious mononucleosis. Following either symptomless infection or mononucleosis the virus is carried lifelong and the individual also has lifelong immunity. Immune T lymphocytes can be demonstrated *in vitro* in assays in which they prevent the outgrowth of transformed cells from B lymphocytes which have been exposed to the virus (regression assays). Under normal circumstances there is thus a balance between virus production and spread and the immune response, while in immunosuppressed individuals the immune system may be unable to prevent virus spread. The T cells of such individuals cannot prevent outgrowth of EBV transformed B cells *in vitro*, and virus can often be isolated from body tissues and secretions such as saliva.

If it is accepted that T cells deal mainly with infections, what relationships does the immune system have to the majority of tumours which do not have an obvious viral cause? Evidence from experimental animals and in man suggests that some tumours do provoke an immune response by the host (see later sections). Such a response would not occur until a stimulatory dose of antigen (a large enough number of tumour cells) was available. Grafts of small numbers of tumour cells may provoke a response which causes tumour rejection while large numbers overwhelm the immune response and grow progressively, but very low numbers of grafted cells may again grow progressively. This phenomenon is termed 'sneaking through'.

Since the grafting of small numbers of tumour cells may be similar to the early phase of growth of a spontaneous tumour from a single cell, much effort has been devoted to the elucidation of the mechanisms by which a nascent tumour manages to grow in the face of a competent T cell immune system. In experimental animals a variety of mechanisms have been demonstrated, including the masking of tumour cell antigen by 'blocking' antibody, the liberation by the tumour cells of soluble antigen, the formation of 'blocking' antigen-antibody complexes, and the development of suppressor T cells. These mechanisms are illustrated in Figure 15.3. Nevertheless the fact that anti-tumour immune responses can be demonstrated in animals suggests that, given sufficient understanding, it might be possible to manipulate the response to prevent blocking or suppression and stimulate an effective anti-tumour response. To do this effectively, it is necessary to know what target antigens the immune system 'sees' on tumour cells and which immune mechanisms are important in tumour cell destruction. While experimental models can provide useful clues, most have utilized tumours induced with viruses or carcinogens. It is important, therefore, to attempt to define the nature of the immune response to spontaneous human tumours both in terms of target antigens and immune mechanisms.

15.4 Human tumour antigens

15.4.1 *Detection by polyclonal antisera*

A great deal of effort has been devoted to attempts to use antibodies to detect new antigens on human tumours (see Chapter 18). A unique

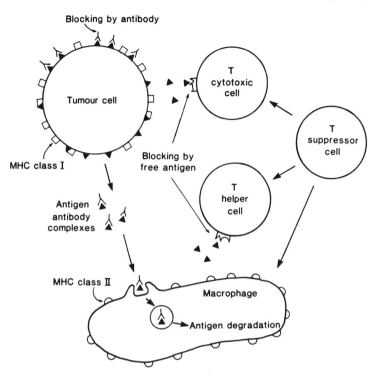

Fig. 15.3 Mechanisms which prevent an effective immune response to a tumour. Antibody masks tumour antigens and free antigen blocks T cell receptors. Antigen–antibody complexes prevent presentation of antigen to T cells and suppressor cells switch off T cell responses.

genetic change in a cell might lead to the expression of a new antigen unique to that tumour—a tumour specific antigen. Such an antigen may provoke a host response but the development of antibodies to it may only be useful to the tumour bearing individual because the same antigen is not found in other tumours, even of the same type. More useful from the point of view of diagnosis or immunotherapy are tumour associated antigens. These are antigens present on or in all tumour cells of a particular type but not found on normal cells. In tumours caused by viruses, proteins coded by the viral genome are effectively tumour associated because they are generally found only in very rare normal cells. In man some lymphomas have EBV antigens and one type of T cell leukaemia has antigens of the human T lymphotropic virus (HTLV-1) which may directly transform T lymphocytes. These are both rare tumours so we must now consider tumour associated antigens of more common tumours.

Early attempts to reveal tumour associated antigens used sera either from tumour patients or from animals deliberately immunized with human tumours. Both types of study have considerable problems. Sera from tumour patients might appear to be ideal reagents but in practice they often have in them antibodies capable of reacting with many types of cells. These include antibodies to blood group antigens, to histocompatibility antigens, and autoantibodies which react with normal as well as tumour cells. To sort out a minor proportion of antibodies specific for tumour antigens is a complex task. It has usually been attempted by absorption analysis in which the serum is incubated with a succession of different normal cell types to remove antibody to them and then tested for reactivity with tumour cells. Such manoeuvres generally dilute the specific antibody and also lead to non-specific loss so that even if the resulting antiserum reacts only with tumour cells it may be so weak that it is difficult to use for identification and characterization of the antigens detected.

Antisera raised in animals, usually rabbits, present similar problems. The rabbit antiserum 'sees' many antigens on a human tumour cell but the majority of these are present on normal cells also. Such sera therefore require extensive absorption to render them specific for tumour cells and it is not surprising that reports of successful production of specific heteroantisera are few in number, nor have they in general been particularly useful in tumour diagnosis or therapy. Some exceptions are mentioned in the next section.

15.4.2 *Detection by monoclonal antibodies*

When the hybridoma method for producing monoclonal antibodies was developed, many investigators realized that monoclonal antibodies might provide reagents for detecting differences between cell types at a molecular level (see Chapter 18). This has indeed proved to be the case and, for example, mouse monoclonal antibodies can distinguish between human leucocytes and all other human cells, between T and B lymphocytes or between different subpopulations of T lymphocytes. The molecules identified by these monoclonal antibodies are differentiation antigens (antigens present on one cell type but not another, or related to the stage of maturation, see Chapter 3) and in some cases have been shown to be involved in functions associated with the particular cell type identified. These results suggested that it should be possible to produce monoclonal antibodies which could distinguish between tumour and normal cells, if differences existed. Differences have indeed been recognized but so far there is no convincing evidence of a specific tumour associated antigen.

One of the few useful polyclonal heteroantisera was raised against acute lymphoblastic leukaemia (ALL) cells. After extensive absorption this serum could distinguish ALL cells from normal lymphocytes or bone marrow. Several monoclonal antibodies have been produced which react in a similar fashion and were therefore considered initially to identify a tumour associated antigen of leukaemia cells (common acute lymphoblastic leukaemia antigen or CALLA). More careful examination of bone marrow showed that a small number of normal cells carried CALLA. Subsequent studies have shown that CALLA is a differentiation antigen transiently expressed on cells early in the B lymphocyte lineage. One category of antigens which can easily be confused with a tumour associated antigen is thus a differentiation antigen expressed only on rare normal cells.

But from the point of view of diagnosis and treatment, CALLA is a very useful antigen. CALLA positive cells are very rare in normal bone marrow (<1 per cent) and are not found in peripheral blood so that their presence can be used to monitor disease. Furthermore, because CALLA is not present on stem cells, it is possible to remove CALLA positive cells from bone marrow without damaging the potential of the marrow cells to regenerate a functional haemopoietic system (see Chapter 18). This, therefore, is an example of a normal differentiation antigen which for practical purposes may be regarded as a tumour associated antigen.

There are a number of other examples of differentiation antigens which provide similar possibilities. Many antibodies raised against carcinomas recognize heavily glycosylated surface glycoproteins. These antigens are often restricted to particular epithelia or specialized cells within an epithelium. Tumour cells expressing the antigens can therefore often be detected when the tumour spreads outside the primary site. This has been exploited in detecting small metastases of breast cancer in the axillary lymph nodes and metastatic lung cancer cells in bone marrow.

Another category of antigens which can appear tumour associated are those which are expressed in dividing cells only. Some monoclonal antibodies raised against tumour cell lines appeared initially to distinguish between tumour and normal cells. More extensive studies showed that these antibodies also detected an antigen present on normal cells when these were actively dividing. This antigen has now been shown to be the cell surface receptor for transferrin. Transferrin is a serum protein which transports iron required for cell division. The expression of the transferrin receptor is therefore correlated with the cell cycle, not with malignancy. The proportion of cells in a population which express transferrin receptors may therefore indicate how many cells are actively dividing. By no means all cells in a tumour divide, but in general the greater the percentage of dividing cells the more rapid will be the growth of the tumour. In a study of lymphomas it was indeed found that the more rapidly progressive tumours did have a higher proportion of transferrin receptor positive cells. The transferrin receptor is therefore useful in indicating the prognosis in tumour patients.

While the transferrin receptor is widely distributed on actively dividing normal cells, other differentiation antigens which appear on dividing cells are restricted to certain cell types. One example of this is the receptor for interleukin 2. This is expressed on T lymphocytes (and some B lymphocytes) after these have been activated by contact with antigen. Some T cell tumours express this receptor and, as in the case of CALLA, for practical purposes it may be regarded as a tumour associated antigen because normal T cells have been replaced by the malignant population. This has encouraged attempts to treat some patients with antibodies to the receptor.

Well before the advent of monoclonal antibodies, conventional heteroantisera were used to define a rather different category of tumour associated antigens to which monoclonal antibodies have now been raised: these are differentiation antigens with a restricted tissue distribution and are expressed during foetal life but not found in the adult (oncofoetal antigens). Certain tumours, however, re-express these antigens. Two examples have been studied particularly extensively: carcinoembryonic antigen (CEA) and alpha foetoprotein (AFP). The former is found in foetal intestine and in colonic tumours, whereas the latter is found in foetal liver and adult liver tumours.

Both antigens can be detected in the serum of tumour patients and sensitive immunoassays for their detection have been developed, but neither has proved satisfactory for diagnosis. In the case of CEA, this is because it is difficult to establish normal and abnormal levels since, in contrast to earlier data, more recent results have shown that many different tumours produce CEA and that levels may also be raised in a variety of non-malignant conditions. In the case of AFP, raised levels are associated with liver cancer but also with other liver diseases and false negative results are sometimes obtained. Both CEA and AFP are probably most useful in monitoring the effects of treatment on CEA or AFP producing tumours. A fall in the serum level occurs following successful treatment and a rise may be detectable before clinical recurrence of tumour. Antibodies to both CEA and AFP have been used also in studies of tumour localization and immunotherapy (see Chapter 18).

It is notable that there are no solely tumour associated antigens, but studies of cellular oncogenes suggest that tumour cells do express altered proteins (Chapters 10, and 12) so that tumour associated antigens should exist. Why then are they not detected? Several explanations may be offered. First, if the genetic changes in a tumour are unique to that tumour the antigen would be tumour specific. While this might provoke a host response, the specific antibody in a polyclonal antiserum may be difficult to detect especially as it would only react with that particular tumour. Second, cell bound surface antigens may provoke a T cell rather than antibody response (see on). Third, attempts to detect tumour antigens with heteroantisera, even using monoclonal antibodies, are likely to be difficult because of the large number of foreign proteins seen by the immunized rabbit or mouse. In spite of this there have been some reports of detection of human tumour specific antigens with monoclonal antibodies. These are of course difficult to confirm because the antibody reacts only with the immunizing tumour. Such antibodies are of use for diagnosis or therapy only in the original patient and may be most useful in studying genetic changes in tumour cells. In the foreseeable future the most useful antibodies are likely to be those against differentiation antigens with a restricted distribution which are also expressed on tumour cells. How these can be exploited is discussed in Chapter 18.

15.5 Cell mediated immune responses to tumours

15.5.1 Cell transfer experiments

The discovery that rejection of foreign tissue grafts was mediated by T lymphocytes stimulated attempts to identify the immune mechanisms responsible for protection against tumours in animals. The early experiments were performed *in vivo* by passive transfer; lymphocytes or serum from a donor animal immune to a tumour were transferred into a genetically identical but non-immune host which was then challenged with the same tumour. In such experiments, both cells and serum could sometimes transfer immunity. Antibody is most effective against leukaemia cells while lymphocytes could protect against solid tumours (usually carcinogen induced fibrosarcomas). The reason for this may be that leukaemia cells generally remain within the blood or lymph so that the cells are easily reached by antibody. In contrast carcinoma or sarcoma cells are extravascular and antibody may not always easily penetrate the tumour (see Chapter 18) while lymphocytes are able to leave blood vessels and enter the tumour tissue.

More detailed analysis of the mechanisms responsible for tumour protection by cells depended on technical advances. When separation of T and B lymphocytes became possible, these populations could be passively transferred before challenge with tumour and, in later experiments, a similar approach was used to study the roles of the T helper and T suppressor/cytotoxic subsets in tumour immunity. These methods are cumbersome and time consuming and it is difficult to assess the contribution of host non-immune cells to the anti-tumour response. More importantly, they cannot be applied to studies of tumour immunity in man so that another technical advance was required before further progress could be made.

15.5.2 In vitro *cytotoxicity*

The first method which allowed the study of the effect of lymphocytes on tumour cells *in vitro* was the colony inhibition technique. In the original method, lymphocytes were mixed with tumour cells and seeded in culture dishes. After several days the lymphocytes can be washed out of the dish leaving adherent tumour cells behind. By this time each tumour cell originally seeded will have divided several times, forming a colony. After appropriate staining these colonies can be counted with the naked eye. If lymphocytes from immune animals are used, there is a reduction in the number of colonies compared to controls. The reduction may reflect either death of some tumour cells or inhibition of growth. This test was the forerunner of others in which the lymphocytes and tumours were incubated for a shorter time (48 hours) and surviving single tumour cells counted microscopically. A further development was to label the tumour cells with a radioisotope and measure cell death by the release of the radiolabel into the medium. These cytotoxicity assays could of course be applied to human cells provided that appropriate target tumour cells could be obtained. Tumour material is often available from cancer patients at operation and it is possible to disperse this into a suspension of single cells. Generally tumour cells obtained in this way will survive long enough in tissue culture for cytotoxicity assays to be performed. In addition, a proportion of tumours explanted *in vitro* can be grown into permanent cell lines. These lines may retain phenotypic characteristics of their cell of origin for long periods of culture.

The early data obtained from colony inhibition assays using tumour cells and lymphocytes from cancer patients showed that human tumour cells could be killed by autologous (self) lymphocytes. Surprisingly the apparent specificity of the cytotoxicity differed from that found in animals. In man lymphocytes from a patient with a lung tumour could kill lung tumour cells but not colon, breast or other target cells from other individuals. In animals in contrast the cytotoxicity was specific for the original tumour only. Subsequently much of the human data was invalidated by a study in which the lymphocytes from a large number of tumour patients and normal individuals were tested on a panel of target cells of varying origin. The results showed that all lymphocytes could kill most *in vitro* grown target cells. This type of cytotoxicity came to be called natural killer (NK) activity because prior immunization was not required.

15.5.3 *Natural killer cells*

Much effort has been expended in the identification of the cells responsible for NK activity, their relationship to other lymphocytes, their biological role, and the identification of the antigens recognized by them on target cells. Only the first question can be answered with any confidence. NK cells have a characteristic phenotype. They are larger lymphocytes than most T and B cells and have characteristic cytoplasmic granules (large granular lymphocytes). They share surface antigens with T lymphocytes and also with monocytes. There are also some surface molecules unique to NK cells. Just as their phenotype makes it difficult to determine their origin so is it difficult to assign these cells a definite function though various possibilities have been suggested; for example, that they regulate haemopoiesis, or are an early non-specific response system for combating viral infections. Because they can kill many tumour cell lines, NK cells have also been suggested as playing a role in surveillance against tumours.

Irrespective of their exact function, NK cells have made it very difficult to study specific immune responses to human tumours using cytotoxicity assays. A further problem not at first appreciated is posed by the necessity for antigens to be seen by T cells in association with self MHC antigen (genetic restriction). Even if tumour specific immune T lymphocytes are present in a patient, they would be expected to kill only the patient's own tumour or another tumour carrying the same tumour antigen and the correct MHC antigen. NK cells in contrast show no genetic restriction. It is therefore very difficult to perform adequately controlled experiments to reveal specific T cell immunity, especially as this is likely to be a weak effect since in any patient with a growing tumour the immune response must have been overwhelmed or suppressed. To overcome these technical problems and amplify a weak specific response, tumour immunologists have attempted to use the *in vitro* boosting method developed for studying T lymphocyte responses to non-tumour antigens.

15.5.4 In vitro *boosting of T cell immunity*

In both experimental animals and man it has proved possible to restimulate immune T lymphocytes *in vitro* with foreign MHC antigens (in a mixed lymphocyte culture) or antigens such as tetanus toxoid or influenza virus. The stimulated T cells proliferate and express receptors for the growth stimulatory factor IL2. Long term growth of the cells is possible if the T cells are alternately exposed to their specific antigen and more IL2. In principle very large numbers of antigen specific T cells can be grown in this way from a single cell. Cloned T cell populations have been used in studies of T lymphocyte function, to examine how T cells interact with monocytes and B lymphocytes, the nature and number of lymphokines produced by different types of T cells, the role of T cell surface molecules in T cell function, and the specificity of T cell responses to antigen. In principle, therefore, T cell clones which respond to tumours can be used to determine the nature of antigens in a tumour which can be recognized by the host T cells. In practice the technical problems are formidable. T lymphocytes from all donors do not seem to grow equally well and in experiments on tumour immunity the amount of antigen for stimulation and assay of the T cells may be limited, unless the tumour cells can be grown as a permanent line. Although it is often possible to stimulate a patient's T cells and then grow these as a poly-clonal population, it has often proved difficult to obtain clones. Never-theless some information on the specificity of tumour reactive T cells has been obtained.

In the earliest studies in man intriguing results were obtained. Two sorts of T lymphocyte lines were grown. Cytotoxic lines were able to kill autologous tumour cells but not others of the same type while T cells which proliferated in response to tumour (presumed to be helper/inducer cells) could respond to autologous and other tumours of the same type. These results suggested that the proliferating T cells might be recognizing tumour antigens processed and displayed in association with MHC antigen by accessory cells (monocytes). Cytotoxic T cells in contrast see only autologous tumour because only this has the correct tumour and MHC antigens (Fig. 15.4). In these early experiments the T cells were not cloned so that the dominant specificity in the population would be observed. Results with T cell clones have revealed further complexity.

When a set of clones which could proliferate in response to a lung tumour extract was examined, it was found that individual clones reacted in a variety of ways. They might react to autologous tumour extract only, all lung tumour extracts, extracts of any dividing cell, all autologous extracts or extracts of tumour but not normal tissue. While the antigens detected by these clones have not been identified in molecular terms, the results suggest that part of the T cell response to a tumour may be against tumour specific or tumour associated antigens but much of the response is to normal tissue components. The tumour response may thus be partly an autoimmune response, perhaps induced by the breakdown of tissue caused by tumour growth.

A rather different result was obtained when cytotoxic clones reacting to melanoma cells were analysed. Some of these seemed to be able to kill all melanoma targets but not most other cells. The target structure for these T cells has been partially characterized as a highly glycosylated molecule

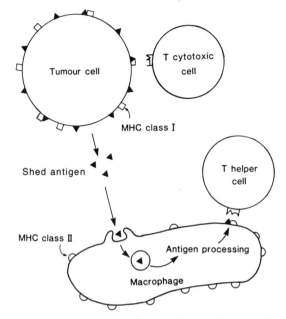

Fig. 15.4 Presentation of tumour antigen to T lymphocytes. Tumour antigen may be displayed in association with MHC Class I antigen (□) on the cell surface so that it is recognized directly by cytotoxic T cells or processed by macrophages and displayed with MHC Class II antigen (◠) to stimulate T helper cells.

on the surface of melanoma cells. Whether T cells recognize this target using the same type of receptor that normally sees antigens in association with self MHC antigens is not clear, but it is intriguing that the specificity of these killer T cells is similar to that observed in the earliest experiments in humans using the colony inhibition assay.

While many questions remain to be answered it is clear that the T cell response to tumours is complex in terms of the variety of molecules recognized on the tumour cells and the different types of T cells activated during the response. As techniques improve it is likely that many more tumour reactive clones will be obtained and that these will increasingly be used to identify molecules in tumours to which the host can respond. Some of these molecules may be sufficiently restricted in their tissue distribution to be useful in diagnosis or therapy.

15.6 Immunodiagnosis and immunotherapy

15.6.1 *Immunodiagnosis*

Ideal reagents for immunodiagnosis or immunotherapy would discriminate absolutely between tumour and normal cells. In addition they would distinguish between benign and malignant tumours. However, as discussed earlier, most if not all antibodies raised against tumours identify differentiation antigens. Nevertheless, antibodies can be useful in cancer diagnosis just because they identify differentiation antigens and thus the origin of a cell. Panels of monoclonal antibodies are finding a role in pathology and haematology laboratories where they are used to improve the identification and classification of tumours. For example in the diagnosis of acute lymphoblastic leukaemia (see Chapter 3) antibodies have allowed clear distinctions to be made between T and B cell forms of the disease which have very different prognoses with conventional chemotherapy. Identification of bad prognosis patients is important because it is sensible to try new forms of therapy in individuals with little chance of survival with current treatment.

Monoclonal antibodies are also useful in identifying the origin of tumour cells when this is difficult by conventional histological methods; antibodies to cytoskeletal proteins (cytokeratins), epithelial membrane antigens and leucocyte antigens can usually identify the origin of metastatic tumour cells even if these are cytologically undifferentiated. This has important implications for the management of the patient because secondary carcinoma is often chemotherapy resistant while lymphoid tumours are often sensitive.

Monoclonal antibodies are also being used in attempts to localize tumours *in vivo* (see Chapter 18).

15.6.2 *Immunotherapy*

Immunotherapy is treatment by immunological means. In active immunotherapy the tumour bearer's own immune system is stimulated to respond to the tumour while in passive immunotherapy, immune cells or their products are given. Table 15.4 summarizes the possibilities. The aim of treatment in cancer is to eliminate the tumour without harming the host. Because immune responses are highly specific, immunologists have long hoped that immune cells or antibodies might be used in this way. Unfortunately, as discussed earlier, few cells or antibodies are truly tumour specific so that some side effects on normal cells must be expected. Nevertheless many experiments have been carried out. Since the use of monoclonal antibodies is discussed in detail in Chapter 18 only other means will be considered here.

Attempts to treat tumours by active immunization (Table 15.4) with tumour, or the administration of immunostimulating agents, have met with little success. It could be argued that this is because the presence of a growing tumour blocks immune effector mechanisms (see Fig. 15.3). This may be untrue because even when immunization has been tried after conventional treatment to reduce tumour load, it has still not been

Table 15.4 Immunotherapy

Approach	Method	Agent
Non-specific		
Local, active	Intra-tumour injection	BCG[1], viruses
Systemic, active	Immunostimulants	BCG, MER[1], *C. parvum*[1], Levamisole
Systemic, passive	Mediators or lymphokines	Thymic factors, interleukins, interferons
Specific		
Systemic, active	Immunization	Tumour cells or extract+ adjuvant
Systemic, passive	Specific factors	Transfer factor
	Serotherapy	Polyclonal or monoclonal antibodies, coupled to drugs, radioisotopes or toxins
	Cells	*In vitro* grown specific T cells
Ex vivo	Bone marrow purging	Antibodies+complement or antibodies coupled to magnetic beads or toxins

[1] BCG, Bacille Calmette-Guerin, a non-pathogenic strain of tubercle bacillus. MER, the methanol extraction residue of BCG. *C. parvum, Corynebacterium parvum*. BCG, MER and *C. parvum* all have adjuvant activity.

successful. A more likely explanation for failure of active immunization is that there are few host lymphocytes capable of responding to tumour antigens. Because the results of active immunization have been disappointing and yet some tumour responding T cells can be detected *in vitro*, experimenters have tried to expand these populations for therapeutic use. What then are the possibilities and difficulties of this approach?

First, the technical difficulties of isolating and growing large numbers of tumour specific T cells are formidable. *In vitro* responses to tumour cells or extracts are weak, presumably reflecting a low frequency of responding T cells, and while a few groups have succeeded in isolating tumour reactive clones, it has proved extremely difficult in most cases to grow large numbers of cells. Unfortunately the factors governing the extent of growth *in vitro* of T cell clones are not yet understood but may include the genetic makeup of the donor as well as the type and state of differentiation of the responding T cells. Other problems remain, not the least being the possibility that the *vitro*–grown T cells may not migrate normally *in vivo* and thus the majority may fail to reach a tumour site. Data concerning the *in vivo* function of T cell clones in experimental animals are conflicting, but at least in some cases protection against tumour challenge has been observed. Much more experimental data on the most effective type of T cell, the most effective way to use them, and how best to induce and grow tumour immune cells, needs to be gathered before this type of therapy becomes a practical proposition. It is also likely to be extremely expensive!

While the use of immune cells for immunotherapy has not progressed very far, their secreted products (lymphokines) are now becoming available. The techniques of molecular biology have made it possible to produce sufficient quantities for *in vivo* studies of these substances which are normally secreted in minute quantities during immune responses. So far the most extensively studied lymphokines are the interferons, a family of glycoproteins which were first identified because they inhibit the replication of viruses. Interferons also inhibit cell division and stimulate NK activity. All of these properties suggested that they might have therapeutic effects on tumours. A number of clinical trials on different types of tumour have been carried out and it is clear that interferons are not strikingly effective anti-tumour agents for treatment of most tumours. Some effects have been documented for certain rare tumours, and in experimental models; however, it may be that further research will better define when interferons can be useful and how they should be combined with other treatments. Data on the anti-tumour effects of other lymphokines are scanty but the genes for several of these have been cloned (IL2, tumour necrosis factor, lymphotoxin) and material will shortly become available for therapeutic use. All of these agents suffer from the problem of non-specificity, that is, they are equally likely to have effects on normal as well as malignant cells.

15.7 Conclusions

The advent of the hybridoma technique for production of monoclonal antibodies has provided reagents to identify and purify molecules present in lymphocytes, other normal cells or tumour cells. The techniques of molecular biology make it possible to isolate the genes coding for these molecules, to sequence them and, if required, to produce the molecule *in vitro*. These are powerful techniques for investigating the function of the immune system and for attempting to define how tumour cells differ from normal cells. The immune system also provides a model for studying the growth and differentiation of cells. Lymphocytes can be readily obtained even from humans, and are readily cultured *in vitro*. In the long term it is likely that immunologists may contribute more to cancer research by providing research tools and insights into cell function than by experiments on immune responses to tumours, which may well turn out to be illusory.

In the more immediate future the use of monoclonal antibodies in immunodiagnosis and immunotherapy is likely to expand. For therapy, human monoclonal antibodies would be advantageous since rodent antibodies provoke an antibody response to the foreign protein which limits the duration of treatment. So far it has proved difficult to produce human antibodies of a desired specificity with any regularity and in large quantities. Genetically engineered hybrid antibodies, part mouse part human, may be an alternative solution.

The next few years are likely to see many studies of the effect of purified lymphokines. While it seems unlikely that most of these will provide 'magic bullets' which will be tumour specific, these agents do have powerful biological effects and an understanding of these will contribute to elucidating the mechanism of regulation of growth and differentiation in cells.

I have left to the end an area in which immunology may well contribute to cancer treatment, or rather prevention. It is clear that a number of viruses play a role in the induction of tumours. These include hepatitis B virus in liver cancer, EBV in Burkitt's lymphoma and nasopharyngeal cancer, papillomaviruses in genital tumours and HTLV-1 and 2 in some lymphoid tumours (see Chapter 9). Prophylactic immunization against these and perhaps other as yet undiscovered agents is likely to prevent or reduce the incidence of these tumours. Already hepatitis B vaccine is available and under trial; much effort is also being expended on a vaccine to EBV. As is the case with infectious disease, prophylactic immunization rather than treatment may be the immunologists most direct contribution to the reduction of cancer mortality.

Further reading

Hood, L., Weissman, I., and Wood, W. (1984). *Immunology* (2nd Edition). Benjamin/Cummings, Menlo Park, California.

McMichael, A. J., and Fabre, J. (1982). *Monoclonal antibodies in clinical medicine.* Academic Press, London.

16

The local treatment of cancer

I. S. FENTIMAN

16.1 How tumours present

Almost all patients with cancer seek treatment because of abnormalities which arise as either a direct or an indirect result of the malignant process. When carcinoma cells invade connective tissue there may be a stromal reaction producing fibrosis. Thus in organs such as the breast or thyroid this may manifest itself as a palpable lump made up of malignant cells and fibrous tissue whereas in tubular organs like the oesophagus or colon, tumour induced fibrosis may result in stricture formation so that the passage of contents is impeded or obstructed. Malignant cells may infiltrate blood vessels leading to a local haemorrhage and thus produce, for example, blood stained sputum in the case of bronchial carcinoma or blood in the urine (haematuria) from cancers of the kidney or bladder.

All of these symptoms may arise from non-malignant causes but act as a signal to the physician that further investigation is justified. Our knowledge of cancer biology suggests that by the time the cancer becomes detectable (at say a volume of 1 ml) it contains about 1×10^9 cells, and there is a high probability that tumour metastasis has occurred. To increase the chance of cure, it is necessary to diagnose tumours earlier or, better still, to diagnose tumours in which spread through the basement membrane has not occurred as in, so called, *in situ* carcinomas (see Chapter 1). One of the aims of screening programmes is to diagnose asymptomatic carcinomas. This has been shown to be of value in preventing deaths from carcinoma of the uterine cervix by means of cervical smears. Despite this, there is little evidence that most other forms of screening for cancer actually result in a diminished mortality. Urine cytological testing in aniline dye workers has not affected the natural history of bladder cancer, nor has screening for gastric carcinoma produced any attributable reduction in mortality among the Japanese in whom this is a common malignancy (see Chapter 4).

In Britain the most frequent tumours are in the lung but chest X–rays have not been of value for early diagnosis. In contrast to these negative results, a positive benefit has been demonstrated in screening for breast cancer. A large study in New York showed a diminished mortality from breast cancer in women over 50 years old who were examined clinically and radiologically, compared with others who received only routine medical followup. Since this study, there have been many arguments over the cost effectiveness of screening, without any adequate data being presented. Studies which are at present being conducted in Britain and Canada may yield more information on the respective benefits of mammography, breast self examination, education, and dietary advice on reduction of fat intake.

16.2 Diagnosis of cancer

The clinical diagnosis of cancer may be made by inspection and palpation of superficial tumours such as those of skin, tongue, and breast. In addition, with the use of appropriate instruments (endoscopes), many internal cancers may be visualized and biopsied. These include tumours of the larynx, bronchus, oesophagus, stomach, colon, rectum, uretha, and bladder. However, to detect many of the more deeply located tumours, a variety of imaging techniques may be required.

16.2.1 *Radiography*

Although plain X–rays may be of benefit in suggesting a diagnosis of lung or bone cancer, there is little difference in density between normal and malignant tissue and thus radio–opaque contrast medium is often necessary to delineate tumours. Many cancers of the upper and lower gastrointestinal tract may be demonstrated by either barium meals or enemas, with tumours being seen as strictures, ulcers, or filling defects (regions from which the radio–opaque material is excluded).

The demonstration of certain cancers requires more sophisticated administration of contrast medium through a needle (cannula), either intravenously or intra-arterially. A bladder carcinoma may be seen after an intravenous urogram. In this procedure, the radio–opaque dye is injected intravenously and is concentrated in the kidneys and excreted in the urine; radiographs of kidney and bladder are then taken. For visualization of a renal carcinoma, injection of the material directly into an artery (arteriogram) may be necessary. These techniques involve not only radiation exposure but also the risk of allergic reactions to contrast media and haemorrhage after arterial cannulation. For these reasons radiologists have attempted to develop other techniques.

16.2.2 Computerized tomography (CT) scanning

This relatively new and still expensive technique which uses computerized interpretation of multidirectional radiation beams enables the construction of transverse sectional X-rays of skull, thorax, abdomen, and pelvis, albeit with a moderate radiation exposure but without the need for any invasive technique. CT scanning may be of particular value in demonstrating tumours and lung lesions that are poorly visualized by plain radiography.

16.2.3 Ultrasound scanning

The use of ultrasonic waves permits the demonstration of lesions as small as half a centimetre in diameter. This is achieved without any radiation exposure, so that multiple ultrasonic examinations may be performed without danger. The technique is of use in differentiating between fluid filled (cystic) and solid masses, particularly in the liver, kidney, pancreas, and ovary; some cystic masses may be aspirated after localization.

16.2.4 Cellular diagnosis

Although a cancer may be strongly suspected on clinical and radiological grounds, the diagnosis cannot be said to have been made with certainty until cytological or histological confirmation has been obtained. Without this pathological proof of malignancy, treatment cannot be properly planned, therapeutic procedures cannot be compared, nor can any prognostic estimate be made accurately. It is likely that many of the past claims for cancer cure were due to the spontaneous regression of inflammatory lesions mimicking malignancy. Only under the most exceptional

circumstances should any patient be treated for cancer without pathological confirmation of the diagnosis.

16.2.5 *Cytology*

In this technique, cells from the suspected or potential malignant site are
removed, smeared onto a slide, stained, and examined by an experienced
cytologist. Malignant cells may be recognized by alterations in cell size
and shape, together with changes in nuclear morphology (see Chapter 1).

16.2.5.1 *Exfoliative cytology.* The examination of cells which have been
shed is termed exfoliative cytology and may be applied to cells from the
uterine cervix, sputum or urine. When malignant cells are identified cytologically this is an indication for further investigation.

16.2.5.2 *Aspiration cytology.* Cells are aspirated from the suspected
tumour through a fine needle attached to a syringe. This technique is now
in widespread use in the evaluation of breast lumps. It should be stressed
that because the topography of the aspirated cells cannot be determined
it is not possible to differentiate between *in situ* and infiltrating carcinomas. In addition, occasional false positive cases have been reported. For
these reasons and because of the shortage of trained cytologists, histopathology is still the mainstay of diagnosis for the majority of solid
tumours.

16.2.6 *Histopathology*

This is of value in confirming the diagnosis of cancer and also for providing information on tumour differentiation (Grade) and extent of spread
(Stage). Tissue is obtained either as a sample of the tumour (incision
biopsy), or by complete removal of the tumour (excision biopsy). The
method of processing the tissue will depend upon the urgency with which
a diagnosis is required. Thus, as part of a planned major procedure, an
incision biopsy may be taken and the tissue immediately frozen in solid
carbon dioxide to allow rapid sectioning by microtome after which the
sections are stained and examined. Using this frozen section technique, a
definite diagnosis of malignancy may be obtained within 10 minutes of
biopsy, and the proposed operation can be performed secure in the
knowledge that the pathological diagnosis is correct.

There are, however, certain disadvantages in the use of frozen section.
First, the frozen section method is suboptimal for the preparation and
staining of tissue for examination, so that the pathologist may be pressur-
ized into making a hurried decision on a less than perfectly prepared
slide. Second, under some circumstances the 'smash and grab raid'
approach to cancer surgery may mean that the patient has not had full

staging investigations prior to surgery, so that a major curative surgical procedure may be performed under circumstances in which the cancer has already disseminated. Finally, but most importantly, many patients are profoundly disturbed by the prospect of a major procedure such as permanent colostomy (in which the large bowel opens onto the abdominal wall) or mastectomy being performed without an opportunity for them to discuss treatment options with the surgeon. Although frozen section techniques are still widely used for the diagnosis of cancer, it has become increasingly popular for the specimens to be processed more slowly to preserve the tissue architecture and to allow fuller investigation and examinations.

16.2.6.1 *Paraffin section.* In the laboratory the tissue is fixed, usually with formalin. This procedure takes approximately 24 hours, after which the tissue can be dehydrated, embedded in paraffin wax and then sliced with a microtome; then the wax is removed and the slide usually stained with haematoxylin and eosin (H and E stain). This entire procedure takes approximately 48 hours but does provide better material for examination. Furthermore the examination of multiple specimens allows determination of the extent of the tumour and possible lymphatic and venous tumour invasion.

16.2.6.2 *New approaches.* The H and E stain has been the cornerstone of histopathological technique, and usually allows the pathologist to reach a definite conclusion on the tumour type. There are, however, circumstances in which this is not possible, particularly with poorly differentiated tumours which may display none of the morphological features of the tissue of origin. Under these circumstances the pathologist may be unable to determine whether the tumour is a carcinoma, a melanoma, a sarcoma, or a lymphoma.

The recent development of monoclonal antibodies (see Chapters 15, and 18) to characterize specific cell markers has enabled pathologists to use more informative staining techniques. Use of the immunoperoxidase method or other enzyme linked assays allows the demonstration of cell specific determinants, so that differences between morphologically similar tumours may be found. In some cases, e.g. lymphomas, the correct histological diagnosis allows the appropriate therapy to be given.

16.3 Staging

Staging is an assessment of the extent of spread of a particular tumour and this estimate may be made in two ways: rather crudely by clinical examination, and more accurately by laboratory methods. Even the latter methods lack sensitivity so that micrometastatic spread cannot be detected.

16.3.1 *Clinical staging*

The accuracy of clinical staging depends upon a combination of anatomical features, physical characteristics of the individual patient, and the experience of the examining clinician. Even under optimal circumstances the clinical staging can be very crude. For instance, palpation of the axillary lymph nodes of patients with breast cancer may give a 30 per cent false negative and 30 per cent false positive assessment of metastatic spread. For superficial tumours of the testis, lymphatic drainage is to the para-aortic lymph nodes, which may remain impalpable unless grossly enlarged even in a thin individual. However, despite drawback of this nature, clinical staging is still the most widely used system because it does enable some kind of comparison of cases treated in different centres, not all of which may have access to sophisticated staging techniques. The main international system is the TNM classification (see Chapter 1). Individual components of the TNM system can be quite complex but use of this does allow staging to be performed (Table 16.1).

Stage I and II tumours are usually deemed operable and therefore suitable for local treatment. Stage III tumours are inoperable but may be treated by a combination of radiation and surgery, whereas Stage IV tumours are incurable by local techniques.

16.3.2 *Other staging investigations*

Choice of the most appropriate staging investigations for a particular tumour depends upon knowledge of topographical anatomy, together with the most likely pattern of spread of metastases. Thus gastrointestinal carcinomas spread early to the local lymph nodes and this is followed by venous embolism into the hepatic portal system resulting in liver metastases. In contrast, breast cancer rarely metastasizes early to the liver but, because of early blood borne spread, secondary tumours are more likely located in bone or lung.

The simplest staging investigations are blood tests to determine haemoglobin and white cell count. Bone marrow metastases may manifest as a leukoerythroblastic anaemia, or tumour cells may be detected in bone marrow smears. Routine blood tests include measurements of electrolytes and bone and liver derived enzyme levels which may be elevated in response to metastatic disease. Finally, most patients have a plain chest X–ray to exclude gross disease of the lung, pleura, and ribs.

Table 16.1 TNM staging

Stage	Clinical manifestations
I	small localized tumour
II	spread to local lymph nodes
III	large local tumour and/or spread to further lymph nodes
IV	presence of distant metastases

16.3.3 *Radio-isotopic scans*

The principle underlying these scans is that radioactively labelled compounds are selectively taken up by particular organs, and thus by means of a gamma camera a scintiscan may be obtained. The presence of either filling defects or areas of increased uptake may suggest the presence of metastatic disease. Cancers of the lung, thyroid, prostate, breast, and kidney have a particular tendency to spread to bone and therefore a bone scan is usually performed in the investigation of patients with these tumours. Abnormalities are usually revealed as areas of increased uptake (hot spots) which indicate regions of increased bone turnover. X–rays are then necessary to determine whether the hot spots result from metastatic disease or from degenerative disease (osteoarthritis) or trauma (old fractures).

Patients with gastrointestinal tumours usually are investigated by either a liver ultrasound or radioisotopic scan depending upon local circumstances. By this means, hepatic metastases as small as 0.5 cm may be identified.

16.3.4 *Lymphangiography*

To visualize the lymph nodes draining certain tumours, a lymphatic vessel is cannulated and an iodine containing contrast medium is injected, after which tumour deposits may be recognized as filling defects. By means of an injection in the foot, the lymphatics draining a melanoma in the leg may be demonstrated and, as the dye passes centrally, the lymph nodes draining the testis, prostate, and bladder may also be visualized. Unfortunately, lymphangiography has not been shown to be of any value in imaging the lymph nodes draining tumours of breast, lung, and gastrointestinal tract.

16.3.5 *Operative staging*

Although it is possible to stage accurately certain tumours preoperatively, for the majority of common cancers this information only becomes available after a pathologist has examined the surgical specimen. It can then be determined whether the cancer has penetrated the wall of an organ such as the oesophagus, stomach, colon or rectum. Furthermore because the operative procedure will have cleared appropriate surrounding tissue, the presence or absence of metastases in the local lymph nodes can also be confirmed. With this information a more accurate prognosis can be made, as for example of cancer of the rectum for which the Dukes staging system is used (Table 16.2).

Table 16.2 Dukes staging system for cancer of the rectum

Stage	Description	Proportion of patients (%)	Crude 5-year survival (%)
A	Cancer not infiltrating through rectal wall	15	80
B	Tumour spread through rectal wall	35	60
C	Spread to local lymph	50	25

16.4 Treatment

In the discussion of local treatment of cancer it is important to stress that, although such methods cannot achieve cure in patients with micrometastatic disease, there are those in whom the disease can be eradicated by local means. If inappropriate treatment is given to such patients their survival may be unnecessarily compromised.

16.4.1 *Which cancers are curable?*

There are two groups of cancers which should always be curable. First, there are the *in situ* carcinomas in which there is no invasion. The second group are cancers which locally infiltrate but have a minimal tendency to metastasize, and these include the basal cell carcinoma of the skin (rodent ulcer) and the sacral chordoma (a tumour of the lower spine derived from embryonal cells). Provided that rodent ulcers are widely excised or adequately irradiated then cure is possible, but failure to achieve local clearance or destruction of the tumour results in an inexorable ulcerative process producing surrounding tissue destruction. As many of these lesions are located on the face, a very unpleasant disfigurement occurs after suboptimal treatment.

Sacral chordoma, which is a rare tumour, is another example of a locally invasive cancer which does not usually metastasize. Unfortunately because of its pelvic location and propensity to invade surrounding nerves and viscera, the tumour may be only curable by very extensive surgery, the Procrustean measure of hemicorporectomy. Although this might result in a clinical cure the end result will daunt the majority of patients. This extreme case does illustrate one of the most difficult aspects of cancer surgery. What is the patient prepared to accept in order to have a high probability of cancer cure? Thus, Dukes Stage A rectal cancers may be cured by excision of the rectum and anus leaving the patient with a permanent colostomy, but for some patients this is unacceptable and so a non-curative but anal sphincter conserving procedure may be performed. Although there are patients who can be predictively cured, in the majority of solid tumours our present patho-logical and biochemical methods are insufficiently precise to determine those that will be cured by local treatment.

16.4.2 *En bloc resection*

This remains the fundamental technique in cancer surgery. The aim of en bloc resection is to remove the tumour, its draining lymphatics, lymph nodes, and sufficient normal tissue to clear widely the margins of tumour. By this means it is hoped that the tumour bearing field can be removed. The underlying assumption is that tumour cells invade local lymphatics and are retained in local lymph nodes before blood borne spread occurs. While this is sometimes true, unfortunately the presence of metastases in lymph nodes may often be a manifestation of micrometastatic disease elsewhere. En bloc resection for certain gastrointestinal tumours requires technically difficult reconstructive surgery with an associated risk of postoperative complications and death. Thus although a small number of patients with tumours in the pancreas may be cured by excision of the head of the pancreas, duodenum, and common bile duct, the results of this treatment overall are no better than much simpler palliative procedures.

16.4.3 *Radiotherapy*

The results of treatment of many tumours by radiotherapy are as good as those obtained surgically. Because such results may be obtained without the pain of surgery and sometimes with less disfigurement, this may be a more acceptable option for many patients, although there is still a wide-spread lay prejudice that radiotherapy is only used for the treatment of incurable cancers. There are two main techniques of radiotherapy, external or interstital.

External radiotherapy is nowadays usually megavoltage from either linear accelerators or Cobalt sources in the form of X–rays and gamma rays. By this means, deeply located lesions such as oesophageal or bronchial carcinomas may be treated without excessive radiation damage to the skin and adjacent normal organs, by giving the total dose in fractions.

Interstitial radiation gives a large local dose to the tumour from implanted radioactive sources such as radium or iridium. This technique is widely used in the treatment of head and neck cancers to give a high tumour dose but with protection of sensitive organs such as the lens and spinal cord. Sometimes a combination of interstitial radiation and external radiotherapy may be given to treat the potentially malignant peritumour field as well as the tumour. Radiation sources may also be inserted into body cavities and this form of intracavitary therapy has been particularly useful in the treatment of certain gynaelogical malignancies. How radiation kills cancer cells selectively is not fully understood, but all dividing cells are particularly sensitive to radiation damage and consequently rapidly proliferating tumour cells are especially vulnerable, but one of the drawbacks of radiation treatment is that therapeutic doses may also kill dividing cells of normal tissues.

16.4.4 *Combined approaches*

To treat cancer with less disfigurement or with greater efficacy, combined approaches using surgery, radiotherapy, and sometimes chemotherapy are becoming more prevalent. Hodgkin's disease is one example of a lymphoma which was previously incurable but is now for many a curable disease. A diagnosis is usually made by surgical excision of an enlarged lymph node, followed by an operation in which the spleen is removed and para-aortic lymph nodes are biopsied; in addition, liver and bone marrow biopsies may also be taken. By this means, the extent of spread of the disease can be fairly accurately determined, so that radiotherapy fields can be planned as can appropriate cytotoxic chemotherapy.

Bone marrow transplantation is a local procedure which is used as an adjunct to systemic therapy of tumours such as small cell carcinoma of the lung. Marrow is removed from the patient and stored during the period of treatment in which dosages of cytotoxic agents are given to achieve the maximal tumour cell kill. Such dosages also destroy all potential blood forming cells in the marrow. After therapy has ceased the marrow is reinfused in order that haemopoetic function can be restarted (see Chapter 18).

Another example of the combined approach is for follicular carcinoma of the thyroid. After the diagnosis has been made histologically, a total thyroidectomy is performed. This is followed by a thyroid scan using a radioactive isotope of iodine I^{131} which is selectively taken up by normal and neoplastic thyroid cells. If thyroid cells persist, a thyroid destroying dose of I^{131} is given. This is followed by regular thyroxine administration both to supply physiological requirements and also to inhibit any persistent thyroid activity.

One of the more important recent uses of a combined approach has been in the treatment of breast carcinoma. For many years the treatment of this disease was by some form of mastectomy often followed by radiotherapy. For many patients this was an unacceptable mutilation and may have been responsible for delay in presentation to the physician. In the new combined approach, the tumour is excised and the tumour bed implanted with plastic tubes which are subsequently loaded with iridium[192] wire. At the same time the axillary lymph nodes are resected en bloc through a small separate axillary incision. Treatment is completed by external beam radiotherapy to the entire preserved breast and adjuvant treatment may be given if necessary depending on the result of the axillary nodal histology. It is hoped that this combined regimen will be an effective treatment and also an improvement in the quality of life resulting from conservation of the breast.

16.4.5 *Palliative treatment*

Many patients either present with advanced cancer, or develop recurrences after what was hoped to be curative treatment. Local treatment may still play an important role in the palliation of symptoms so that, even in the presence of proven metastases, the local tumour may be excised or irradiated to prevent unpleasant symptoms such as bowel obstruction, haemorrhage or ulceration. In addition, symptomatic metastases may be amenable to local treatment so that bone secondaries may be irradiated not only to relieve pain but also to prevent pathological fractures. The pleural space is a common site of metastases from lung, breast, and ovarian lesions and this may give rise to a pleural effusion which by compression of the underlying lung produces shortness of breath. Good relief of this symptom may be obtained by drainage of the fluid and installation of talcum powder. This stimulates a fibrous reaction that obliterates the pleural space and hence prevents reaccumulation. Similarly, intraperitonal installation of cytotoxic agents or insertion of peritoneovenous shunts may prevent reaccumulation of ascitic fluid due to carcinomas of the ovary or bowel.

Certain tumours, such as those arising from the breast, prostate or uterus, may be hormonally sensitive. Significant remissions may be achieved in patients with advanced disease by removing the source of such endocrine stimulation. Thus breast cancer metastases may be palliated by ovarian excision (oophorectomy) and prostatic malignancy may regress following testicular excision (orchidectomy). Further remissions may be achieved by surgical removal of the adrenal or pituitary glands. However, such surgical procedures are used infrequently nowadays since comparable results may be obtained using hormonal therapy which does not have the serious side effects of major endocrine surgery (see Chapter 13).

16.5 The problem areas

Certain tumours, such as those arising from the lung, pancreas and ovary, almost invariably present at a stage beyond that curable by local means. It is therefore necessary to delineate high risk groups when possible and to develop markers which can identify early malignant change. With the exception of lung cancer, the present epidemiological methods have not been able to identify patients at high risk of other common tumours, nor have sufficiently sensitive biochemical markers been developed to detect early disease, except in the rare choriocarcinoma, a tumour of the uterus that produces a hormone (chorionic gonadotropin) that is easily detected in the blood. A reduction in the level of the hormone indicates a response to treatment.

It would be expected that skin cancers should be detectable at an early stage and therefore be curable. Many are, but unfortunately one type, malignant melanoma, behaves in a very aggressive manner with the prognosis related not to the surface area covered but to the depth of invasion. Despite producing a cell specific marker, the pigment melanin, this has not been found to be of value in early detection or in monitoring of disease. Surgery may sometimes be curable but recurrence is resistant to radiotherapy, and attempts at immunotherapy or infusion of cytotoxic drugs into blood vessels to an affected limb have not affected disease progression.

The tumours grouped together as breast cancer provide a continuum from those cured by local treatment to those with widespread metastases at presentation. Unlike many tumours in which the five year survival is an accurate indicator of cure rate, breast cancer recurrence and tumour associated deaths occur up to 30 years after diagnosis. The major determinants of prognosis in breast cancer are tumour grade, size, and axillary nodal involvement, but none are able to predict those patients who will survive more than 15 years. The only indicator of long term survival is age at diagnosis which probably relates to age associated mortality.

Our present ability to predict the outcome in patients with cancer is very limited. New approaches to the characterization of tumours, together with an increased understanding of physiological and pathological differentiation, may yield information of great clinical importance. More sensitive techniques in the detection and monitoring of cancer are necessary so that local treatment may be used when appropriate but also combined with other methods of management for patients in whom local measures are unable to control the progress of the disease.

Further reading

Dukes, C. E. (1957). Discussion on major surgery in carcinoma of the rectum with or without colostomy, excluding the anal canal and including the recto-sigmoid. *Proceedings of the Royal Society of Medicine* **50**, 1031.

Fentiman, I. S., Cuzick, J., Millis, R. R., and Hayward, J. L. (1984). Which patients are cured of breast cancer? *British Medical Journal* **289**, 1108–11.

Hayward, J. L., Winter, D. J., Tong, D., Rubens, R. D., Payne, J. G., Chaudary, M. A., and Habibollahi, F. (1984). A new combined approach to the conservative treatment of early breast cancer. *Surgery* **95**, 270–4.

Isherwood, I., and Forbes, W. St. C. (1980). CT scanning—the body. In: *A textbook of radiology and imaging* pp. 1297–304. (ed. D. Sutton) (3rd Edition) **Vol. 2.** Churchill Livingstone, Edinburgh.

Johannesson, G., Geirsson, G., and Day, N. (1978). The effect of mass screening in Iceland 1965–74 on the incidence and mortality of cervical carcinoma. *International Journal of Cancer* **21**, 418.

Shapiro, S. (1977). Evidence on screening for breast cancer from a randomized trial. *Cancer* **39**, 2772–82.

Whipple, A. O. (1946). Observations on radical surgery for lesions of pancreas. *Surgery, Gynaecology and Obstetrics* **82**, 623–31.

17

Chemotherapy

J. S. MALPAS

17.1 Introduction

Chemotherapy is a relatively new method of treating cancer. The tradition of treating cancer with surgery had been in existence for over a century, and radiotherapy had been used for at least a quarter of a century before chemotherapy made its appearance in the middle of the Second World War. Malignant disease, such as leukaemia, which was generalized when it first presented, or tumours which had become disseminated, were incurable up to that time. Chemotherapy gave a first promise of cure.

The development of analogues of mustard gas and their profound effects on the lymphoid system suggested that they might be effective in treating lymphomas or tumours of the lymphatic system. The use of these agents, which were called radiomimetic drugs, as they were very similar to radiotherapy in their effect, was already quite advanced when the second success was reported in 1948 with the use of the anti-metabolic agent amethopterin in the treatment of childhood lymphoblastic leukaemia. In the next decade, a 'golden age' for the discovery of and introduction to clinical use of alkylating agents and anti-metabolites, a wide range of common and rare malignancies were treated with these agents.

It was soon apparent that for a drug to be successfully introduced for use in the clinic, it was necessary to progress through a series of tests. Initially, its toxicity and the effects on various organs were established by testing in small animals. Toxicity in the liver or kidneys, for example, could be assessed, and these features looked for carefully when it was first administered to patients. The sequence of events in clinical trials will be discussed in more detail later, but essentially, Phase I studies of drugs establish the dose, route of administration, excretion pattern, and salient toxic features. Once this information is available, Phase II studies, in which patients with a variety of malignancies receive the drug, are carried out, and the spectrum of tumours that are sensitive to the agent can be defined. More advanced studies, sometimes called Phase III studies, allow for in depth evaluation of patients, usually being treated for one form of malignancy, in which the effect of the new drug plus the best established previous method of treatment is compared to a control group of patients in a randomized manner, the control group having the previously most successful form of treatment. The difficulties, errors and constraints on the introduction of new drugs will be discussed in more detail at the end of this chapter.

17.2 Classification of chemotherapeutic drugs

Using this approach, a whole range of clinically effective drugs was made available over the next two decades. Some of these act directly on tumour cells whereas others must be activated by metabolic processes, either in the tumour cells or in organs such as the liver. A list of some of the most important drugs is given in Table 17.1. Increasing knowledge of the mechanism of cell division was being gained *pari passu* with the introduction of these agents. In the hope that greater knowledge of how these agents worked would enable them to be used more effectively clinically, questions as to whether they were active on the dividing cell and, if this was so, whether they were active at a particular stage of cell division, became of great interest.

It is possible to divide drugs into those that are not active only on dividing cells, those that are active on dividing cells and affect a very particular phase of cell division (phase specific drugs), and those that effect all or most of the phases of the cell cycle (Table 17.2).

The particular phases where some of these drugs act are shown in Figure 17.1. Whatever the mode of action of the chemotherapeutic agent, a very important finding is that it destroys malignant cells according to

Table 17.1 Anticancer drugs

Classification	Drug
Alkylating agents	Mechlorethamine Busulphan Chlorambucil Cyclophosphamide Melphalan Thiotepa
Antimetabolites	Methotrexate 6-mercaptopurine Thioguanine 5-fluorouracil Cytosine arabinoside 5-azacytidine
Plant alkaloids	Vinblastine Vincristine VP-16
Antibiotics	Actinomycin D Doxorubicin Bleomycin Daunorubicin Mithramycin Mitomycin C
Nitrosoureas	Carmustine Lomustine Semustine Streptozotocin
Enzymes	L-asparaginase
Random synthetics	*Cis*-platinum diammine dichloride Dacarbazine Dibromomannitol Hexamethylmelamine Hydroxyurea Mitotane Procarbazine

first order kinetics; in other words the same proportion of cells is killed for each dose of the agent.

It is very important to recognize that chemotherapeutic drugs damage normal tissues as well; indeed, if they were non-toxic to normal tissues,

Table 17.2 Phase and cycle specific drugs

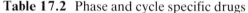

Phase specificity	Acts on	Drug
S phase specific	DNA synthesis	Methotrexate Cytosine arabinoside Hydroxyurea
Relatively S phase specific	DNA, RNA and protein synthesis	5-fluorouracil 6-mercaptopurine
Cycle specific	DNA at all phases of cycle	Nitrogen mustard Nitrosourea Cyclophosphamide

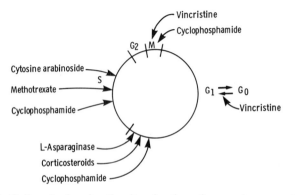

Fig. 17.1 Cell cycle showing the site of action of some phase specific drugs.

cancer would have been cured long ago. The only reason that chemotherapy is feasible is that normal tissues recover fully, and somewhat more rapidly, than the tumour cells. It is on this narrow difference in behaviour that practical clinical chemotherapy rests.

From the point of view of the practising clinician treating patients, the contribution that the knowledge of the kinetics of cancer cells and the effect of the drug on the cell cycle has made has been disappointing, probably because human tumours are very different in their behaviour from the rapidly growing experimental animal tumours in which the proportion of dividing malignant cells in the tumour is very high.

A more helpful classification, based on the mode of action of particular groups of agents, is probably of more immediate help (Table 17.3). The remarkable feature about this table is the wide variety of sources for chemotherapeutic agents. Some were produced deliberately

Table 17.3 Groups of chemotherapeutic agents

Class of compound	Examples	Tumours against which drug is most active
Antifolic compounds	Methotrexate	Acute leukaemia Choriocarcinoma
Antipurines and pyrimidines	6-mercaptopurine 5-fluorouracil	Acute leukaemia Breast cancer
Alkylating agents	Melphalan Cyclophosphamide Busulphan	Myeloma Lymphoma Chronic myeloid leukaemia
Sex hormones	Oestrogens Androgens	Prostate cancer Breast cancer
Steroids	Corticosteroids	Leukaemia Lymphoma
Antitumour antibiotics	Actinomycin Anthracyclines Daunorubicin Doxorubicin Mitomycin	Wilms' tumour Leukaemia Lymphoma
Plant extracts	Vinblastine Vincristine Vindesine	Hodgkin's disease Leukaemia

on the basis of interfering with the metabolic pathway, but many were discovered by pure chance—vincristine, for example, in the search for a new anti-diabetic agent, procarbazine in the development of a tranquillizing drug, and the anti-tumour antibiotics were often discovered in the search for new anti-bacterial agents. Furthermore, the source of these drugs gives very little indication of the likelihood of activity against a particular tumour.

17.3 Drug toxicity

Information on toxicity is most useful to the clinician when considering the choice of chemotherapeutic agents for cancer therapy. Toxicity can be divided into that occurring shortly after administration, that which is somewhat delayed, and the very long term toxic effects. Before a drug or combination of drugs is administered to a patient, the gain in terms of clinical benefit must be balanced against these toxicities, examples of which are shown in Table 17.4. The table has been arranged to show the common non-specific toxicity that may be encountered with most therapeutic agents. Specific toxicities are shown on the right hand side of the table. The clinician must know in detail the general and specific toxicities of all the chemotherapeutic agents that he uses.

17.4 Principles of chemotherapy

It is important to be quite clear about the reason for giving a cytotoxic drug or combination of drugs. From experience we now know that it is possible for chemotherapy to cure various malignancies. Children with acute leukaemia, Wilms' tumour, soft tissue sarcomas, lymphomas, and other tumours are curable. Adults with acute myelogenous leukaemia, lymphoblastic leukaemia, non-Hodgkin's lymphoma, Hodgkin's disease, and teratoma of the testis are potentially curable. These drugs, therefore,

Table 17.4 Drug toxicity

Common	Special
Immediate (within hours)	
Nausea and vomiting	Haemorrhagic cystitis (cyclophosphamide)
Phlebitis	Radiation recall (actinomycin)
Hyperuricaemia	Fever (bleomycin)
Renal failure	
Early (days to weeks)	
Reduction in white blood cells (leucopenia)	Paralytic ileus (vinca alkaloids)
Reduction in blood platelets (thrombocytopenia)	Pancreatitis (asparaginase)
Hair loss (alopecia)	Cerebellar disorders (high dose cytosine arabinoside)
Diarrhoea	Ear toxicity (platinum)
Delayed (weeks or months)	
Anaemia	Peripheral nerve damage (vinca alkaloids)
Aspermia	Inappropriate ADH (cyclophosphamide)
Liver cell damage	Jaundice (6-mercaptopurine)
Fibrosis of lung	Adrenal deficiency (busulphan)
Late (months to years)	
Sterility	Liver fibrosis (methotrexate)
Testicular or ovarian atrophy	Brain damage (methotrexate)
Second malignancies	Bladder cancer (cyclophosphamide)

have to be given to the limits imposed by toxicity, on a definite schedule, which may have to be tailored around other methods of treatment such as surgery or radiotherapy.

In some tumours, cure cannot be realistically contemplated, and in these patients effective drugs or drug combinations may be able to extend useful life considerably. Good examples are breast carcinoma, ovarian carcinoma, small cell carcinoma of the bronchus, and myeloma.

There are some forms of malignant disease where it is known that there has been no improvement in the duration of survival since chemotherapy was introduced, but the quality of life has been immeasurably improved. Such a disease is chronic granulocytic leukaemia, where the median duration of survival is still only about 34 months some 30 years after busulphan was introduced for the condition, but patients lead normal lives during most of the course of the disease, and the benefit of what is palliative therapy is immense.

Finally, there are occasions when chemotherapy may be used as an effective palliative agent in a tumour which has been previously treated with radiotherapy or surgery. The bone pain associated with disseminated breast cancer may be rapidly relieved, the fearful symptoms of strangulation occasioned by a large carcinoma in the region of the trachea may be dispelled in a few hours by the injection of nitrogen mustard. These beneficial effects should not be underrated.

17.5 Administration of chemotherapeutic drugs

17.5.1 *Combination chemotherapy*

From time to time in the clinic it is very evident that a tumour will not respond to a chemotherapeutic drug which is usually effective in the condition, or possibly, after a period of time in which the tumour has responded, it again becomes unresponsive. This phenomenon of resistance will be discussed in more detail later. An immediate practical solution has been to add a second drug, which ideally would not have the same toxicity. Such an example was the so called 'induction' therapy for acute lymphoblastic leukaemia in children. Vincristine and prednisolone were both found to be effective in producing remission, and when given singly, achieved remission in about half the patients; that is, they could return the child to normal health with no clinical evidence of leukaemia, a normal blood count, and a bone marrow test in which the leukaemic blast cells had gone. When the two drugs were combined, this percentage rose to over 90 per cent. Futhermore, as the drugs had very different toxicities, this was achieved without great hazard. In this instance the anti-tumour effect doubled, but the toxicity did not.

Addition of even more drugs was found in some tumours to be more

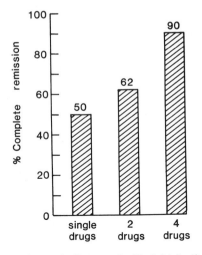

Fig. 17.2 Improvement in remission rate in Hodgkin's disease as the number of drugs used in combination increases.

effective. An example of response rates to one, two, and then four drugs in Hodgkin's disease is shown in Figure 17.2. In both acute lymphoblastic leukaemia in children and in Hodgkin's disease, this considerable increase in remission rate has been accompanied by a notable increase in survival (Fig. 17.3).

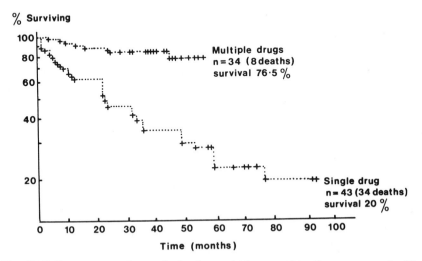

Fig. 17.3 Improvement in survival using multidrug combinations compared with the use of single agents in Hodgkin's disease.

The latest adult tumour to show sensitivity to this approach is teratoma of the testis, the commonest tumour of young men between the ages of 20 and 35. This may be cured, even when it is disseminated, by a combination of vinblastine, bleomycin, and *cis*-platinum. It is probable that, in the case of Hodgkin's disease and teratoma of the testis, the multi drug combination prevents the emergence of any drug resistant strains of tumour cells, a feature which is not seen in many other tumours.

The response to the application of multiple drug regimens in the case of bladder carcinoma and bowel carcinoma has not been so successful, and more effective agents are awaited.

17.5.2 Adjuvant chemotherapy

This form of chemotherapy was first introduced into the treatment of Wilms' tumour, a tumour of the kidney in young children, on the assumption that metastases were already widely disseminated when the patient was first seen. This hypothesis considered that these metastases are composed of a few cells, which have an increased mitotic rate and a good blood supply, so that although they are not detectable they are nevertheless very susceptible to the action of chemotherapeutic agents. More recently, this degree of sensitivity has been queried, but nevertheless, when this hypothesis was tested in Wilms' tumour, it was shown that survival had increased considerably. With surgery and radiotherapy, survival was seen in only about 40 per cent of patients. Given 'adjuvant' therapy, that is, treatment directed at the micrometastases from the time of presentation of the tumour, led to an increase in survival, which is now regularly seen in most clinical series at between 85 and 90 per cent. This principle has been applied, with considerable success, to other childhood tumours. It has been much less successful in adult solid tumours, but this is only to be expected, since the response to chemotherapy of most carcinomas affecting adults is much less satisfactory.

17.5.3 Sanctuary sites

A major problem in the administration of anticancer agents is that they may not always be distributed throughout the body. Thus, in the induction of remission in children with acute lymphoblastic leukaemia, the drugs vincristine and prednisolone do not enter the meningeal spaces surrounding the brain and spinal cord, certainly not in sufficient concentration to be tumoricidal. This was responsible for the high frequency of relapse seen with the meningeal leukaemia in these children, until it was demonstrated in the early 1970s that the administration of methotrexate directly into the meningeal space, combined with cranial radiotherapy, could eliminate these cells lodged in so-called 'sanctuary sites'. There is considerable argument as to whether there are other sanctuary sites, such as the testes of boys who have lymphoblastic leukaemia, or localized peritoneal areas in women with ovarian cancer.

17.5.4 *Principles of high dose therapy*

Studies on experimental tumour systems have shown that for some drugs, alkylating agents for example, the number of tumour cells that are killed is directly related to the dose of the drug that is given. There is also evidence that the emergence of drug resistance is also related to the intensity of the initial drug therapy, and that resistance is far less likely to develop if effective drugs are given in high dosage early in the course of the disease. Drug resistance most often develops if repeated small doses of drug are given over a long period of time. The range of drugs that can be used in the clinic for high dose therapy is limited. There are two kinds: one in which there is a specific antidote to the drug (for example, metho-trexate, where the patient may be 'rescued' by the use of a specific agent, citrovorum factor or folinic acid), and the other, in which the dose limit-ing toxicity is such that the patient can be supported through the period of the acute damage to normal tissues produced by the drug. An example of the latter is the alkylating agent melphalan, which in normal circum-stances is very toxic to bone marrow, but has no other deleterious effects, even when quite high doses are given. If bone marrow is removed, and stored before the drug is given, it can be replaced as soon as the drug has been excreted. Repopulation of the bone marrow follows, and the patient's blood count recovers rapidly. Drugs which may be useful in high dose therapy include cyclophosphamide, cytosine arabinoside, and new drugs such as etoposide. Use in the clinic is still at a relatively early stage, but it appears that increased response rates and possibly increased length of survival may be seen in some children treated in this way, and in adults who, for example, are being treated for the plasma cell tumour myeloma. Further studies will be necessary before the usefulness of high dose chemotherapy can be properly assessed.

If high dose chemotherapy or a combination of this procedure and whole body irradiation prove to be effective, it becomes even more important to improve methods for removing any tumour cells from the bone marrow which had been removed and stored. Intensive research is now going on in an attempt to do this. Physical methods for removing tumour cells have not been very successful, but new methods using monoclonal antibodies are now being tried. In one technique, tumour associated antibodies are attached to magnetic beads. Tumour cells adhere to the antibodies and the beads are then removed by passing the cell suspension through a magnetic field induced by powerful electro-magnets. In another technique a toxic material, ricin, is coupled to the monoclonal antibodies so that the drug is delivered only to the tumour cells. The use of this technique in chemotherapy is discussed in detail in Chapter 18. Another approach is to use a drug, 4-hydroxyperoxycyclophosphamide. This is related to cyclophosphamide but, unlike its parent compound, does not require activation by passage through the liver *in vivo,* but can be safely incubated with human bone marrow *in vitro.*

There is now great interest in the extension of chemotherapy using these manoeuvres, but it is not yet possible to say whether the approaches will be useful.

17.6 Drug resistance

As with many other illnesses, a patient may not respond to a drug when it is given, or possibly, having responded, after a short time ceases to do so. In the clinic, failure to respond may be simply that the patient has not taken the drug (failure of compliance), and although this seems unlikely to occur in the management of cancer, surprisingly, studies have shown that some patients do not take the drugs, and even children are not given the oral medication for their leukaemia by their parents. If the drug has been taken, it may not be absorbed. There is a large variation in the rate of absorption of melphalan, for example, between different individuals. Even if the drug is absorbed, it may not reach the appropriate site, as seen already in the case of meningeal leukaemia. Although all these phenomena could be included in a discussion of resistance, what the chemotherapist and biochemist is most interested in is the reason why a cell becomes resistant. This topic is discussed in detail by Stark and Calvert (see Further reading).

Biochemical resistance will be discussed generally, and then a more detailed description of resistance in the case of the drug methotrexate will be considered. It can be shown that the uptake into the cell of certain drugs can gradually decrease with repeated exposure. Examples of this are found in cells treated with methotrexate, actinomycin or the anthracyclines.

Antimetabolites (see Table 17.1) work by competing with certain enzymes. If these enzymes are rendered inactive, more enzyme may be produced by the cell or alternative pathways found. For example, the dihydrofolate reductase content of cells becoming resistant to methotrexate increases. A similar increase also occurs with the enzyme asparaginase synthetase, when resistance develops after treatment with L-asparaginase, which acts by destroying the enzyme, thus depleting the cell of the essential amino acid asparagine. There is also evidence that the affinity of the drug for the target enzyme may be reduced.

Many drugs, particularly antimetabolites, require activation if they are to be effective. In resistant cells the activating enzyme may be reduced.

Thus, decreased phosphoribosyl transferase may impair the activity of 6-mercaptopurine and 6-thioguanine. A similar effect has been shown where two enzymes, uridine phosphorylase and kinase, are reduced, thus impairing the activity of 5-fluorouracil.

Increased inactivation of drugs by the tumour cells may also be the cause of resistance. Cytosine arabinoside, one of the most effective drugs in the treatment of acute non-lymphoblastic leukaemia, may be rendered ineffective by the production of deaminase by the leukaemic cells. It can be shown in the patient that the use of grams of cytosine arabinoside, rather than milligrams, can again induce remission in patients whose leukaemia had become resistant to the smaller dose. Although the subject of metabolic pathways and cells is immensely complicated, there is good evidence that some resistance is due to acquired enhancement of various alternative pathways providing the tumour cell with necessary intermediate metabolites.

Few of these mechanisms would explain the resistance to alkylating agents, where it has been shown that various enzymes, including the nucleases, are recruited during the development of resistance, to aid in DNA repair.

17.7 Methotrexate resistance as a model

Methotrexate acts principally during the S phase of the cell cycle by inhibiting the enzyme dihydrofolate reductase which is necessary for the production of an essential metabolite, tetrahydrofolate, necessary for DNA synthesis. Probably no other chemotherapeutic drug has been so intensively studied with regard to the development of resistance. Some of these studies have already been considered. The different rate of transmembrane passage in resistant and nonresistant cells has been shown, and the relationship between sensitivity and rate of uptake of methotrexate has been demonstrated in murine leukaemia cells. Two mechanisms, one active and one passive, have been demonstrated, and the presence of this latter mechanism forms the basis for the use of therapy with high dose methotrexate. The whole subject of membrane permeability has become much more complicated since the discovery of a single surface protein associated with a genetic change in the cell, the p-glycoprotein. This glycoprotein has a mol. wt. of 170 000 daltons. The higher the concentration of p-glycoprotein, the greater the degree of resistance which occurs to transport of a wide variety of unrelated chemical substances across the membrane. When very resistant cells have been produced in the laboratory expressing a high level of p-glyco-protein, it has been shown that this high degree of resistance can be conferred on drug sensitive cells by DNA mediated gene transfer (see Chapter 10 for methods of gene transfer).

Another fundamental finding necessary to the understanding of resistance to methotrexate is the ability of even a small amount of the enzyme dihydrofolate reductase to stimulate enough thymidylate synthesis for cell activity. Thus, unless there is a continuous presence of free drug, synthesis will start again. Consequently, even minor changes in binding or the ability to produce more dihydrofolate reductase will profoundly affect the action of the drug, and render it ineffective. While drug binding to reductase has been found to be related to resistance in mouse leukaemias, the evidence for this in man is weak. What has been shown more recently is that with the steady increase in exposure to methotrexate, amplification of the gene controlling formation of the enzyme occurs, and homogeneously staining regions (see Chapter 11) on a specific marker chromosome can be seen to be increased in the resistant cell. This resistance, which comes about as the result of gene amplification, may of course be occurring in both normal cells and tumour cells, and only appears under selective pressures. It is possible that mechanisms for resistance which develop to other antimetabolic drugs are of this nature.

The spontaneous occurrence of drug resistance in malignant tumour cells is of such fundamental importance that it is not too great an exaggeration to say that the future for chemotherapy depends on its understanding and exploitation. Normal cells never become resistant to chemotherapy, a fact of equal importance to our understanding of the differences between normal and malignant cells.

17.8 Clinical trials

The vast array of synthetic and non-synthetic compounds which might be effective in cancer chemotherapy has led to the definition of some common sense principles of assessment, so that time, expense, and other resources are not used wastefully.

The introduction of a new agent, whether it has been developed in the pharmaceutical industry or university laboratory, is preceded by a time-consuming and expensive series of toxicity trials in animals. A Phase I trial on a human subject is designed to determine the best route of administration, the features of the pharmacokinetics such as the routes of excretion and rapidity of excretion, and details of toxicity such as dose limiting toxic side effects, and the range of toxic effects that may occur. Many patients may have had previously all the conventional treatment available, so that the response may be minimal. Even so, a response in one patient in a consecutive series of, say, 14 or 15 patients who have been previously treated, would encourage a Phase II study.

Phase II trials concentrate on the clinical response, and these are defined in Table 17.5. In Phase II trials, the drug is given to patients who

Table 17.5 Criteria for response in solid tumours

Response	Criteria
Complete response	Complete disappearance of all demonstrable disease
Partial response	More than 50 per cent reduction in the sum of the products of the longest perpendicular diameters of tumour with no disease progression elsewhere
No response	No change or less than 50 per cent reduction
Progression	Increase in size of tumour at any site

have a variety of different tumours. Some will have already been previously treated. The aim of the trial is to determine the spectrum of activity of the agent. It very often happens that the tumour chosen is one that responds relatively infrequently to a chemotherapeutic agent of any kind, and in this case, so called 'randomized Phase II trials' are justified, in which the overall response to the new agent is compared on a random basis with the ones used previously. Phase II studies give more information about toxicity and the possible therapeutic benefit of the drug. Their chief danger is that they underestimate the efficacy of the drug, and may deter its investigation in the more difficult Phase III studies.

A great deal has been written about the advantages and disadvantages of randomized trials. Penicillin, for example, would not have needed a randomized study to show its efficacy. Unfortunately, because of the less dramatic effects of most anticancer agents, benefit is not easily detected, and physicians have been misled by small non-randomized studies. What is also quite apparent is that carefully conducted randomized studies can occasionally produce contradictory answers. This is most likely to be due to the fact that the two populations, the patients treated with the new drug and the controls who have been treated with the standard regimens, differ in some subtle and perhaps unrecognized way that biases response. The only way in which this bias can be eliminated in a randomized Phase III study is by recruiting large numbers of patients. The question is then whether one is ethically justified in doing this; if the difference is small, perhaps the answer doesn't matter, and a large number of patients may be locked into a trial which may contribute relatively little to knowledge about the disease and its management.

It is very tempting in this case to turn to comparing results with 'historical' controls. It is very difficult to conclude that the historical controls are ever matched adequately. If nothing else has changed, the physician will have improved his ability to manage the condition under investigation (or at least one would hope so). Criticisms about variation in the general supportive care, ancillary services such as blood transfusion, treatment of bacterial infections, etc. are valid, but are less likely to be true in the case of a Unit which admits a lot of patients suffering from one particular disease, and where the supportive care is relatively unchanged over a number of years. Any marked improvement in response or survival is then probably a true finding, and has the advantage that any new modification can be built into the therapeutic programme quite rapidly. New methods of analysing data are now being studied. This activity, and the debate on how one should measure what is done, will certainly be welcomed, for the critical attitude that it encourages is our only real hope for continued progress.

17.9 Conclusion

It will be seen that the agents currently employed in the treatment of cancer are imperfect, achieve their effects by methods which are poorly understood, and may produce lasting damage to normal tissues. Despite this, the number of patients who are being cured of their cancers as a result of chemotherapy is increasing gradually every year. By 1990 it is estimated that one in every 2000 young adults reaching the age of 21 will have been cured of cancer. This is a remarkable achievement when it is remembered that it has occurred within the space of one professional lifetime.

Further reading

Calman, K. C., Smyth, J. F., and Tattersall, M. H. N. (1980). *Basic principles of cancer chemotherapy*. Macmillan Press, London.

Morfardini, S., Brumer, K., Crowther, D., Olive, D., MacDonald, J., Eckhardt, S., Whitehouse, J., and Redd, D. (eds.). *Manual of cancer chemotherapy* (3rd edition). UICC Technical Report Series, Vol. **56**, UICC, Geneva.

Stark, G. R., and Calvert, H. (eds.) (1986). Drug resistance. *Cancer Surveys* **5**, No. 2.

For detailed information on specific topics, consult the following specialized review series.

Seminars in oncology. Grune and Stratton, 111 5th Avenue, New York, N.Y. 1003, USA.

Cancer treatment reports. Public Health Service, National Institutes of Health, National Cancer Institute, Bethesda, Maryland 20205, USA.

Monoclonal antibodies and therapy

EDWARD J. WAWRZYNCZAK and PHILIP E. THORPE

18.1 Introduction

Antibodies are proteins made by higher animals when infected with bacteria, viruses or other foreign substances. They are secreted into the blood by plasma cells as part of a complex immune response against the invading 'organism' (see Chapter 15).

Animals in the laboratory similarly can produce antibodies against a wide range of foreign molecules that need differ only slightly in structure from the animal's own molecules to be immunogenic. Thus, homologous proteins from closely related species may stimulate antibody production. Tumour cells often bear surface molecules which are immunogenic in the natural host or in other animal species. By immunizing animals with preparations of tumour cells, antisera can be raised that contain antibodies recognizing the various antigens found on the tumour cell surface. Antibodies that bind to normal cells can then be removed from the antiserum by suitable absorption procedures leaving behind those antibodies that react strongly with tumour cells.

Attempts to use these antibody preparations for cancer therapy have been disappointing. This is partly because the antiserum contains many antibodies with different specificities, which increases the likelihood of cross reaction with normal cells, and partly because the anti-tumour antibody is diluted with a large excess of antibodies with irrelevant specificity. In addition, the anti-tumour antibodies are often difficult to purify in adequate quantities and preparations from different animals are not equally effective. These problems were largely overcome by the technique devised by Kohler and Milstein for immortalizing and cloning individual antibody forming cells. Each clone of cells produces a single type of antibody called a 'monoclonal antibody' having a single type of antigen binding site. These cells can be grown up in large numbers allowing the reproducible manufacture of the monoclonal antibody in essentially unlimited amount and in a highly pure state. Such antibodies have a number of important uses in the diagnosis and therapy of cancer (see Chapters 3, 16, and 17).

One application of monoclonal anti-tumour antibodies is to identify the type of malignant cell by analysing the tumour cells with a panel of monoclonal antibodies against different antigens. This helps the clinician to decide the most appropriate course of treatment. Second, antibodies can be used to measure the levels of soluble antigens which some tumour cells shed into the blood (see Chapters 15, and 17). Third, anti-tumour antibodies injected into the patient can selectively concentrate within the tumour tissue. If the antibodies are radiolabelled, then it is possible to identify the sites of the primary tumour and large metastatic deposits within the body from the radiation that they emit. Moreover, anti-tumour

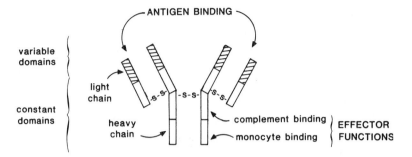

Fig. 18.1 The structure of IgG.

antibodies injected into a patient can exert specific therapeutic effects by stimulating the various defence systems of the body to attack the tumour. Similarly, powerful cell poisons can be attached to the antibody which then carries the poison to the tumour cells and kills them. Lastly monoclonal antibodies can be used to remove malignant cells or T lymphocytes from bone marrow *ex vivo* as part of the treatment of leukaemia and other malignant diseases. Here, we review the present and possible future applications of monoclonal antibodies in the therapy of cancer.

18.1.1 *Antibody structure and function*

The antibody molecule, in its simplest form, consists of four polypeptide chains linked by disulphide bonds: two identical 'heavy' chains and two identical 'light' chains (Fig. 18.1). Each heavy chain consists of a variable domain and three or four constant domains, whereas the light chain consists of a variable domain and a single constant domain. The variable and constant domains of one light chain fold over the variable and first constant domain of one heavy chain to give an 'Fab' arm which contains a single antigen binding site and hence, each antibody molecule has two reactive sites (bivalent). The other constant domains of the heavy chain constitute the 'Fc' portion which mediates the effector functions of the antibody according to the immunoglobulin (Ig) class to which it belongs.

The variable region domains contain 'framework' regions and 'hypervariable' regions. Framework regions of the primary sequence are very similar in antibodies of the same class and are believed to include amino acid residues that are concerned with maintaining the three dimensional structure of the domain. Within hypervariable regions there is much greater diversity of the amino acid sequence between antibodies of the same class. It is principally the spatial distribution of these amino acid residues that determines the individual antigen binding specificity of an antibody molecule. The antigen-binding sites of antibody molecules constitute unique structures that can be distinguished immunologically and are called 'idiotypes'.

Immunoglobulin classes are defined according to the kind of heavy chain the molecule contains. There are five major types of heavy chain, γ. μ, δ, α and ε, which differ in their constant domains, and two types of light chain, κ and λ. The most abundant immunoglobulin in the bloodstream is IgG. It exists as a monomer with two γ chains and either two κ or two λ chains, which have a combined mol. wt. of 150 000 daltons. In humans, there are four IgG subclasses, IgG1, IgG2, IgG3 and IgG4, which have closely related constant domains encoded by different genes. In the mouse and rat, the subclasses are IgG1, IgG2a, IgG2b and IgG3. IgM (containing μ chains) exists in the bloodstream as a pentamer of subunits linked by a joining or J chain and having a combined mol. wt. of 900 000 daltons. Each of the subunits resembles an IgG monomer except for the presence of an extra constant domain on the heavy chain to which the J chain attaches. IgD (together with IgM) is present on the surface of B lymphocytes and acts as a receptor for the antigen. IgD, IgA, and IgE are minor components of serum.

Antibodies of different classes and their subclasses activate different effector mechanisms in the animal (see Section 18.4) and may differ in their activity as anti-tumour agents depending on which effector mechanism is the most active against any particular tumour. Since it is the Fc portion that activates the effector arm of the immune response, the intact antibody molecule is needed for immunotherapy. For radio-imaging or targeting of cytotoxic agents, however, only the antigen binding portion of the antibody is needed and so it is possible to use antibody fragments, i.e. Fab or F(ab')$_2$ generated by the proteolytic action of papain or pepsin respectively (Fig. 18.2).

18.1.2 *Monoclonal antibodies*

When an antigen binds to a B lymphocyte bearing surface immuno-globulin that recognizes the antigen (in the presence of macrophages, helper T cells, and their soluble products), it triggers proliferation and gives rise to a clone of cells all of which, when mature, secrete the same antibody. A single antigen usually stimulates many different B cells. Thus, an immunized animal produces many different antigen specific antibodies. Since normal B lymphocytes soon die out in culture, there was no way to obtain an individual clone of B cells secreting a single kind of antibody until Kohler and Milstein ingeniously preserved the specific antibody-producing characteristics of individual B lymphocytes by converting them into continuously growing tumour cell lines. Their procedure has three stages (see Fig. 18.3).

In the first stage, a suspension of lymphocytes is prepared from the

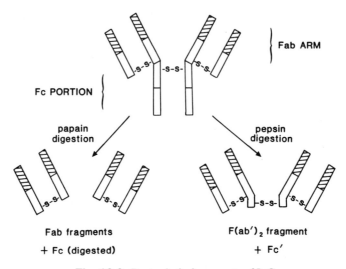

Fig. 18.2 Proteolytic fragments of IgG.

spleen of a suitably immunized animal, usually a mouse or rat. These lymphocytes are mixed with 'myeloma' cells in the presence of an agent such as polyethylene glycol, which causes the cells to fuse together. A myeloma is a malignant plasma cell tumour whose cells secrete immunoglobulins. The myeloma cell lines used for fusion are variants that have been selected for a number of useful characteristics, including resistance to 8-azaguanine (see on), inability to synthesize or secrete immunoglobulin encoded by the myeloma genes, high fusion rates, and stable growth in culture or in rodents. The fusion of a splenic B lymphocyte with a myeloma cell gives rise to a hybrid cell called a 'hybridoma'. This hybrid inherits both the capacity of the myeloma partner for continuous proliferation and the capacity of the B lymphocyte partner to synthesize and secrete the specific antibody.

In the second stage of the protocol, hybridoma cells are isolated from unfused myeloma cells in the fusion mixture by drug selection. This step is necessary because myeloma cells often divide more rapidly than hybridoma cells and would soon outgrow them in culture. Normally, myeloma cells cannot grow in the presence of 8-azaguanine. However, the variant myeloma cells used for fusion are resistant to this drug because they lack hypoxanthine phosphoribosyl transferase (HPRT), an enzyme which catalyses a step in the synthetic pathway from hypoxanthine to purines (see Chapter 7). These resistant myeloma cells use alternative synthetic pathways for DNA synthesis and replication. Accordingly, the cell mixture is grown in medium containing hypoxanthine,

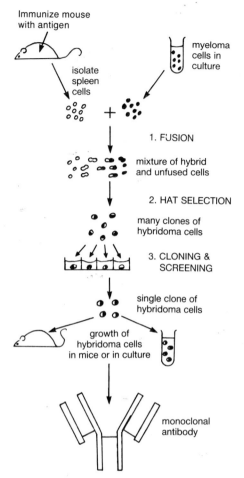

Fig. 18.3 Production of monoclonal antibody.

aminopterin, and thymidine (HAT). Aminopterin blocks the main pathway of purine and pyrimidine synthesis so that the myeloma cells (lacking HPRT) are unable to grow. The hybridoma cells divide normally since they have HPRT activity contributed by the parental splenic B lymphocyte and can use hypoxanthine as a substrate for DNA synthesis. Unfused splenic B lymphocytes do not grow in culture and only the hybridoma cells persist when cultured continuously in the HAT selection medium.

Finally, the mixture of purified hybridoma cells is screened to identify and isolate individual hybridoma clones which secrete an antibody that binds the antigen of interest. This is usually done by diluting suspensions of hybridoma cell mixtures into individual wells of plastic microtitre plates so that each well contains, on average, less than one cell. Clones of cells are allowed to grow and the cell supernatants are assayed for the presence of specific antibody by immunochemical techniques. Cells of clones that secrete such an antibody can be recloned by the same limiting dilution procedure and rescreened until truly monoclonal cell suspensions are obtained. An alternative way to isolate individual clones is to disperse hybridoma cells in agarose mixture and pick out the individual clones that grow.

Hybridoma cell lines can be grown up in large numbers either in tissue culture or as tumours in mice. If grown in tissue culture, the monoclonal antibody can be purified from the culture medium by passing it through a column of anti-mouse Ig or anti-rat Ig coupled to an inert matrix. The bound monoclonal antibody is then eluted from the column, usually with buffers of high or low pH or high salt. If grown in animals, the antibody is extracted from the blood and peritoneal fluid of the animal by standard methods but, in this case, the monoclonal antibody is contaminated with normal Ig which copurifies with the antibody.

18.1.3 *Human monoclonal antibodies*

One factor that limits the usefulness of rodent monoclonal antibodies for cancer therapy in patients is that the antibodies themselves are immunogenic in man. Human monoclonal antibodies would be less immunogenic because they would have the same constant domains as normal human immunoglobulins. However, the hypervariable region of human antibodies would still be immunogenic because it is complementary in structure to the antigen and must therefore itself be foreign. The production of human monoclonal antibodies is more difficult than that of murine monoclonal antibodies for a number or reasons. First, mouse myeloma cell lines are not ideal fusion partners for human B lymphocytes because mouse:human hybrid cells tend to lose the human chromosomes encoding the antibody molecule during prolonged growth in culture. Second, there are at present few human myeloma cell lines which fuse with human B lymphocytes to produce hybridomas that secrete monoclonal antibodies in useful amounts. Third, immune B lymphocytes are difficult to obtain from man although such cells may be extracted from within and around tumour sites in patients. This problem may be solved by the techniques now being developed for immunizing human B lymphocytes with the antigen *in vitro*. Finally, not all human:human hybrid cells grow as tumours even in immunologically-deficient mice. Other ways of immortalizing human antibody forming cells are also being sought; for example, B lymphocytes can be transformed into continuously growing cell lines by infecting them with viruses such as the Epstein Barr virus.

18.1.4 *Genetically engineered antibodies*

Recently, genetic engineering techniques have been used to construct vectors with altered immunoglobulin genes. When a suitable non-producing mouse myeloma cell is transfected with one of these vectors, it expresses the manipulated genes and is able to secrete the modified antibody. Thus, it is possible to create antibodies in which the variable region domains of the heavy and light chains are encoded by genes of a mouse antibody-secreting myeloma and the constant region domains are encoded by human genes. These 'chimaeric' antibodies have the antigen binding specificity of the antibody produced by the parental mouse myeloma and effector functions determined by the Fc portion of the human molecule. Such advances may overcome some of the difficulties associated with the production of human monoclonal antibodies since genes could be isolated from unstable hybridoma lines and preserved within the vector system.

In an extension of this approach, Neuberger and his colleagues replaced the constant region domains in the Fc portion of a mouse anti-body with a nuclease from *Staphylococcus aureus*. The resulting bifunctional chimaeric molecule retained both antigen binding ability and nuclease activity. This example demonstrates the promise of these techniques for combining the antigen recognition properties of anti-bodies with novel effector functions. For cancer therapy, it would be useful to produce chimaeric molecules made with proteins that possess cytotoxic activity. However, not all the factors which determine the correct folding and assembly of antibody molecules, or indeed of chimaeric antibodies, are understood. The *S. aureus* nuclease is a secreted monomeric protein which contains no disulphide bonds and is easily refolded after denaturation. Many of the best candidates for fusion do not have these useful properties and it is not clear whether present methodology will allow more complex polypeptides to be incorporated into bifunctional antibodies in a biologically active form.

18.2 Tumour associated antigens

18.2.1 *The tumour cell surface*

The plasma membrane of normal cells is a mosaic consisting of different glycoproteins and glycolipids which are partially embedded in a fluid lipid bilayer. Some membrane molecules serve a transport function, others are involved in cell to cell contact, and many act as receptors for growth and differentiation factors. Some of these molecules are shared by many cell types while others have a more restricted distribution, occasionally being limited to a single cell type or even being only transiently expressed at a particular stage of cell maturation.

When a normal cell becomes malignant, it continues to express many of the cell surface molecules that are characteristic of its normal counterpart. However, these 'normal' molecules can be expressed in abnormal amounts. The malignant cell can also express cell surface molecules that are not produced by the parent cell, for example, viral antigens or antigens normally expressed only during embryological development. Although these antigens may not be tumour specific, they can often be highly selective for particular types of tumour cells (see Chapter 15).

When a malignant tumour cell is injected into an animal of another species, the animal produces a mixture of antibodies against those cell surface components which it recognizes as foreign. The immunogenic determinants (epitopes) of glycoproteins can be structures formed by either the amino acid residues or by the carbohydrate side chains. Only the carbohydrate component of glycolipids tends to be antigenic, however, since the lipid component is sequestered within the membrane bilayer.

18.2.2 *Target antigens*

It is the rule rather than the exception that a monoclonal antibody against a tumour associated antigen binds to some normal cells in addition to the target cell. The normal tissue may express either the same antigen as the tumour cell or a molecule structurally related to that recognized by the antibody. This is not a serious problem for tumour imaging provided that the normal cells have an anatomical distribution that does not obscure the image of the tumour cells. For therapy, however, binding to normal cells reduces the amount of antibody that reaches the tumour and also increases the risk of damage to normal tissues.

Antibodies that react with normal tissues may still be used for therapy in a number of situations. First, this is possible if the normal tissue is not life sustaining; for example, tumours of lymphoid origin can be attacked using antibodies against antigens on T or B lymphocytes because the healthy lymphoid cells that are killed by the treatment are soon replaced by new cells which emerge from the bone marrow. Second, the normal tissue may express the target antigen at a much lower density than the malignant cells and so escape damage. For example, leukaemic cells induced by human T cell leukaemia virus, HTLV-1, have 10- to 100-fold more surface receptors for interleukin 2 than do normal T lymphocytes. Similarly, malignant cells often proliferate more rapidly than normal cells and so express a relatively high level of the transferrin receptor and other molecules needed for cell division. Lastly, anatomical barriers can some-times prevent the antibody from gaining access to the normal tissue bear-ing the target antigen. An example of this is the carcinoembryonic antigen (CEA) which is often expressed by colonic carcinoma cells. CEA is also found on the luminal epithelial cells of the gut but anti-CEA antibody injected intravenously rarely traverses the gut wall to reach the normal cells.

Tumour associated antigens can arise in a number of different ways (Fig. 18.4). CEA is one example of an 'oncofoetal' antigen that is normally associated with foetal cells of the same cellular lineage as the tumour cell and reflects the tendency of malignant cells to become more primitive. A second type of tumour associated antigenic determinant is found on molecules which are structural variants of normal cellular products. The p97 antigen associated with melanoma is structurally related to sero-transferrin and lactotransferrin. Mutant proteins can result from random mutations in the DNA of the cell sustained after exposure to chemical carcinogens or ionizing radiation. Thus, each individual rodent fibro-sarcoma induced by exposure to 3-methylcholanthrene has a different unique antigen. Cells transformed by some oncogenic viruses synthesize mutant proteins that are apparently related to the normal products of certain cellular genes. Of these, a number are expressed at the cell surface, for example the truncated avian epidermal growth factor (EGF) receptor on cells transformed by avian erythroblastosis virus (see Chapters 10, and 12).

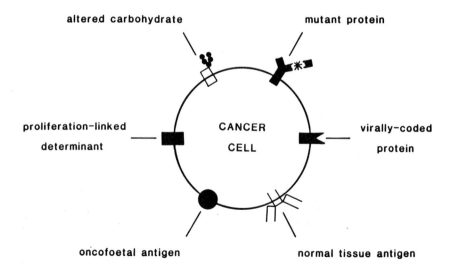

Fig. 18.4 Target antigens.

A large number of the monoclonal antibodies which detect tumour associated antigens recognize unusual carbohydrate portions in glycoproteins and glycolipids. These antigens result from derangements in the pathways of the tumour cell which synthesize oligosaccharide side chains. Human tumours which display characteristic glycolipid structures include melanoma (GD3), Burkitt's lymphoma (Gb3), Hodgkin's leukaemia (asialo GM2 and Gg3) and cancers of neuroectodermal origin. A glycolipid related to the Le^a blood group antigen is present on human foetal intestinal cells as well as on gastrointestinal adenocarcinomas. Changes in carbohydrate expression on the cell surface may also reveal cryptic (masked) antigens.

18.2.3 *Problems of targeting to tumour associated antigens*

Only a proportion of the cells in a tumour have the capacity for self renewal and are truly malignant. In some diseases, such as chronic granulocytic leukaemia, these clonogenic malignant cells represent only a small proportion of the tumour mass. Although the bulk of cells which carry the target antigen can be successfully imaged using antibodies, in therapy it is imperative that the antibodies reach and kill the clonogenic subpopulation. However, it has proved difficult to identify these rare cells and demonstrate that they also bear the target antigen.

In the heterogeneous tumour cell population, some cells express only low amounts of the target antigen and may escape being killed because less antibody binds to them. If these cells are clonogenic, the tumour will regrow. Moreover, as tumour cells continue to proliferate, mutant malignant cells that lack the target antigen frequently emerge. Thus, there are foci of cells within the primary tumour and its metastatic progeny which cannot be recognized by the antibody. This presents a serious obstacle to successful imaging or therapy that can sometimes be countered by using 'cocktails' of monoclonal antibodies which recognize several different tumour associated antigens.

The cells of a tumour which express high levels of the target antigen may also evade being coated by antibody in a number of ways. First, some antigens, which are loosely associated with the cell membrane, are shed from the tumour cell surface. The antigen in the circulation can then form complexes with the antibody and this greatly reduces the quantity of antibody that actually reaches the tumour cells. Second, the host's immune system may raise its own antibodies against the tumour associated antigen which then coat the malignant cells and 'mask' the antigen from the murine monoclonal antibody. Lastly, antibody may be physically prevented from gaining access to the majority of cells within the tumour. Thus, the most accessible tumour cells are those which surround the blood capillaries.

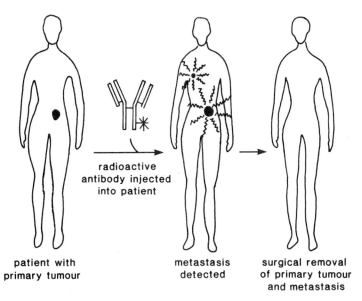

patient with
primary tumour

radioactive
antibody injected
into patient

metastasis
detected

surgical removal
of primary tumour
and metastasis

Fig. 18.5 The principle of radioimmunolocalization.

18.3 Tumour imaging

18.3.1 *Principles*

Tumour imaging is a procedure which allows the clinician to identify both primary and secondary sites of tumour growth in a patient and to estimate the overall tumour burden without recourse to surgery. An anti-tumour antibody labelled with a radioactive isotope, usually ^{131}-Iodine (^{131}I), is injected into the patient intravenously and, after allowing the antibody time to localize within the tumour, the patient is scanned using a radiation detector called a gamma camera. A computer compiles an image of the radioactivity detected in the patient's body and colour codes it according to the intensity of the radiation. Zones of high radioactivity in the regions of the body that are not expected to accumulate the anti-body or its metabolites indicate the possible presence of a tumour. This is illustrated in Figure 18.5. In combination with other clinical evidence, these results can help determine the most appropriate form of surgical, radiological or chemotherapeutic treatment.

The principle of radioimmunolocalization was first demonstrated by experiments in which tumour-bearing animals were injected with radio-labelled polyclonal antibodies directed against malignant cells. The concentration of anti-tumour antibodies in the tumour typically reached levels up to four times higher than those in miscellaneous normal tissues. The absolute amount of radioactivity associated with tumour increased in the first few hours after injection reflecting the time taken by the antibody to get out of the bloodstream and to diffuse to the site of the tumour. Maximal specific uptake by tumour is generally reached between one and four days after injection. Most of the antibody that is not cleared remains in the blood and extravascular compartment. Consequently, there is a background of radiation, particularly in blood rich organs such as the liver and spleen. Tumours in these sites are not easy to detect unless the image is corrected for background radiation (see on).

18.3.2 *Clinical studies*

The first clinical study using radioimaging to detect tumour tissue was reported by Goldenberg *et al.* in 1978. Patients were injected with ^{131}I-labelled anti-CEA antibodies and were then scanned after an interval of 24–72 hours. To correct the image for the non-specific background of radiation, a subtraction technique was used. Before injection of ^{131}I-antibody and scanning, patients were injected with ^{99m}-Technetium (^{99m}Tc) either bound to human serum albumin or free as pertechnetate, ^{99m}TcO$_4^-$. After computer subtraction of the ^{99m}Tc-image from the ^{131}I-image, areas of specific antibody uptake were highlighted.

A number of groups have now used anti-CEA antibodies to image a total of several hundred human carcinomas. Similarly trophoblastic tumours and germ cell tumours expressing human chorionic gonadotropin (HCG) or alpha foetoprotein (AFP) have been imaged using labelled anti-HCG antibodies and anti-AFP antibodies respectively. There have been only a few reported uses of radiolabelled murine monoclonal antibodies for imaging of tumours: colorectal cancer using anti-CEA antibodies; ovarian and breast cancer with antibodies against human milk fat globulin (HMFG) and melanoma using anti-p97 antibody and its Fab fragments. Figure 18.6 shows an example of tumour imaging in a patient. These clinical trials have identified a number of problems that limit the usefulness of the technique.

The first limitation of present radioimaging techniques is that not all tumours are detected. The amount of radioisotope which reaches tumour sites is small, generally 1–2 per cent of the amount injected, and so small tumour masses are poorly resolved. In practice, the tumours which are routinely diagnosed have diameters of at least 1 cm but metastatic microfoci, which may be more relevant to the long term survival of the patient, are unlikely to be detected. Even the larger tumours escape detection if they express a low level of the target antigen or if they are poorly vascularized. For these tumours, computerized tomography (CT) scans (see Chapter 16) give more reliable results. A further problem is that intravenously injected antibody cannot normally penetrate sanctuary sites in the body such as the brain.

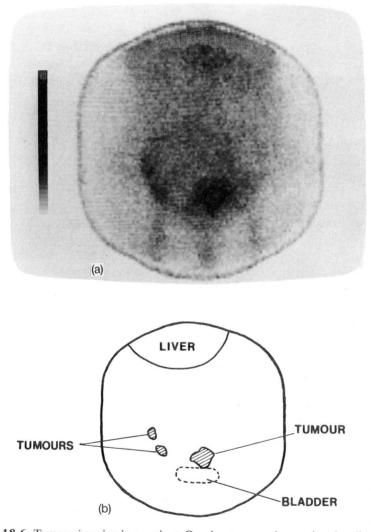

Fig. 18.6 Tumour imaging in a patient. Ovarian tumours in a patient localized by a monoclonal antibody H17E2 labelled with ^{123}I. This antibody recognizes a placental-type alkaline phosphatase associated with ovarian tumours of epithelial origin.

A second limitation of radioimaging is that areas of high radioactivity which are free of tumour are detected. These false positives occur when immune complexes formed in the blood are trapped by the liver and when free ^{131}I released from the antibody is eliminated from the blood-stream predominantly into the kidneys, urinary bladder, stomach, and intestine. Accumulation of iodine by the thyroid gland is usually blocked by co-administering Lugol's iodine or potassium iodide. Subtraction of the background radiation does not always eliminate false positives. The radiation emitted by ^{99m}Tc has a lower energy than that of ^{131}I and penetrates tissue more poorly, resulting in the appearance of 'halo' effects in the image of the ^{131}I radioactivity after subtraction.

18.3.3 *Recent developments*

The sensitivity of tumour detection is improved by using radionuclides with better imaging characteristics than ^{131}I and by better methods for removing background radiation. ^{131}I has too high an energy for optimal imaging with current gamma cameras; radiation with an energy of 0.2–0.4 MeV is most suitable. Its half-life is rather long (8 days) so that the patient's normal tissues are excessively exposed to radioactivity and the decay process also produces potentially harmful beta-particles. ^{131}I is being superseded by other isotopes of iodine (^{123}I) and by radionuclides that have shorter half-lives, better energy characteristics and emit no beta particles (Table 18.1). The radioactive metal ions of indium (^{111}In) and

Table 18.1 Isotopes for imaging

Isotope	Energy of principle γ emission (MeV)	Half–life (hours)	Method of coupling to antibodies
^{131}I	0.36	192	direct
^{123}I	0.16	13	halogenation
^{111}In	0.17, 0.25	67	chelation
^{67}Ga	0.09	78	

gallium (^{67}Ga) can now be stably coupled to antibodies by means of chelating molecules.

Background radiation due to the residue of circulating radiolabelled antibody can be cleared in a number of ways. First, synthetic lipic vesicles called 'liposomes' coated with anti-mouse immunoglobulin bind mouse monoclonal antibodies in peripheral blood and accelerate their clearance probably because liposome particles are rapidly removed by cells of the reticuloendothelial system. Second, clearance can be enhanced by the injection of a second antibody directed against radiolabelled antibody. Lastly, the use of F(ab')$_2$ or Fab fragments may improve tumour discrimination since antibody fragments are cleared from the circulation much more rapidly than intact Ig. Moreover, since these antibody fragments lack the Fc portion, there is less non-specific accumulation of radioactivity by the reticuloendothelial system.

A new approach to background subtraction depends on the slower rate of loss of radioactivity from tumour tissue as opposed to normal tissue. A series of scans is taken at intervals after injection of the radiolabelled antibody. Zones in the body where the antibody persists show up as 'hot spots' of radiation. This techique avoids the imaging problems associated with the use of a second radionuclide.

Finally, the use of a single photon emission computerized tomography, analogous to CT scanning using X irradiation, may allow a better discrimination between valid and false positive tumour images. The computer constructs images of transverse sections of the patient's body and allows examination of putative tumour sites from several angles.

18.4 Immunotherapy

18.4.1 Mechanisms of tumour cell killing

The goal of antibody mediated immunotherapy is to treat cancer patients with anti-tumour antibodies that will bind selectively to tumours and bring about the destruction of malignant cells either directly or by stimulating the natural defence mechanisms of the recipient.

An antibody can be directly cytotoxic (or, more accurately, cytostatic) if it binds to and inactivates a cell surface molecule which is necessary for survival or proliferation. For example, an anti-transferrin receptor antibody can inhibit the growth of human tumour cells both *in vitro* and in athymic mice. Other antibodies which might directly suppress tumour growth are those against the receptors for interleukin 2, EGF, and platelet derived growth factor (see Chapter 12) which are particularly abundant on certain types of tumour cell. Such examples are rare; antibodies themselves do not usually kill cells and need some accessory mechanism to do so.

There are two main ways by which antibody molecules bound to the surface of a cell can activate host defence mechanisms (Fig. 18.7).

18.4.1.1 *Complement mediated cytotoxicity.* Complement is the name given to a series of proteins (C1–C9) present in serum in inactive form. The C1q complement component binds to the Fc part of cell bound antibody and triggers a cascade reaction in which several of the remaining complement components are activated by proteolytic cleavage. The other complement proteins (C5b–9) then form a 'membrane attack complex' which inserts into the cell membrane and induces lysis.

COMPLEMENT   PHAGOCYTOSIS

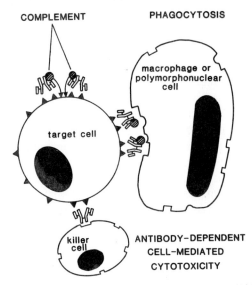

Fig. 18.7 Antibody mediated mechanisms of cell killing.

18.4.1.2 *Antibody dependent cell mediated cytotoxicity.* Several distinct types of defence cells kill antibody coated cells *in vitro* and it is presumed that they also do this *in vivo*. The effector cells include poly-morphonuclear cells (e.g. neutrophils), macrophages, and a type of mono-nuclear cell called the NK (or natural killer) cell which is present in lymphoid tissues but which lacks mature T and B lymphocyte markers (see Chapter 15). All these cells adhere to antibody coated cells by means of receptors for the Fc portion of the immunoglobulin molecule. Polymorphonuclear cells and macrophages also have receptors for the C3 component of complement. If the antibody is of a type that binds complement, this gives dual recognition which strengthens the adherence of the effector cell to the target cell. The various effector cells then kill the target cell by phagocytosis or direct lysis.

The heavy chain class or subclass of the monoclonal antibody deter-mines which effector systems are activated. With monoclonal antibodies raised in the mouse, IgGs of all major subclasses can elicit cell mediated cytotoxicity, whereas IgA and IgM cannot. By contrast, IgM is the most powerful activator of complement whereas IgG2a, IgG2b, and IgG3 fix complement weakly, and IgG1 not at all. The therapeutic effect of an antibody therefore depends on which host defence system is most effective at killing tumour cells.

18.4.2 *Studies in experimental animals*

The feasibility of immunotherapy has been demonstrated by several studies in experimental animals. For example, Bernstein and his colleagues showed that up to 3×10^5 leukaemia cells transplanted into mice could be eliminated by intravenous injection of antibody against the Thy1.1 surface antigen expressed by the leukaemia cells. When mice carrying 3×10^6 tumour cells subcutaneously were treated in the same fashion, the mice were not cured, apparently for two reasons. First, antigen positive leukaemic cells coated with antibody were not killed by the host. Second, antigen negative leukaemia cells were detected in the spleen, suggesting that antibody therapy had prevented the spread of antigen positive tumour cells but that a mutant subpopulation of tumour cells lacking the antigen had escaped. Other studies have tested mouse antibodies against human tumour associated antigens in mice carrying xenografts of human tumour tissue. In general, significant regression of the transplanted tumour was only observed in animals with small tumour burdens, a situation very different from the clinical situation in human patients with spontaneous tumours and large tumour cell burdens. IgM antibodies were generally ineffective in these *in vivo* studies. Mouse antibodies of the IgG2a and IgG2b subclasses were the most effective and have since been used for Phase I clinical trials in humans.

18.4.3 *Clinical trials*

Mouse monoclonal antibodies have been used to treat patients suffering from a variety of advanced malignant diseases. Only tumours of the haematopoietic system have responded well to this treatment and there has been one outstanding success.

Miller *et al.* raised monoclonal antibodies against the idiotypic determinants of the neoplastic cells of a patient with a type of B cell lymphoma called 'follicular lymphoma'. In this form of cancer, a single clone of B cells proliferates and so all the cells of the tumour bear surface Ig with the same idiotype. Since each clone of normal B lymphocytes in the body expresses a molecule with a unique antigen binding site, the idiotype of the surface Ig of the lymphoma cells provides a unique tumour specific target antigen. Tumour regression occurred after repeated intravenous infusions of the anti-idiotype monoclonal antibody and continued when treatment was stopped, leading to a complete remission (see Fig. 18.8). The mechanism of this remarkable therapeutic effect is obscure, however. It is possible that the malignant cells were not killed by the patient's defence systems but that the antibody directly suppressed their proliferation in a manner analogous with the way in which anti-idiotypic antibodies normally control the proliferation of cells that produce antibody in response to an antigenic stimulus. In support of this notion is one recent observation that, of 12 patients treated in a similar fashion with anti-idiotypic antibodies, those with the largest number of T cells infiltrating the tumour showed the best response.

More typically, in therapeutic trials against lymphomas and leukaemias,

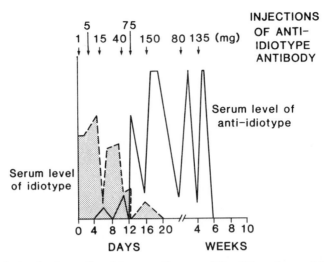

Fig. 18.8 Antibody-mediated immunotherapy of B cell lymphoma. The effect of anti-idiotypic antibody on the level of serum idiotype in a patient with B cell lymphoma (see text). The onset of tumour regression coincided with the antibody induced clearance of serum idiotype.

the infusion of anti-tumour monoclonal antibodies lowered the number of tumour cells in the blood but only transiently. For example, Miller and Levy treated a patient with advanced cutaneous T cell lymphoma with monoclonal antibody against the Leu-1 antigen, a normal T cell differentiation antigen. Continued treatment reduced but did not completely remove circulating Leu-1 positive cells and the tumour cells in the patient's lymph nodes grew unchecked. Similarly, in acute leukaemia, Ritz and his colleagues obtained no long lasting benefit by treating patients with a monoclonal antibody against the common acute lymphoblastic leukaemia antigen (CALLA). The temporary improvements observed may reflect an inherent limit to the capacity of host effector mechanisms to kill large numbers of tumour cells. It is known, for example, that the capacity of the hepatic reticuloendothelial system to clear antibody coated tumour cells from the blood can become saturated. The tumour deposits in the lymph nodes may have been more resistant than tumour cells free in the circulation because they were less accessible to the antibody. Alternatively, the lymph nodes may have contained too few effector cells; immunotherapy using monoclonal antibodies relies on the patient being able to destroy the antibody coated tumour cells and it is likely that the effector systems of a patient with advanced malignant disease will have been compromised either by prior therapy or by the disease itself.

Several problems undermining the therapeutic value of the anti-tumour antibodies arose during the clinical trials. These included hypersensitivity reactions to the murine protein in some patients, and transient fevers apparently caused by the presence in the circulation of substances released from dying tumour cells. More seriously, patients who were not severely immunosuppressed produced antibodies that bound to and neutralized the injected mouse monoclonal antibodies thus making further therapy with the antibody pointless. This problem could be limited by giving antibody therapy in combination with immuno-suppressive drugs. On the other hand, if host defence systems are necessary for a therapeutic effect, immunosuppression may prevent tumour destruction. The effectiveness of the antibody treatment was also reduced by the formation of complexes between the infused antibody and target antigens shed from the tumour cell surface. In some patients, this occurred even with target antigens that are not normally shed at high levels because the tumour cell destruction which followed attachment of antibodies and subsequent attack by host effector systems itself tended to raise the systemic level of free antigen. There is no good solution to the problem of antigen shedding.

Another serious obstacle encountered in the clinical trials was the phenomenon of antigenic modulation. Some cell surface components, when cross linked by antibodies, are actively internalized by the cell in a matter of minutes or are shed from the cell surface. This reduces the number of molecules of the target antigen available for binding by the antibody and may allow the cell to escape killing since the modulated antigen is only reexpressed when antibody is no longer present some days later. There are a number of ways to bypass the effect of antigenic modulation. First, not all surface components are subject to modulation and so a non-modulating antigen would be the preferred target. Second, treatment with antibody can be tailored to maximize the chances of killing the tumour cell. For instance, repeated infusions of antibody can be scheduled to coincide with the reappearance of the antigen that occurs once the antibody has cleared. Lastly, since the cross linking of target antigens that leads to modulation is a consequence of the bivalency of the antibody molecule, the way to avoid this problem may be to use monovalent anti-tumour antibodies.

Monovalent antibodies have been produced in two ways. Limited proteolysis of bivalent rabbit antibodies yields Fab/c fragments which contain a single antigen binding site (Fig. 18.9). Alternatively, hybrid cells, made by fusing B lymphocytes with a myeloma, secreting Ig light chains manufacture a proportion of antibodies with only one functional antigen binding site (Fig. 18.10). The heavy chain has an equal chance of combining with the irrelevant myeloma light chain or the splenic light

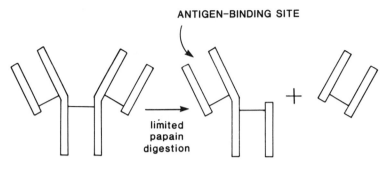

ANTIGEN–BINDING SITE

limited
papain
digestion

+

rabbit antibody

monovalent
Fab/c fragment

Fab fragment

Fig. 18.9 Fab/c fragments of rabbit IgG.

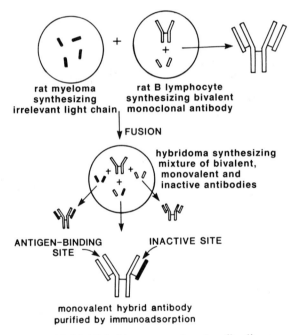

rat myeloma
synthesizing
irrelevant light chain

rat B lymphocyte
synthesizing bivalent
monoclonal antibody

FUSION

hybridoma synthesizing
mixture of bivalent,
monovalent and
inactive antibodies

ANTIGEN–BINDING
SITE

INACTIVE SITE

monovalent hybrid antibody
purified by immunoadsorption

Fig. 18.10 Hybrid rat monoclonal antibodies.

chain so that about half of the antibody molecules produced by the
hybrid will contain one Fab arm that can bind the target antigen and one
which cannot. These monovalent antibodies have normal Fc regions and
so are able to activate host effector systems. Since twice as many monovalent antibodies can, in theory, bind to the cell surface, their therapeutic
effect might be greater than that of bivalent antibodies. However, the

strength or 'avidity' of binding to the cell surface is greater for a bivalent antibody molecule than for a monovalent one, since both arms of the bivalent antibody contribute to the energy of binding.

18.5 Targeting of cytotoxic agents

18.5.1 *Principles*

In general, the anti-cancer drugs now in clinical use do not discriminate between malignant and normal cells (see Chapter 17). Most exert their effects on dividing cells so that tumour growth is inhibited but the dose of drug which can be used is limited by its toxicity to the normal tissues of the body which need to divide frequently, e.g. gastrointestinal epithelium and the haematopoietic cells of the bone marrow.

The aim of drug targeting is to deliver the cytotoxic drug to the tumour and only expose the rest of the body to a low level of the drug, so preventing harm to normal tissues. Several systems for drug delivery have been explored. One approach is to package the drug in liposomes which are then coated with the anti-tumour antibody. The liposomes attach specifically to tumour cells *in vitro* and kill them, probably by fusing with the cell membrane and discharging their drug content into the cell. Unfortunately, *in vivo*, the large size of the liposomes causes them to be engulfed by phagocytic cells in the bloodstream. The anti-tumour effects of drug loaded liposomes in experimental animals have thus been unremarkable. Attempts to endow cytotoxic agents with target specificity by simply linking them directly to the antibody have been more successful. Drugs of low molecular weight, radionuclides, toxins of bacterial and plant origin, and cell surface active agents have all been coupled to specific antibodies and the conjugates found to exert selective cytotoxic effects.

18.5.2 *Chemotherapeutic drugs with intracellular sites of action*

In early studies, non-covalent complexes made by physically adsorbing chlorambucil to anti-tumour antibodies were found to kill appropriate tumour cell targets in tissue culture and in mice more efficiently than the free drug or antibody alone. The anti-tumour effects were later shown to be due not to drug targeting but to synergism between free drug and antibody after dissociation of the complex. The synergy probably arises because the drug impairs the cell's capacity to repair plasma membrane damage caused by the antibody and complement.

To prevent dissociation, covalent bonds have been used to link several anti–cancer agents (e.g. adriamycin, daunomycin, methotrexate, and vindesine) directly to anti-tumour antibodies. In most cases, the cytotoxicity of the conjugate to target cells *in vitro* exceeded that to cells lacking the target antigen, but the cytotoxic potency of the conjugate was invariably low. These drugs have intracellular sites of action and enter cells by simple diffusion or active transport. Once linked to the antibody, however, they cannot enter the cell by their usual route. Antibody-drug conjugates bind to target antigens on the cell surface, enter the cell in endocytic vesicles and are degraded by enzymes when the vesicles coalesce with lysosomes (see Fig. 18.11). Thus, the low potency of these conjugates may have been because too few drug molecules had originally localized at the cell surface to enter by this route or because drug release by lysosomal enzymes was inefficient.

Much progress has been made in devising ways to accelerate the rate of drug release once internalization has taken place by increasing the susceptibility of the covalent linkage between drug and carrier to hydrolysis. Daunomycin directly linked to albumin is not released by lysosomal enzymes but if a proteinase sensitive peptide spacer is interspersed between the drug and the carrier, drug release occurs rapidly. Similarly, acid labile linkages between drug and antibody can improve potency, presumably because the drug dissociates from the conjugate when exposed to the acidic milieu of the lysosome.

Only about 10 drug molecules can be attached covalently to an antibody molecule without diminishing its antigen binding capacity. To raise the potency of antibody drug conjugates, a carrier molecule such as human serum albumin, poly-L-glutamic acid or dextran can be used.

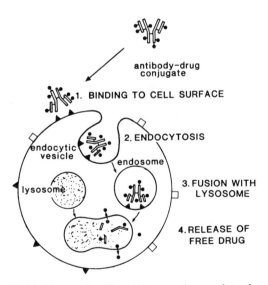

Fig. 18.11 Entry of antibody drug conjugates into the cell.

Such conjugates are more effective anti-tumour agents *in vitro* and *in vivo*. For example, Tsukada and his co-workers induced long term remission in 60 per cent of rats with hepatoma by intravenously administering daunomycin dextran coupled to anti-AFP antibodies. The effect was specific since daunomycin alone, daunomycin-dextran plus antibody in unconjugated form, or control conjugates of irrelevant specificity were all less effective.

18.5.3 *Radionuclides*

Radionuclides such as ^{131}I or ^{32}-phosphorus (^{32}P) are attractive cell killing agents for targeting because they emit high energy beta particles which have path lengths (2 mm for ^{131}I, and 6 mm for ^{32}P) that span many cell diameters. This is important for two reasons. First, the radioisotope does not need to be internalized to kill the cell. Second, the emissions can kill cells which surround the targeted cell, allowing the destruction of neighbouring malignant cells which do not bear the target antigen and of cells in poorly vascularized tumours. Radionuclides also irradiate normal tissues as they circulate through the body in conjugated form and as metabolites. For effective use, the antibody radionuclide conjugate should localize well within tumour and not be retained within normal tissues. The recent improvements in methods for tumour imaging (Section 18.3) offer ways in which non-specific irradiation during therapy can be minimized.

Alpha particles may be more effective cytotoxic agents since they dissipate more energy than beta particles in a path length of only one or two cell diameters, and therefore have an exceedingly powerful cytotoxic action. So far, suitable alpha emitters have proved too unstable to exploit for this purpose. An alternative is to target atoms of a non-radioactive isotope of boron (^{10}B) to cells. When this nuclide is subsequently irradiated with low energy thermal neutrons, it undergoes nuclear fission liberating a high-energy alpha particle *in situ*. Unfortunately, thermal neutrons penetrate tissues so poorly that this approach to targeting seems to have limited application.

18.5.4 *Cell surface active agents*

A number of substances have a potent disruptive action on cell membranes. These include enzymes from snake venom and bacteria which cleave phospholipids, agents which form pores in membranes by binding cholesterol, and other agents whose mechanism of action is less well understood. Phospholipase C coupled to antibodies against mouse erythroleukaemia cells lysed leukaemic but not normal spleen cells *in vitro* but no results have yet been reported *in vivo*. Similarly, a conjugate of the C3b-like glycoprotein of cobra venom linked to a monoclonal antibody against human melanoma cells induced immune cytolysis of melanoma cells *in vitro* by activating complement.

18.5.5 *Toxins and related proteins*

Bacterial toxins (e.g. diphtheria toxin) and the plant toxins, ricin and abrin, are extremely potent; a single molecule appears to be sufficient to kill a cell if it enters the cytoplasm. These toxins have a similar molecular architecture, each consisting of two polypeptide chains, A and B, joined by a single disulphide bond and they bind to virtually all cells of higher animals by means of the B chain. The membrane-bound toxin is taken into the cell by endocytosis and the A chain is then somehow translocated across the membrane of the endocytic vesicle into the cytoplasm where it inactivates the cell's machinery for protein synthesis.

When targeting a toxin to a cell, the objective is to confer upon it the specificity of the antibody without attenuating the capacity of its A chain to enter cells and inhibit protein synthesis. Attempts have been made to achieve this aim by targeting intact toxins, toxin A chains only, and members of a group of ribosome inactivating proteins which act in a manner seemingly identical to the A chains of abrin and ricin. Conjugates between antibodies and toxins or their fragments are known collectively as 'immunotoxins'.

Immunotoxins made from intact toxins indeed prove to be outstandingly powerful cytotoxic agents for cells with appropriate antigens, often matching or even surpassing the potency of the native toxin *in vitro*. Since the B chain of the toxin can still bind to non-target cells, these immunotoxins are highly poisonous and show little evidence of selective cytotoxicity. The non-specific and undesirable binding properties of conjugates made with intact ricin or abrin (which bind to galactose-containing oligosaccharides on the cell surface) can be blocked *in vitro* with high concentrations of galactose or lactose. In animals, however, lactose is excreted rapidly and cannot protect the animal against non-specific toxicity. For therapy in animals, a permanent or semipermanent blockade is needed. Intact ricin conjugates in which the galactose binding site of the toxin is apparently sterically (spatially) hindered by the antibody moiety show improved anti-tumour effects *in vivo* but, for reasons that are not understood, retain high toxicity to animals.

The most widely used way to eliminate non-specific binding is to link the isolated A chain of the toxin directly to the antibody. The coupling is usually accomplished by introducing into the antibody a cross linker that can form a disulphide bond with the free sulphydryl group of the A chain so that the A chain can be released from the conjugate by reduction in the cell after endocytosis (see Fig. 18.12). A chain immunotoxins are

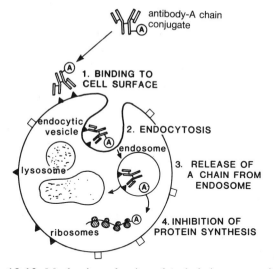

Fig. 18.12 Mechanism of action of A chain immunotoxins.

almost wholly selective in their toxic effect upon target cells in tissue culture and, in several studies, have produced impressive anti-tumour effects *in vivo*. One of the most dramatic therapeutic effects was obtained by Vitetta and her colleagues, who induced prolonged remissions in mice with advanced lymphocytic leukaemia by administering a ricin A chain immunotoxin in conjunction with total lymphoid irradiation and splenectomy.

The main problem with A chain immunotoxins is that their toxicity to target cells varies greatly depending on the antigenic determinant recognized, the type of target cell, and its stage in the cell cycle. The reasons underlying these differences are not understood but are presumed to reflect the pathway by which the A chain immunotoxin enters the cell and the influence of the metabolic status of the cell upon that process. This variable cytotoxicity contrasts with the consistent and generally superior toxicity of conjugates made with the intact toxins. The cell-killing effect of weakly cytotoxic ricin A chain immunotoxins can be markedly enhanced *in vitro* by free ricin B chain, suggesting that the B chain also plays a role in facilitating the entry of the A chain portion of the conjugate into the cytoplasm of the cell. A recent finding with therapeutic potential is that toxicity is also potentiated by a 'piggyback' treatment with a B chain immunotoxin directed against the A chain immunotoxin. In addition, the weak cytotoxicity of some A chain immunotoxins is enhanced *in vitro* by the use of agents which elevate endosomal (Fig. 18.12) and lysosomal pH such as ammonium chloride, chloroquine or monensin.

Many plants have been found to contain proteins that inhibit protein synthesis on eukaryotic ribosomes. These single chain proteins are similar in size and action to the toxin A chains and are probably evolutionarily related but they are virtually non-toxic to intact cells because they lack the equivalent of the B chain for binding to the cell surface. Gelonin, the ribosome inactivating protein from *Gelonium multiflorum*, acquires potent and specific cytotoxic activity after its covalent linkage to the monoclonal antibody, anti-Thyl.1. Pokeweed antiviral protein, from *Phytolacca americana*, and saporin, from *Saponaria officinalis*, are likewise rendered cytotoxic when conjugated with this antibody. A great advantage of using the single chain inhibitors over the toxin A chains is that they are safer to handle in quantity and need not undergo the same rigorous purification to exclude traces of intact toxin or contaminating B chain.

In the future, it will be possible to use genetically engineered toxins for targeting. The structural gene which encodes a non-toxic fragment of diphtheria toxin has been cloned and expressed in *Escherichia coli*. This toxin fragment retains the enzymic activity that disrupts protein synthesis but not the site which allows binding to the cell surface. It is expected that the B chain portion of this modified toxin, once attached to a specific antibody, will retain its ability to insert into the membrane of the target cell and will assist the A chain to enter the cell and kill it. Similar manipulations are envisaged for other toxins.

Several problems which reduce the therapeutic value of immunotoxins have been encountered in animal studies. First, there is evidence that some of the linkages used to attach toxic proteins to antibodies are labile in the animal, probably as a result of enzymic action or premature reduction of the disulphide bond. Second, the mannose-containing carbohydrate moieties of ricin and abrin are recognized by cells of the reticuloendothelial system which then rapidly clear the immunotoxins from the bloodstream. Clearance can be prevented if the toxins are deglycosylated by chemical or enzymic methods. Third, the toxic proteins are immunogenic. Fortunately, since the single chain inhibitor proteins appear to be immunologically distinct from the toxic A chains and from one another, it should be possible to avoid immunological neutralization during therapy by using a series of several immunotoxins made from different inhibitors. Alternatively, it may prove possible to manipulate toxin genes to produce functional proteins which have altered antigenic determinants and are not neutralized when given to patients who have been immunized against the toxin. Lastly, subcutaneous tumour cells have proven more difficult to attack than tumour cells that are free in the bloodstream or peritoneal cavity, suggesting that the major strength of immunotoxins may be in their ability to locate and destroy metastatic tumour microfoci rather than to treat sizeable tumour masses.

18.5.6 *Clinical trials*

A few attempts to treat human malignancies with cytotoxic agents linked to polyclonal antibodies have been reported. Patients with disseminated malignant melanoma received multiple injections of goat anti-melanoma antibodies to which chlorambucil had been adsorbed non-covalently. A few patients showed regression of cutaneous and nodal metastases, but treatment had to be discontinued when they developed anaphylactic reactions to the globulin. Tumour regression was also observed in a child treated with a covalent conjugate of chlorambucil and an antibody against neuroblastoma.

Pilot studies, in which patients were given antibodies radioiodinated to high specific activity, produced evidence of tumour regression with few toxic side effects. For example, Carrasquillo and his colleagues treated patients with advanced metastatic melanoma with ^{131}I-Fab fragments of two antibodies against melanoma associated antigens, p97 and 'high molecular weight antigen'. In some patients, a stabilization or transient reduction of tumour size was observed but most developed an antibody reaction against the mouse globulin that precluded further treatment. The other problems encountered were complexing of antibody with circulating p97, dissociation of the conjugate, and poor localization of the radio-labelled antibody within the tumour.

The anti-tumour effects that have been demonstrated experimentally *in vitro* and in simple animal models have promoted a view of cytotoxic conjugates as 'magic bullets' that can be fired directly at tumour cells. The complexity of the interactions between immunotoxins and both normal and malignant cells within the host shows this to be an over-simplification. The usefulness of immunotoxins as therapeutic agents is limited partly by factors dependent on the antibody part of the conjugate:antibody clearance, shed antigen, and cross reactivity with non-malignant cells. The attachment of the toxic protein introduces additional considerations such as immunogenicity and the stability of the linkage to the antibody. As with any new form of therapy, targeted drugs must evolve through the process of design, testing, and redesign. In the absence of clinical data, it is too soon to judge the true value of these agents.

18.6 Bone marrow transplantation

18.6.1 *Principles*

A number of malignant diseases, including leukaemia and lymphoma, respond to high dose chemotherapy and whole body irradiation. This treatment is not more widely adopted because it destroys the haemato-poietic stem cells of the patient's bone marrow. The limited treatment with drugs and radiation that can be given to the patient may not eradicate all tumour cells and frequently the patient relapses. If higher and potentially curative doses of radiochemotherapy are to be used, the bone marrow of the patient must be reconstituted after treatment (see Chapter 16).

There are two ways to do this. In autologous bone marrow transplant-ation, a sample of the patient's own marrow is removed before therapy and later reimplanted on completion of the treatment. With diseases such as leukaemia or lymphoma, the marrow is infiltrated with malignant cells and so it is imperative to clear the marrow of these cells before it is returned to the patient. The alternative method, allogeneic bone marrow transplantation, is to give the patient normal bone marrow from another individual. In this case, the donor and recipient must be matched for histocompatibility antigens in order to reduce the risk of provoking graft versus host disease (GVHD), a life threatening complication that results from the attack of host cells by T lymphocytes in the allograft. GVHD is a common occurrence even with closely matched donors and recipients. The solution to this problem is to remove or kill the T lymphocytes in the marrow of the donor before it is infused into the patient.

18.6.2 *Methods for purging bone marrow*

The aim of bone marrow purging is to eliminate malignant cells from autologous marrow grafts or T lymphocytes from allogeneic marrow grafts and leave intact the haematopoietic stem cells. This has been made possible by using antibodies recognizing antigens that are present on malignant cells or T lymphocytes but absent from the stem cells. Three approaches have been used clinically.

The first method is complement mediated cytolysis of antibody coated cells. In one study of patients receiving matched allogeneic grafts, Prentice and his co-workers pretreated the donor marrow with two mouse anti-T cell monoclonal antibodies of the IgM class and followed this by two incubations with rabbit complement. This eliminated more than 99 per cent of the T cells and prevented acute GVHD in all 13 evaluable patients. In a study by Bast and his colleagues, the bone marrow of 16 patients with common acute leukaemia was purged with a monoclonal antibody against CALLA in combination with rabbit complement. After therapy and reimplantation of the treated autologous bone marrow, six of the patients have remained in complete clinical remission for over one year. The action of complement is rapid but one serious drawback is the inherent variability between different batches of rabbit complement. This means that each preparation has to be screened for its ability to lyse cells in the presence of antibody and for lack of toxicity in the absence of antibody.

The second method for purging bone marrow uses monoclonal antibody toxin conjugates. These were recently used by Filipovich and her colleagues with two patients undergoing marrow transplantation for acute lymphoblastic leukaemia in third remission. Bone marrow cells from a histocompatible sibling were treated with a cocktail of anti-T cell antibody ricin conjugates in the presence of lactose (to prevent non-specific binding to normal cells via the ricin B chain), then washed to remove the immunotoxin and finally infused into the patient. The treated marrow was successfully grafted and no symptoms of toxicity or GVHD were evident. It seems likely that immunotoxins will also be clinically useful for removing malignant cells from the bone marrow of patients for whom a suitable donor cannot be found. The method is straightforward and the immunotoxins can be prepared in large batches that are stable over many months.

A third technique has been developed by Kemshead and his group to remove neuroblastoma cells from bone marrow. Tumour cells in the isolated marrow are first coated with a cocktail of several mouse monoclonal anti-neuroblastoma antibodies and then with a second layer of sheep anti-mouse Ig antibodies bound to polystyrene microspheres containing magnetite. The tumour cells can be removed by passing the marrow between the poles of a series of magnets (Fig. 18.13). The separation procedure removed 99.9 per cent of tumour cells from the bone marrow of patients. The cells which passed through the separation apparatus were free from polystyrene microspheres and were grafted successfully in four patients. The advantage of this approach is that the same antibody magnetite beads can be used to withdraw tumour cells coated with any mouse monoclonal antibody or with cocktails of antibodies.

Clinical trials in lymphocytic leukaemia and neuroblastoma patients clearly demonstrate the value of bone marrow purging using monoclonal antibodies. It is unclear whether the procedure will be of value in the treatment of other malignant diseases in which there is bone marrow involvement. To be successful, intense radiochemotherapy must eradicate all the clonogenic tumour cells in the patient's body or reduce them to a number which can be contained by the patient's immune and other defence mechanisms when they recover from the effects of the treatment. Other diseases that are responsive to radiochemotherapy and in which benefit might be expected from more intense treatment are lymphoma, oat cell carcinoma of the lung, carcinoma of the breast, testis and ovary, and paediatric malignancies such as Wilms' tumour.

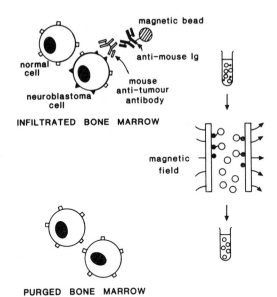

Fig. 18.13 Bone marrow purging using magnetic beads.

18.7 Prospects

Conventional chemotherapeutic or radiotherapeutic regimens often fail
to cure patients because they do not kill all malignant cells. One reason is
that the dose needed to eradicate the tumour is usually so large that the
patient's own tissues would be severely damaged. The usefulness of monoclonal antibodies or antibody-conjugates for therapy is also limited by
the extent to which they cross-react with, and harm, normal tissues. The
molecular characterization of tumour associated antigens may, in the
future, help to elucidate the basis for cross reactivity of some anti-tumour
antibodies and indicate whether improvements in selectivity can be
obtained, for example, by raising antibodies against other epitopes of the
target antigen. Furthermore, new tumour associated antigens, such as the
products of oncogenes, may prove to be tumour specific.

A second factor contributing to the failure of conventional chemotherapy is that cells insensitive to the drug evolve from the tumour cell
population during treatment (see Chapter 16). Antibody mediated
therapy has to contend with the same problem since tumours normally
contain a proportion of cells that lack the target antigen or express it at a
low level. Similarly, a proportion of tumour cells expressing a high level of
the target antigen may escape being killed by antibody conjugates either

because they are resistant to the action of the cytotoxic agent or because they lack the mechanism to internalize the conjugate and to release the toxic moiety. It may be possible to prevent the outgrowth of resistant tumour cells by administering conventional drugs in conjunction with antibody conjugates provided that the way in which resistance to the conjugate develops does not also make the cells more resistant to the drug.

Tumour cells within solid tumours are less accessible to antibody because antibody molecules may only permeate the tumour to a depth of a few cell layers from the vasculature. Unless antibodies or antibody conjugates can gain access to the core of solid tumours and other sanctuary sites, they may be effective only against smaller deposits of tumour cells such as metastatic microfoci. It may be possible to kill cells in the solid tumour core with antibody radionuclide conjugates. Alternatively, the permeability of these tumours might be increased by agents that cause inflammatory damage or that disrupt cell to cell contacts and the extracellular matrix.

18.8 Conclusion

Monoclonal antibodies have revived earlier optimism for the prospect of treating cancer by immunotherapy. Anti-tumour monoclonal antibodies are now being evaluated in patients whose tumours are resistant to conventional forms of therapy. The main value of such trials is to ascertain the side effects of the therapy, and an accurate evaluation of the therapeutic benefit will only emerge when trials are conducted in patients with disease at a less advanced stage.

The principle of using antibody molecules as carriers of cytotoxic agents that have no inherent tumour cell specificity is likely to be extended to other biologically active molecules such as interferons and inducers of cell differentiation. New developments in hybridoma technology and genetic engineering will allow the manipulation of the structures of immunoglobulins, toxins, and enzymes, and the creation of novel antibody molecules with characteristics desirable for cancer therapy. The potential of these sophisticated techniques is likely to be fulfilled in concert with advances in our understanding of the fundamental biological processes that determine the origin and development of malignant disease.

Further reading

Barbieri, L., and Stirpe, F. (1982). Ribosome-inactivating proteins from plants: properties and possible uses. *Cancer surveys* **1**, 489–520.

Collier, R. J., and Kaplan, D. A. (1984). Immunotoxins. *Scientific American* 7, 44–52.

Lennox, E. S. (ed.) (1984). Clinical applications of monoclonal antibodies. *British Medical Bulletin* **40**, No. 3.

McMichael, A. J., and Fabre, J. W. (eds.) (1982). *Monoclonal antibodies in clinical medicine.* Academic Press, London.

Miller, R. A., Maloney, D. G., Warnke, R., and Levy, R. (1982). Treatment of B-cell lymphoma with monoclonal anti-idiotype antibody. *New England Journal of Medicine* **306**, 517–22.

Neuberger, M. S. (1985). Making novel antibodies by expressing transfected immunoglobulin genes. *Trends in Biochemical Sciences* **10**, 347–9.

Olsnes, S., and Pihl, A. (1982). Toxic lectins and related proteins. In: *Molecular action of toxins and viruses* pp. 51–105 (eds. P. Cohen, and S. van Heyningen). Elsevier Biomedical Press, New York.

Prentice, H. G., Blacklock, H. A., Janossy, G., Gilmore, M. J. M. L., Price-Jones, L., Tidman, N., Trejdosiewicz, L. K., Skeggs, D. B. L., Panjwani, D., Ball, S., Graphakos, S., Patterson, J., Ivory, K., and Hoffbrand, A. V. (1984). Depletion of T lymphocytes in donor marrow prevents significant graft-versus-host disease in matched allogeneic leukaemia marrow transplant recipients. *Lancet* **i**, 472–6.

Treleaven, J. G., Gibson, F. M., Ugelstad, J., Rembaum, A., Philip, T., Caine, G. D., and Kemshead, J. T. (1984). Removal of neuroblastoma cells from bone marrow with monoclonal antibodies conjugated to magnetic microspheres. *Lancet* **i**, 70–3.

Uhr, J. W. (1984). Immunotoxins: harnessing nature's poisons. *The Journal of Immunology* **133**, i–x.

19

Some conclusions and prospects

ROBIN A. WEISS

19.1 Understanding carcinogenesis

It is evident from the foregoing Chapters that we are on the threshold of gaining major insight into the nature of cancer. The excitement in this field derives from the realization that a finite, analysable set of genes is involved in carcinogenesis. These are the genes collectively called oncogenes (see Chapter 10). Their identification has brought together seemingly distinct areas of cancer research such as chemical and radiation carcincogenesis (see Chapters 7, and 8), oncogenic viruses (see Chapter 9), chromosome anomalies (see Chapter 11), and growth factors (see Chapter 12). While it is possible that oncogenes may also underlie some of the specific inherited predispositions to cancer (see Chapter 5), they have been chiefly identified in association with the mutation and rearrangement of genes during carcinogenesis; in other words cancer is usually the result of genetic changes in somatic cells.

The somatic mutation hypothesis of cancer has a venerable pedigree. The notion that carcinogenesis involves genetic change dates from the turn of the century when Boveri identified chromosomes as the repository of genetic material and speculated on chromosome imbalance in cancer. The link between mutation and cancer was first drawn by Muller in 1927, who demonstrated the mutagenicity of ionizing radiation in fruit flies (radium and X-rays were already known to cause cancer). Later Auerbach showed that a carcinogenic chemical, mustard gas, also induced mutations, and it now appears that the great majority of chemical carcinogens or their active metabolites are mutagens (see Chapter 7).

Thus the concept that certain stages in carcinogenesis, in particular initiating events, were mutational has been firmly embedded in our thinking about cancer for many decades. But this gave no indication as to which genes became altered, or indeed whether the same genes were regularly affected. It was thought that the accumulation of mutations might allow otherwise recessive traits to appear, by removing the action of some of the very large number of genes involved in cellular control processes. The recent studies of oncogenes has focused attention on just 20 out of the 50 000 or so genes in the human genome.

The repeated identification of the same set of genes—whether captured by retroviruses, or revealed by DNA transfection, DNA amplification or chromosome rearrangement—indicates that these genes are of major importance in understanding cancer. Moreover, oncogenes are active genes, and tend to be expressed in a dominant manner. Mutation may cause overexpression of a normal protein or normal levels of expression of an altered protein, but in each case the gene products contribute positively to the neoplastic phenotype. This contrasts with the earlier assumption that deletion of active genes led to cancer, that normality is dominant and cancer recessive.

Carcinogenesis is, of course, a much more complicated, multistep process than the activation or mutation of a single oncogene (see Chapters 1, and 7). Mutated oncogenes are not clearly dominant over their normal alleles, and expression of several different oncogenes may act synergistically in producing the malignant phenotype (see Chapter 10). Moreover, some somatic cell hybrids between normal and malignant cells have a normal phenotype.

Nevertheless, the evidence that identifiable proteins encoded by onco-genes contribute to neoplastic transformation is a major step forward in our understanding of cancer, and suggests new means of treatment by blocking the function of such proteins.

It remains to be seen whether 'anti-oncogenes' exist, genes whose products are essential for the maintenance of normal regulatory processes. These genes will be much more difficult to identify. But their action in the fine regulatory network of cell proliferation should prove to be equally interesting, and may possibly allow new modes of intervention in cancer.

The somatic mutation hypothesis of cancer presupposes the clonal origin of the cells comprising the malignant population. Clearly, a mutation or genetic change occurring in one cell can only be passed on to that cell's linear descendants, i.e. its derivative clone. By and large, where cancers have been amenable to analysis, clonality has been upheld. For example, there is a polymorphism for an enzyme coded by an X linked gene which happens to be relatively common in black people. Following inactivation of one or other of the X chromosomes early in female development, each cell will express only one form of the enzyme. Thus normal tissues display a fine mosaic of cells expressing one or other enzymic form (see Chapter 5). Fialkow's studies show, however, that the malignant cells in a tumour usually express one form of the enzyme only, demonstrating the clonal derivation of the tumour cells after X chromosome inactivation has taken place.

Other evidence also points to a clonal evolution of tumour cells at early stages of carcinogenesis. In chronic granulocytic leukaemia, a chromosome translocation (the 'Philadelphia' chromosome) involving the *abl* oncogene (see Chapters 3, 10, and 11) is present in the majority of apparently normal and premalignant cells of the blood, indicating that a clonal stem cell carrying the translocated chromosomes has populated almost all the bone marrow before malignancy appears. Experimental chemical carcinogenesis in mouse skin indicates that a *ras* gene is mutated in codon 12 in premalignant stages of papillomatosis (see Chapters 7, and 10), again indicating clonality.

It is not clear, however, that all premalignant changes are clonal in origin. Pathologists frequently recognize 'field changes' in tissues which look abnormal and from which a malignant tumour may emerge (see Chapter 1). For example, cancer of the stomach frequently arises in patches of stomach epithelium that have undergone intestinal metaplasia, in which the tissue resembles the epithelium of the intestine rather than the stomach, and this observation has been used in early screening for stomach cancer in Japan where this tumour is common. We do not know exactly what triggers metaplasia and whether such altered patches of epithelium are clonal in origin.

In concluding a discussion on the genetic basis of carcinogenesis one should mention that the clonal nature of the cancer in which mutations in a single cell lead to a malignant cell population is not universally accepted. An epigenetic view of cancer has long been held by the radiotherapist, Sir David Smithers, and more recently by Dr. Harry Rubin. 'Cancer is no more a disease of cells than a traffic jam is a disease of cars', wrote Smithers in 1962, continuing, 'A lifetime study of the internal combustion engine would not help anyone to understand our traffic problems. A traffic jam is due to a failure of the normal relationship between driven cars and their environment and can occur whether they themselves are running normally or not'.

This is an attractive argument, but a deceptive one. The body's environment can be of crucial importance in allowing tumours to develop. Many remain dependent on hormones (see Chapters 13, and 14) and growth factors (see Chapter 12), and possibly the host immune system (see Chapter 15). Local interactions between cells also remain important to all but the most anaplastic tumour cells. Thus the cancer 'seed' requires fertile 'soil' in which to proliferate, as is shown by the relative inefficiency of the process of metastasis (see Chapter 2).

Although thousands of tumour cells may be released from a primary tumour only a very small number will develop into secondary tumours. Nevertheless, the interaction of tumour cells with the host environment is an elective or permissive process of stimulation and response in which an essential lesion always exists in the tumour cell itself. This after all is the basis of surgery, radiotherapy, and chemotherapy (see Chapters 16, and 17) directed to the elimination of the tumour. Drug resistance following chemotherapy is another example of clonal evolution and progression of tumours in which genetic changes within the malignant cell (for example gene amplification) determine the response to and escape from therapy.

Smithers based his views on observations that human tumours, particularly embryonal tumours occurring early in childhood, may occasionally regress spontaneously, and he concluded that the malignant phenotype was reversible. Certainly tumour cells differ from normal cells in subtle ways, such as arrested differentiation (see Chapter 3) in which less malignant behaviour may develop if the tumour cells can be made to follow a normal cell maturation pathway. Indeed there has recently been increased emphasis in introducing so called biological response modifiers into cancer therapy. But the natural history of tumour progression (see Chapter 7) unfortunately promotes the selection of subclones with greater malignant potential.

Is there any experimental evidence for the reversibility of malignancy, as one might expect if carcinogenesis were a non-genetic phenomenon? There are some suggestive findings that merit more detailed investigation. For example, in leopard frogs, isolated nuclei from Lucke carcinoma cells (a kidney tumour induced by a herpesvirus) have been introduced into activated, enucleated eggs. Following nuclear transplantation, a small proportion of the nuclei allowed the development of tadpoles with normal, differentiated tissues, but it has not been unequivocally demonstrated that these nuclei came from tumour cells rather than from the stroma. Mouse teratocarcinomas containing pluripotential embryonal carcinoma cells have been the subject of extensive study as these cancer cells can differentiate into many types of apparently normal cells. The introduction of such cells into the embryonic blastocyst allows incorporation into the inner cell mass, and hence into the embryo. Using genetic markers, it has been shown that the embryonal carcinoma cells contribute to most of the normal tissues of the mouse, although such mice have a higher frequency of teratocarcinoma. It has also been found that the descendants of embryonal cell lines can form a normal germ line, but this remains to be confirmed with fully malignant teratocarcinoma cells. Similarly, crown gall tumours in tobacco plants, which are induced by transfer of a bacterial plasmid, can give rise to normal tissues and to whole plants. Thus heritable normal behaviour can be restored to certain pluripotent cancer cells by transplantation into, or cultivation in, a suitable environment.

These experiments suggest that the cancer phenotype is not inexorably irreversible but do not refute the somatic mutation hypothesis. The karyotypic changes in many tumour cells, the mutagenic properties of most carcinogens, and the alteration of specific genes in oncogenesis, strongly suggest that carcinogenesis involves genetic change in the cells that become malignant. It will be of interest to determine whether activated oncogenes introduced into the germ line of mice cause a genetic predisposition to cancer.

19.2 Prospects for prevention and screening

One of the biggest problems in attempting to reduce the incidence of cancer is that of changing the life style of the people at risk. In the 30 years since it became firmly established that cigarette smoking is causally linked to lung cancer, little progress has been made in reducing cigarette smoking or in stopping new cohorts of youngsters acquiring this addictive habit. Dietary factors (see Chapter 4) may be equally important, though less clearly defined, in human carcinogenesis, particularly in the digestive tract itself, and changing patterns of cancer are evident, such as the decrease of stomach cancer and rise of colorectal cancer. It is difficult to change dietary habits, though the availability of fresh or frozen vegetables in all seasons and the increasing recognition of the importance of dietary fibre must lead to better health.

With occupational cancers due in part to industrial exposure, it is much easier to prevent access to the carcinogens once they have been identified. The recognition of β-naphthylamine as a bladder carcinogen (see Chapter 7) soon led to protection of workers who were exposed to this chemical in the rubber and dye industries. Similar measures are currently being undertaken to reduce exposure to asbestos and related carcinogenic fibres.

One of the brightest prospects for prevention arises from the recognition of viruses as important environmental carcinogens for human cancer (see Chapter 9). As shown in Chapter 4 (Table 4.4), some 10 per cent of cancers in the USA are listed as being possibly attributable to infection, chiefly by viruses. Across the world this percentage is likely to be much higher, as the prevalence of oncogenic viruses has been relatively low in the Western world.

Carcinoma of the uterine cervix is becoming the most common cancer of women, especially in South America. Two recently identified strains of human papillomavirus (HPV-16 and HPV-18) appear to be causally linked to flat cervical warts and neoplasia. It is interesting to note that these agents have not been isolated *in vitro* as infectious viruses; rather they have been identified through molecular genetic techniques so that the viral genes have been cloned before virus isolation. Cervical cancer is a disease easily curable by minor surgery if recognized at an early stage before invasion of the subepithelial tissue of the cervix has taken place. Furthermore the cancer, as well as preneoplastic dysplasia, can be recognized by direct inspection (colposcopy) and by the examination of cervical smears. The advantages of regular screening for cervical cancer are proven in reducing cancer mortality and morbidity. Yet the cost of preventative screening as a public health measure are considerable and to date the awareness of its value is largely restricted to those women least at risk of developing the disease. With the identification of the incriminating virus, the possiblity of developing immunizing vaccines is being actively pursued, though for human papillomaviruses this approach is still in its infancy.

Preventive immunization does appear to be effective in the transmission of hepatitis B virus (HBV). This virus is very prevalent in Africa and Asia. It is associated with primary liver cancer, a rare tumour in the West, but ranking sixth in cancer mortality worldwide. Dietary aflatoxins (see Chapter 7) may also play a role in human liver cancer, but there is strong evidence that HBV is the major causative factor. HBV is typically transmitted perinatally. Protection from infection can be achieved with preparations of pooled antibody to HBV surface antigen administered postnatally, following some weeks later by vaccination with surface antigen itself, soon to be manufactured by recombinant DNA methods. Trials in Taiwan and Japan suggest that the cycle of maternal transmission to infants can be broken by these measures, and hopefully this promises a dramatic reduction in the incidence of liver cancer in 40–60 years' time.

There is intensive research on vaccines to other viruses, such as Epstein Barr virus (EBV) and human T cell leukaemia virus type 1 (HTLV-1), but much development is still required before vaccines can be given preliminary trials. Infection by EBV is ubiquitous, and of the two malignancies associated with EBV, a major risk factor for one, Burkitt's lymphoma, may be malaria. Given the high morbidity and mortality of malaria itself, this is the disease that must be tackled. With EBV, however, it is undifferentiated nasopharyngeal carcinoma (NPC) that causes at least 50-fold more premature deaths than those from Burkitt's lymphoma.

NPC is prevalent among Chinese living in southern China and throughout South East Asia. Like most cancers, NPC is multifactorial in causation, with evidence of a slight heritable predisposition (increased risk with certain HLA haplotypes) and evidence of dietary nitrosamines or nickel salts early in life too. But the presence of EBV genomes in the tumour cells and of raised antibody levels to viral antigens in NPC patients implicates the virus in having the major causative role, and gives hope for future prevention.

Like cervical carcinoma, NPC is readily treatable if recognized at an early stage in its growth. Early diagnosis could soon be introduced in China by mass screening for serum IgA specific to an EBV antigen. The IgA can be recognized in a drop of blood from a pin pricked ear lobe, blotted onto paper. Since EBV IgA is elevated at an early stage of NPC growth, healthy subjects with elevated IgA are then investigated for carcinoma *in situ* and are treated curatively at this stage by simple surgery or radiotherapy. The mass screening for EBV IgA in the communes of southern China promises to be a most effective scheme of preventing cancer deaths.

19.3 Prospects for new treatment

Modern methods of cancer treatment have been reviewed in Chapters 16, 17, and 18. Surgical removal and radiotherapy remain the major treatments for solid tumours, although chemotherapy plays an increasingly important role. The newer physical methods of imaging, employing computerized tomography (CT) and nuclear magnetic resonance (NMR) are proving of great importance not only for diagnosis, but for conformational radiotherapy planning too. Immunological methods of imaging with radiolabelled antibodies (see Chapter 18) are still in a very primitive state compared to CT and NMR but may one day prove to be of greater use for detecting small tumours, especially metastases where the nature of the primary tumour is already known.

There have been very considerable advances in chemotherapeutic treatment (see Chapter 16) especially in leukaemia and in tumours of children and young adults. The major cancers of older patients, such as carcinoma of the breast, lung, stomach, and colon, have been disappointingly refractory to curative chemotherapy.

Much discussion of alternative treatment modalities is devoted to immunological mechanisms (see Chapter 15) and immunological vehicles of targeting cytotoxic agents or toxins to the tumour (see Chapter 18). Monoclonal antibodies that bind to the surface of tumour cells but not to haemopoietic stem cells are already proving to be clinically useful in 'cleansing' bone marrow in autologous transplantation. It remains to be seen whether immunological targeting will be successful in tackling solid tumours *in vivo*, but it seems well worth the current investment in this field.

As with more conventional chemotherapy, a problem with immunologically targeted therapy is the likelihood of resistant clones emerging, especially as tumour cells are known to modulate the expression of cell surface antigens. Perhaps the development of new radionuclides emitting alpha particles will be of most promise with antibody treatment; such nuclides may kill all cells within a short range of the targeted antibodies and the need to translocate antibody or toxin across the cell membrane is obviated. However, as related in Chapter 18, there is a need for more research into appropriate radionuclides for conjugation with monoclonal antibodies.

Where expression of surface antigen is a necessary part of the malignant phenotype, there is more hope for immunotherapy, as cells that express the antigen can be killed, and cells that cease to express it should lose their malignancy. There is a promising lead in using a monoclonal antibody to the interleukin 2 receptor to treat adult T cell leukaemia induced by human T cell leukaemia retrovirus, as the tumour cells grossly overexpress the receptor. The overamplified expression of receptors for epidermal growth factor in many squamous cell carcinomas (see Chapter 12) may also be appropriate targets for immunotherapy. In the next few years, much effort will be made to develop drugs or other reagents that directly and selectively block the function of oncogene products.

A few years ago, great publicity was given to the potential of interferons as anti-tumour therapy. Interferons were originally discovered as endogenous anti-viral agents, but they can promote terminal differentiation or arrest the growth of certain tumour cells too. Now that abundant interferon is becoming available through gene cloning, it is apparent that most cancers are unresponsive and further that high doses of interferon are extremely unpleasant and toxic for the patient. Therefore a disillusionment has set in that has been perhaps exacerbated by the over-enthusiastic claims for interferon before it could be tested in appropriate clinical trials. Yet amid this disappointment, one rare kind of malignancy, hairy cell leukaemia, is responding well to interferon in giving a complete response (regression) in the majority of patients, and interferon has become the preferred means of treatment of these patients. We do not understand why this leukaemia is so sensitive to interferon.

Another endogenous protein, tumour necrosis factor (TNF), has taken the place of interferon in the media as the magic cure–all for cancer. Like interferon, the gene encoding TNF has been cloned so that large amounts of this factor can be manufactured in bacteria. TNF is naturally produced in small amounts by macrophages in response to bacterial endotoxins. It is probably identical to a protein known as cachectin, which is thought to play a role in the wasting of normal tissues (cachexia) seen in many advanced cancer patients. Certain animal tumours are cured by TNF administration and clinical trials are just beginning to ascertain its effect on human malignancy. If it promotes cachexia TNF may do more harm than good, but like interferon it is hoped that some human tumours will be elimiated by this biological product. Preliminary reports suggest that interleukin 2 may also be of value in stimulating the host immune T cell response to some tumours.

Lastly, we should not forget the progress that has been made in recent years in improving palliative treatment, designed not to cure cancer, but to improve the quality of life remaining to the affected individual. Most chronic diseases, such as cardiovascular disease, arthritis, diabetes, etc. are not curable, and we have, perhaps, expected too much of oncologists in hoping for the magic bullet. In the meantime, great advances have been made in symptomatic treatment, pain control, and psychological management. With one quarter of deaths in the Western world attributable to malignant disease, improvements in the care of incurable cancer patients deserves considerable devotion and resources alongside the search for preventive measures and curative treatment.

19.4 Conclusion

Cancer is an exciting field of research, for it presents challenging questions in our basic understanding of cell physiology and development, coupled with the prospect of helping to alleviate a major source of human suffering and death. The study of cancer is multidisciplinary, involving scientists and clinicians in many different specialties. To ensure further progress in combating cancer we must practice what we preach, and be open to the new leads that the cross-fertilization of multi-disciplinary research affords.

Glossary

α-particle The nucleus of the helium atom (charge of $+2$) and mass 4.

abl An oncogene originally discovered in the Abelson strain of murine leukaemia virus. This virus causes pre-B cell tumours, whereas a related feline virus isolate causes sarcomas. The cellular *abl* gene is important in chronic granulocytic leukaemia of humans. The gene product displays tyrosine protein kinase (q.v.) activity.

acentric chromosome A chromosome lacking a centromere and, hence, incapable of attaching to the spindle at mitosis; consequently these chromosomes are randomly distributed between daughter cells at mitosis.

actin A cytoskeletal protein family found in all cell types. In muscle cells it is involved in the contractile function of the tissue.

active immunization Induction of a state of immunity by administering antigen.

acute leukaemia A tumour of the reticuloendothelial system that usually runs a rapid course from disease onset to death.

adduct The addition product between two molecules, e.g. a carcinogen (or its metabolite) and a nucleic acid in DNA.

adenocarcinoma A malignant tumour of glandular epithelium.

adenoma A solid, benign glandular tumour.

adjuvant A substance which increases the immune response to an antigen given at the same time.

affinity Used herein for the degree of binding or interaction, e.g. between a ligand and its receptor, or between an antigen and an antibody specific for that antigen. One can speak of high or low affinity receptors or antibodies.

aflatoxin A toxic food contaminant produced by fungi of the genus *Aspergillus.*

alkylating The process of attaching alkyl (usually methyl or ethyl) groups to a chemical structure such as a DNA base.

allele Short for allelomorph, meaning alternative form of the same gene.

alloantigen Differences which distinguish one individual of a species from another.

allogenic Genetically dissimilar.

allogenic graft (allograft) Graft between genetically dissimilar individuals of the same species.

amino acid One of twenty molecules used as the 'building blocks' of a protein.

anaplasia (dedifferentiation) Loss of differentiated characters.

anchorage independent growth Growth (cell division) in suspension in a liquid or semisolid medium, without attachment to a solid substrate. This form of growth is a property of many tumours.

androgens Steroid hormones secreted by the testis; maintain male characteristics.

aneuploidy The presence of extra chromosomes or the absence of chromosomes, so that the karyotype is neither haploid (q.v.) nor an exact multiple thereof.

antibody A globular protein produced by animals in response to an antigen (q.v.) and which binds specifically to the antigen.

antigen A molecule or part of an organism which is capable of stimulating the formation of antibodies (q.v.)

aromatic amines Polycyclic compounds consisting of hydrocarbon ring structures with at least one nitrogen containing amine group.

ascites Accumulation of serous fluid in the peritoneal cavity.

attenuated virus A virus whose pathogenicity is reduced by passage outside its natural host.

autocrine Self stimulation of a cell through production of both a factor and its specific receptor.

autophosphorylation A process by which a protein has the ability to add phosphate groups to amino acids within the protein (*see also* protein kinase).

auxotroph An organism (e.g. a bacterium) capable of synthesizing from simple nutrients all the complex biochemical compounds needed for its own growth.

axon Process of a nerve cell which carries impulses from the nerve body to a nerve or other target cell.

base change (in nucleotides) *See* mutation.

base The purine or pyrimidine component of nucleotides (q.v.).

B cell B lymphocyte: the immune cells of the lineage that makes antibodies.

benign tumour Tumour which does not invade or metastasize; an absolute distinction from malignant tumours is not possible (*see* Chapter 1).

bracken The fern *Pteridium aquilinum.*

Burkitt's lymphoma A tumour in humans of mature immunoglobulin producing B lymphocytes.

burst forming unit-erythroid (BFU-E) A colony of immature and mature red blood cells growing in a semi-solid medium.

cDNA A complementary (copy) DNA transcribed (q.v.) from an RNA template by the enzyme RNA dependent DNA polymerase (reverse transcriptase).

c-*onc* The cellular gene corresponding to a viral oncogene and sharing close DNA sequence homology. It is thought that the virus 'picked up' the cellular gene by chance.

cannula A hollow needle.

carcinogen A chemical substance, or physical agent such as X-ray irradiation or ultraviolet irradiation, that causes cancer.

carcinogenesis Process of tumour induction and development.

carcinoma A malignant tumour of epithelium.

carrier A host with an asymptomatic infection who serves as a source of infection to others.

chemical repair Conversion of a free radical to a stable molecule (usually by hydrogen atom transfer).

chemotaxis Response of cells or organisms to chemical stimuli: attraction towards is positive and repulsion negative chemotaxis.

chorioallantois Embryonic membrane formed by the fusion of the wall of the allantoic sac to the chorion. It underlies the porous egg shell in birds.

choriocarcinoma Cancer of uterus derived from placental tissue.

cirrhosis Fibrous repair in response to liver damage.

class (of antibody) Antibody class is determined by differences in the structure of the constant part of the molecule. Different classes have different biological functions.

clonal chromosomal aberrations Structural chromosome defects observed in at least two cells within a tumour, or numerical defects observed in at least three cells within a tumour.

clone *(noun)* A collection of cells, organisms, nucleic acid sequences etc. that are all derived from the same ancestor and are thus more or less identical; a population of cells derived from a single cell by division, and so usually presumed to contain the same genetic information subject to the occurrence of mutations.

clone *(verb)* To make a clone of nucleic acid sequence by genetic manipulation, replicating the desired sequence in a microorganism, or to isolate single cells.

codon A sequence of three nucleic acids or bases in DNA that together specify the encoded amino acid. Thus a sequence of DNA codons specifies the amino acid sequence of the encoded protein.

collagenase Enzyme which digests collagen.

colony stimulating factor (CSF) A group of proteins that stimulates the proliferation and differentiation of haemopoietic cells growing as colonies in a semi-solid medium; e.g. M-CSF (q.v.), G-CSF (for granulocytes), GM-CSF (q.v.), multi-CSF, etc.

colostomy Artificial external opening of large bowel.

complement A group of serum proteins which can be activated by cell bound antibody (q.v.) to lyse antibody coated cells.

complete carcinogen An agent, usually a chemical compound, which is able to induce cancer alone, i.e. without the need for subsequent treatment by a tumour promoting agent.

connective tissue (mesenchyme) Supporting tissues, made up of mesenchymal cells, collagen fibres, and interstitial substances. Bone, cartilage, fatty tissue, and blood vessels are specialized forms of connective tissue.

contrast medium X-ray dense material for delineating internal structure.

cytochrome (P450) Iron containing, electron accepting molecule involved in oxidation reduction reactions requiring energy, in this case the oxidative metabolism of carcinogens. P450 defines the characteristic absorption wavelength of a particular cytochrome on which these reactions are dependent.

cytolytic Lysing (killing) cells.

cytopathic Damaging cells, often leading to their death.

cytoskeleton The network of insoluble, multifunctional filaments (e.g. actin, vimentin, cytokeratin) remaining after extraction of cells in detergent.

cytotoxicity Cell killing.

deletion The removal of a segment of a chromosome or gene.

dielectric relaxation time The time required for the molecules in a medium to readjust following passage of radiation.

diethylstilboestrol A powerful, synthetic oestrogen.

differentiation Process of development of new characters in cells or tissues.

differentiation antigen Molecule detected by an antibody on or in one cell type which is associated with state of maturation or position in a developmental lineage.

diploid Having twice the haploid number of chromosomes. Normal human somatic cells are diploid, having 46 chromosomes (23 pairs).

dominant An allele that manifests its effects in heterozygotes (q.v.), i.e. when present in a single dose, as well as in homozygotes. A characteristic determined by a dominant allele.

double minutes Pairs of small acentric chromosomes believed to carry amplified genes.

down regulation The decrease in the number of available (exposed) cell surface receptors following interaction with the specific factor which binds to the particular receptor.

downstream promotion An insertional mutagenic event (q.v.) involving specifically a sequence that promotes gene transcription (hence 'promoter'). For this effect, the promoter must be located before the 5′ end (beginning) of the gene; the promoter is thus 'upstream' and it promotes the transcription of the gene elements that are 'downstream' (or toward the 3′ end).

ectoderm Outer of the three primary germ layers in animal embryos, which develops mainly into epidermis, nervous tissue.

electrophilic Literally, 'electron loving'. Applied to electron deficient chemical compounds which carry a net positive charge and are attracted to chemicals with an excess of electrons with which they bond covalently.

embolus Blood clot, tumour cells or other particles in blood stream.

endocrine Stimulation by factor produced at one site e.g. specific cells in a gland, and acting at a distant site.

endocytosis The process by which molecules bound to specific receptors on the cell surface are internalized by the cell.

endoderm Innermost of the three primary germ layers in the animal embryo which gives rise to the lining of the gut from pharynx to rectum, and derivatives from it such as liver, pancreas, etc., and the respiratory epithelium.

endoscope Optical instrument, passed through an orifice, e.g. mouth, anus, for visualizing internal organs.

endothelium Cells lining blood vessels.

enhancer insertion An insertional mutagenic event (q.v.) involving specifically a sequence that enhances (increases) the level of gene transcription (hence 'enhancer').

epidermal growth factor (EGF) A factor originally described for its mitogenic activity for epidermal cells. It is growth promoting for other cells as well.

epigenetic mechanisms Regulating expression of gene activity but not involving alterations in gene structure.

epithelium Tissue specific surface or glandular cells.

epitope A structural region of an antigen (q.v.) that is recognized by an antibody (q.v.) molecule.

epoxide A derivative of an aromatic (ring structured) molecule in which an oxygen molecule forms a bridge across an opened double bond between two carbon atoms.

epoxide hydrase An enzyme which utilizes an epoxide substrate, breaks open the oxygen bridge and adds one molecule of water to form a diol derivative.

erbA A gene sequence originally found in an avian erythroleukaemia virus as part of a fusion to *erbB* (q.v.). It may not be an oncogene *per se*.

erbB An oncogene originally found in two isolates of avian erythroleukaemia virus. It represents part of the gene for the receptor for epidermal growth factor (EGF, q.v.).

erythroblastosis A leukaemia of red blood cell precursors.

erythrocyte Most mature red cell from which the nucleus has been extruded (in mammals).

erythropoietin A growth factor that stimulates the proliferation and differentiation of erythrocyte precursor cells.

ets An oncogene originally found in an avian myeloblastosis virus (strain E26) fused to the *myb* oncogene (q.v.).

eukaryote Higher organisms whose cells are complex, containing nuclei and other organelles.

exocrine Secreting externally; exocrine glands deliver their secretions to an epithelial surface through ducts.

exon The parts of a gene sequence that are found in the messenger RNA (transcript) molecule which will be used for producing (translating) the protein product of the gene. Parts of the gene not found in the transcripts are known as introns (q.v.).

familial polyposis coli Inherited condition where multiple polyps (small benign tumours) of the colon and rectum develop and which predisposes to colon cancer.

fes An oncogene originally found in a feline sarcoma virus (Gardner–Arnstein strain). The gene product displays tyrosine protein kinase (q.v.) activity.

fgr An oncogene originally found in a feline sarcoma virus (Gardner–Rasheed strain). Its gene product has tyrosine protein kinase (q.v.) activity.

fibrosis Formation of scar tissue.

filling defect A region of an X-ray or scan with absence of medium or isotope often due to the presence of tumour.

fms An oncogene originally found in a feline sarcoma virus (McDonough strain). Its product displays tyrosine kinase (q.v.) activity. This gene may be related or identical to the gene encoding the receptor for macrophage colony stimulating factor (q.v.).

fos An oncogene originally found in two murine osteosarcoma viruses. Its product is found in the nucleus and is more abundant in cells responding to growth factor stimulation, and in amnion and mature monocytes.

fps An oncogene originally found in two avian sarcoma viruses (strains

Fujinami and PRCII). Its product displays tyrosine protein kinase (q.v.) activity.

frameshift mutation A mutation in which, by addition or deletion (other than in multiples of three) of nucleic acids, the reading frame of the triplet code is disrupted. All downstream codons are thereby altered and as a rule no functional protein is produced.

free radical An unstable molecular fragment caused by breakage of a chemical bond in a molecule.

gene activation Generally meant to imply that a dormant gene has been 'turned on' so that messenger RNA is made (transcribed).

gene amplification A mutation event whereby a gene is found in greater than the normal number of copies. Amplification generally involves very long stretches of chromosomes (i.e. many genes) and may occur so that the genes are amplified in number many times. (*See also* homogeneously staining regions and double minutes.)

genetic marker An allele of a gene which follows standard Mendelian segregation and so can be used to study linkage in families or associations with a characteristic within populations.

genome The total genetic material of an organism.

genotoxic An agent that is toxic through its ability to damage DNA. At high levels of damage, this is lethal for the cell.

germ (cell) line Cells which give rise to the sperm or egg (ovum) which transmit genes from one generation to another and are thus potentially immortal. All other cells are somatic and die with the individual. Only mutations in the germ cell line can be passed on to future generations. Also used to designate unaltered gene configurations.

glucocorticoids Steroid hormones secreted by the adrenal cortex for the control of carbohydrate metabolism; they also have anti-inflammatory properties and kill certain types of lymphocytes.

glycolipid A lipid molecule having covalently attached oligosaccharide (q.v.).

glycoprotein A protein molecule having covalently attached oligosaccharide (q.v.).

gonadotrophins Hormones secreted by the anterior lobe of the pituitary (q.v.).

granulocyte White blood cells (various maturation stages include the neutrophils and polymorphonuclear cells) involved in the defence system against foreign matter.

granulocyte/macrophage colony stimulating factor (GM–CSF) A factor that stimulates the proliferation and differentiation of precursor cells of the granulocyte and macrophage lineages. Note that these two lineages share a common precursor cell, one that is already more differentiated than the haemopoietic stem cell (known as the CFUs or pluripotential stem cell) that gives rise to all the blood cells.

HLA The major histocompatibility system of man. It is a complex genetic region coding for two major classes of cell surface determinants involved in the control of immune function. There are also other genes in the region, in particular controlling certain of the complement components.

Ha-*ras* An oncogene originally found in two rodent sarcoma viruses (strains Harvey and BALB). Its product is an enzyme catalysing guanosine triphosphate (GTP). It is a member of a multigene family (Ki-*ras*, N-*ras*, q.v.), members of which are often found in mutated form in tumours.

haematuria Blood in the urine.

haemoccult test A clinical biochemical test which detects the presence of blood in the faeces.

haemopoietic Blood cell forming.

half life The time taken for half a given quantity of a chemical (e.g. radioisotopes, proteins, nucleic acids) to degrade or decay. Short half lives reflect an unstable chemical.

haploid Having one copy of each chromosome as in the gametes. The human haploid chromosome number is 23.

hemicorporectomy Surgical removal of lower half of the body.

hemizygous Having only one copy of a given genetic locus (or of a number of loci in the case of deletions or loss of whole chromosomes).

heteroantiserum Antiserum raised in one animal species against cells or molecules of another.

heterozygous Having different alleles at a given locus on homologous chromosomes.

histocompatibility genes Genes that determine susceptibility or resistance to tissue or tumour transplants.

homogeneously staining region (HSR) Region of a chromosome staining with an intermediate intensity throughout its length and without the normal pattern of light and dark bands.

homologous chromosomes Chromosomes that carry genes governing the same characteristics and that pair during the cell division which produces eggs and sperm. Individuals receive one member of a homologous pair of chromosomes from their father and the other member from their mother.

homozygous Having the same allele at a given locus on homologous chromosomes.

hormone A specific chemical substance produced by cells and carried to other cells or organs, often in the blood, to produce a specific effect at a distance.

hybridization, nucleic acid *See* Northern and Southern blotting/hybridization.

hybridoma A hybrid tumour cell created by the fusion of two or more cells of different type. The term is commonly used to refer to monoclonal antibody producing cells formed by fusion of a sensitized B lymphocyte and a myeloma (q.v.) cell.

hydrophilic Literally, 'water loving'. Describes property of a substance preferentially found in water extracts as opposed to lipids.

hydrophobic Literally, 'water fearing'. Describes property of a substance preferentially found in lipid extracts (such as membranes) as opposed to water.

hyperdiploid Having more than the diploid number of chromosomes.

hyperplasia Increase in number of cells in response to stimulus—a reversible process.

hypertrophy Increase in size of cell or tissue.

hypodiploid Having fewer than the diploid number of chromosomes.

IL1 Interleukin 1. A factor produced by monocytes, involved in immune response reactions of antigen presentation by monocytes to T lymphocytes.

IL2 Interleukin 2. T lymphocyte growth factor (previously called TCGF).

IL3 Interleukin 3. A factor that stimulates growth of early multilineage haemopoietic cells.

immunogen A substance which stimulates an animal to produce antibodies (q.v.).

immunoglobulin An antibody (q.v.) molecule.

immunotherapy A form of therapy in which the host's immune system is activated or augmented, e.g. by the use of anti-tumour antibodies (q.v.).

immunotoxin A hybrid molecule formed by the conjugation of an antibody (q.v.) and a toxic protein.

infectious mononucleosis A disease characterized by an imbalance of the immune cells in the body and a massive proliferation of T cells (q.v.).

inflammation Tissue response to infection or damage.

initiation The primary step in tumour induction caused by a carcinogen.

insertional mutagenesis A mutation caused by the insertion of new genetic material into a normal gene or sequences surrounding it. The term is generally used in relation to integrations of retroviruses (q.v.) into chromosomal DNA, although it applies to other inserted material, including DNA sequences moved from one chromosomal site to another ('transposition').

insulin A hormone produced by cells of the pancreas. It is concerned with the regulation of carbohydrate, fat, and protein metabolism. A deficiency of insulin causes diabetes.

integration Insertion of viral DNA within a host chromosome. First applied to integration of phage DNA in the bacterial chromosome.

interferon A group of proteins produced by cells in response to viral infection and other stimuli. Their effects are complex and include antiviral actions exerted at various stages.

interleukin Substance produced by a cell of the immune system which acts on other cells (*see also* IL1, IL2, IL3).

intravenous urogram X-ray of urinary tract after injection of radio-opaque material which is concentrated in the kidney.

intron The parts of a gene sequence that are not found in the messenger RNA (transcript) molecule which will be used to produce the protein product of the gene. Introns are removed from the initial RNA copy of the gene by a process known as splicing (q.v.).

inversion A chromosomal aberration that arises when two breaks occur in the same chromosome and the region between the breaks is reinserted after a 180° rotation resulting in a reversed gene order.

ionization potential Energy required to liberate a non-nuclear electron from an atom or molecule.

isochromosome A chromosomal aberration in which one of the arms of a chromosome is deleted and the other arm is duplicated. The two arms of an isochromosome are therefore of equal length and contain the same genes.

isogenic Genetically identical.

isogenic graft (isograft) Graft between genetically identical individuals, e.g. between identical twins.

isotope One or two or more atoms having the same atomic number but different mass, e.g. ^{123}I and ^{131}I are radioactive isotopes of iodine.

Kaposi's sarcoma A tumour, possibly arising from endothelial cells, often found as skin lesions, purple or blue in colour.

karyotype The chromosome complement analysed and set out according to size, shape, and banding patterns of each chromosome.

keratinocyte Major epithelial cell type of the skin or epidermis, which contains large quantities of cytoskeletal proteins of the cytokeratin family.

Ki-*ras* An oncogene originally identified in a mouse sarcoma virus (Kirsten strain). It is a member of a multigene family (Ha-*ras*, N-*ras*, q.v.), members of which are often found in mutated form in tumours. Its product is an enzyme catalysing guanosine triphosphate (GTP).

kit An oncogene originally found in a feline sarcoma virus (strain HZ4).

L-*myc* An oncogene identified by gene amplification (q.v.) in a lung carcinoma. Member of the *myc* multigene family.

LET (Linear Energy Transfer) Rate of energy loss to the surrounding medium, in a radiation track (unit: keV/micron).

leukoerythroblastic anaemia Reduction in red cells associated with increase in white cells.

leukosis A proliferative disease of leukocytes.

life span study An ongoing epidemiological study e.g., of excess cancer incidence in atomic bomb survivors from the Japanese cities of Hiroshima and Nagasaki.

ligand The substance with which a receptor acts specifically to form a complex at least transiently.

linkage The presence of two or more genes on the same chromosome causing a tendency of alleles of these genes to be inherited together. Linkage occurs only when the genes are sufficiently close to one another on the same chromosome.

lipid bilayer Description of the membranes of cells, including the plasma membrane, of two apposed layers each containing lipid molecules.

liposome A synthetic lipid vesicle.

locus (plural, **loci**) Position of a gene on a chromosome.

LTR A structure found at both ends of the provirus DNA of a retrovirus (q.v.), hence 'long terminal repeat'.

lymphangiogram X-ray of lymphatic vessels.

lymphocyte White blood cell of the T or B lineage.

lymphokine Substance produced by lymphocytes which acts on other cells (*see also* interleukin).

lymphoma A solid tumour of T or B lymphocytes, e.g. in the lymph nodes, thymus or spleen.

lysosome The cellular organelle which degrades molecules that have been taken into a cell by endocytosis (q.v.).

macrophage White cell found in all tissues which can ingest and break down antigens.

macrophage/monocyte colony stimulating factor (M-CSF) A factor that stimulates the growth and differentiation of cells of the macrophage/monocyte (q.v.) lineage.

malignant tumour Tumour which is capable of invading surrounding tissues and of metastasizing.

mammography X-ray of breast.

marker chromosome Abnormal or rearranged chromosome which can be recognized as a characteristic feature.

megakaryocyte White blood cell that undergoes nuclear division without cell division, leading to a multinucleated cell. It shatters to produce the subcellular entities known as platelets (q.v.) that participate in wound healing.

meiosis Two successive cell divisions from a diploid cell, in which the chromosomes are duplicated only once so that each of the new daughter cells have only half the diploid chromosome number, e.g. in the formation of gametes (sperm and ova).

mesenchyme *See* connective tissue.

mesoderm The germ layer lying between ectoderm (q.v.) and endoderm (q.v.). It gives rise to an epithelial component (epithelium of genital and most of urinary system), striated muscle including heart, and mesenchyme (connective tissue, cartilage, bone, smooth muscle, and blood cells).

met An oncogene originally identified by transfection (q.v.) of DNA from a human osteosarcoma (q.v.) cell line treated with a chemical carcinogen (q.v.).

metaphase The phase of mitosis or meiosis in which the condensed chromosomes attached to the spindle fibres line up on an equatorial plate between the two poles of the cell.

metaplasia Abnormal alteration in the structure of cells.

metastasis A secondary tumour arising from cells carried to a distant site from a primary tumour.

microsome (-al) Subcellular membranous particles with membrane bound enzyme activities, derived from the endoplasmic reticulum, in cell fractionation procedures.

mineralocorticoids Steroid hormones secreted by the adrenal cortex for the maintenance of ion balance, especially Na^+ ions.

mitogen A compound capable of causing cells to divide.

mitosis Process of cell division.

modal chromosome number The number of chromosomes per cell which is found most frequently in a mixed cell population.

molecular excitation A change in the electronic configuration of an atom or molecule (accompanied by absorption of energy).

monoclonal Derived from a single cell.

monocyte Similar cell to the macrophage but found in the blood. Both cells assist in immune responses.

monosomy The presence of only one member of a chromosome pair.

mos An oncogene originally found in a mouse sarcoma virus (Moloney strain). Its gene product has serine protein kinase (q.v.) activity.

mutagen A chemical or physical agent that causes changes in the structure of DNA (mutations).

mutagenesis Effecting a heritable change in a nucleic acid.

mutagenicity The capacity of an agent (e.g. a chemical) to cause DNA mutation.

mutation A heritable change in the genetic material. Mutations in the broadest sense include any change, from a single base pair change in the DNA to substantial deletions or re-arrangements of the DNA even involving major parts or the whole of chromosomes, and including chromosome translocations.

mutation frequency The ratio of mutated cells to normal cells following, for example, radiation (expressed either as per cell irradiated or per cell surviving).

myb An oncogene originally found in two avian myeloblastosis (myeloid leukaemia) viruses. Its product is found in the nucleus. The gene has been activated by adjacent insertion of retroviruses (q.v.) in several rodent myeloid leukaemias.

myc An oncogene originally found in four avian 'myelocytoma' viruses. Its product is found in the nucleus and appears to be a DNA binding protein. It is a member of a multigene family (including L-*myc* and N-*myc*, q.v.).

myeloid Literally, 'of the bone marrow'. However, in speaking of myeloid leukaemia, one is denoting cells of the granulocytic or monocytic lineages.

myeloma A plasma cell tumour.

N-*myc* An oncogene identified by gene amplification (q.v.) in a neuroblastoma. Member of the *myc* (q.v.) multigene family.

N-*ras* An oncogene originally identified as a gene amplified in a human neuroblastoma (q.v.) and subsequently in other tumour types. It is a member of a multigene family (Ha-*ras*, Ki-*ras*, q.v.), members of which are often found in mutated form in tumours.

nasopharyngeal carcinoma Carcinoma of the squamous epithelium of the postnasal space.

natural killer cells Cells that are believed to kill nonspecifically tumour and virus infected cells.

necrosis Tissue death.

neonatal thymectomy Removal of the thymus at birth, leaving the animal without functioning T cells.

neoplasia Tumour growth.

neoplasm Tumour.

neu An oncogene originally identified by transfection (q.v.) of DNA from a rodent neuroblastoma.

neuroblastoma A malignant tumour of neural crest origin. It may arise in any site containing sympathetic nervous tissue but is most commonly found in and around the adrenals.

neuroendocrine system A system of cells widely distributed throughout the body, which produces regulatory peptides. One group acts as hormones on distant organs, or on cells locally. A second group is produced at nerve endings and cells act as neurotransmitters.

neurotransmitter A substance released from the axon terminal (nerve ending) of a nerve cell on excitation which stimulates or inhibits a target cell.

Northern blotting/hybridization A technique wherein RNA is fractionated according to size by electrophoresis in agarose-formaldehyde gels and then the RNA is transferred ('blotted') onto nitrocellulose paper. The RNA is then fixed to the paper by baking and then can be identified by using specific nucleic acid sequences ('probes', these may be RNA or DNA) of a particular gene or part of a gene ('hybridization'). This technique allows identification of genes being expressed (i.e. transcribed into RNA), quantitation of levels expressed, etc.

nucleotide The unit component of a nucleic acid comprising a base (q.v.), a sugar, and a phospate group.

oestrogens Steroid hormones secreted by the ovary; maintain female characteristics.

oligosaccharide A structure composed of three or more sugar residues covalently attached to protein in glycoproteins (q.v.) and glycolipids (q.v.).

oncogene Literally, a gene causing cancer. Oncogenes were identified by their presence in cancer causing viruses, where their function is critical for viral transforming properties.

osteolytic Bone destroying.

osteosarcoma A malignant tumour of bone composed of proliferating spindle cells which directly form tumour osteoid.

P450 A class of enzymes involved in oxygenating various compounds, the mono-oxygenases or mixed function oxidases.

PAP test Named after Papanicolaou who devised a staining method for cells shed (or scraped) from the surface of epithelial tissues; particularly used for the routine screening of uterine cervix for cancer cells.

palliation Treatment to ease symptoms.

papilloma A benign tumour usually on a surface, with a frond like structure.

paraaortic Alongside the aorta.

paracentesis Puncture or tapping of a fluid filled space with a hollow needle to draw off the contained liquid.

paracrine Stimulation of a cell through interaction with a substance produced by a neighbouring cell.

parasitism A relationship in which one member (the parasite) benefits at the cost of the other (the host). (*See also* symbiosis.)

partial hepatectomy Surgical removal of part of the liver.

particle accelerators Machines which emit pulses or continuous beams of high energy particulate radiation (cyclotrons, Van de Graaff accelerators, Betatrons, etc.).

passive immunization Immunity acquired by receiving immune cells or antibody.

penetration Passage of a virus from outside to inside the host cell.

phagocytosis The process by which large particles or cells are engulfed by cells of the reticuloendothelial system (q.v.), such as macrophages.

phenotype The combination of characteristics expressed by a particular cell or type of cell.

phorbol ester A variety of compounds originally isolated from plants that are active as tumour promoting (q.v.) agents in multistep carcinogenesis assays.

phosphorylation The process of addition of phosphate groups to a protein (*see also* protein kinase).

pituitary gland (hypophysis) A small gland at the base of the brain with two main lobes, anterior (adenohypophysis) and posterior (neurohypophysis). The anterior lobe produces hormones which control secretion in sex glands, thyroid, adrenal etc. The posterior lobe secretes other hormones which are formed in nerve cells in the hypothalamus. These hormones influence blood pressure, water balance etc.

plasma cell A fully differentiated B lymphocyte synthesizing and secreting antibody (q.v.).

plasma The fluid component of blood.

platelet A subcellular component of the blood formed from megakaryocytes (q.v.) concerned with blood clotting; release mitogens at the site of the wound.

platelet derived growth factor (PDGF) A factor in platelets (q.v.) that is mitogenic for cells at the site of a wound (e.g. endothelial cells, q.v.). Part of the gene for PDGF has been captured by a simian sarcoma virus in which it is known as *sis* (q.v.).

pleural effusion Fluid in the pleural space (surrounding the lungs) in abnormal amounts.

polyclonal Derived from more than one cell.

polycyclic hydrocarbons A class of organic chemicals consisting of carbon and hydrogen molecules arranged in a series of linked ring structures.

polymorphism The occurrence of two or more alleles for a given locus in a population where at least two alleles appear with frequencies of more than one per cent.

polyp A tumour projecting from a surface, usually epithelial.

prednisolone A powerful, synthetic glucocorticoid.

progestins Steroid hormones secreted by the ovary during the menstrual cycle and pregnancy.

promoter insertion An insertional mutagenic (q.v.) event involving specifically a sequence that promotes gene transcription (hence 'promoter'). *See also* downstream promotion.

promotion Stages following initiation; may be caused by specific non-carcinogenic promoting agents.

prostaglandins A group of compounds of similar structure found in the prostate (hence the name) but now known to be widely distributed in the body and affecting blood vessels, nervous system, uterus, etc.

protease Protein digesting enzyme.

protein kinase An enzyme that adds phosphate groups to amino acids (generally serine, threonine and tyrosine); the process is known as phosphorylation (q.v.).

protein kinase C A serine and threonine protein kinase (q.v.) important in the cell's response to growth factor stimulation.

protooncogene The normal cellular counterpart of a gene identified as causing a tumour (c-*onc* and v-*onc*, q.v.).

provirus The intracellular double-stranded DNA form of the retrovirus genome, either free or integrated.

proximate metabolite/carcinogen The carcinogen or its metabolite which undergoes metabolic or spontaneous conversion to a further derivative, the ultimate metabolite/carcinogen which binds to the target macromolecule, usually DNA.

pseudogene A gene thought to be permanently inactive. Many lack introns (q.v.) compared to related genes that are active. May have arisen by gene duplication events.

RBE (Relative Biological Efficiency or Effectiveness) The ratio of absorbed doses of two different types of radiation required to give the same level of effect.

RNA dependent DNA polymerase *See* reverse transcriptase.

RNA splicing A maturation process that removes internal sequences from polyribonucleotide chains (splicing, q.v.).

radiation fractionation Exposure to radiation over two or more periods separated by intervals of time.

radioimaging A technique that uses radioactive substances to visualize sites within the patient's body, e.g. the sites of tumour.

radionuclide An atom which undergoes spontaneous decay with the release of radiation. Radionuclides can be used for the radioimaging (q.v.) or therapy of cancer.

radioprotector A chemical substance that reduces the biological effects of radiation.

radon A chemically inert radioactive gas: a product of radium disintegration.

raf An oncogene originally identified in a murine sarcoma virus (strain 3611). Its product has protein kinase (q.v.) activity.

receptor A structural molecule that binds to a specific factor (e.g. hormone, vitamin, antigen, etc.). These may be found at the cell surface (cell surface receptors, membrane receptor) or within the cytoplasm (cytosolic receptor).

recessive An allele that is expressed only when present in the homozygous or hemizygous state (compare with dominant).

recessive mutation A mutation which is not expressed in the phenotype if it is balanced by a corresponding normal gene on the homologous chromosome, i.e. it is expressed only when both homologous genes are affected or if one is deleted.

recombination Process of exchange of genetic information between two homologous chromosomes, presumed to occur through breakage of both chromosomes at homologous sites followed by reunion after exchange. Also can occur between other RNA or DNA molecules (as with viruses).

rel An oncogene originally found in an avian reticuloendotheliosis (q.v.) virus.

restriction endonucleases Enzymes produced by bacteria that cut double-stranded DNA by recognizing a specific sequence of nucleotides (q.v.).

reticuloendothelial system 'Defence cells'. A diffuse system of phagocytic cells involved with the clearance of foreign proteins, immune complexes, large particles, and cells from the bloodstream.

reticuloendotheliosis A proliferative disease of reticuloendothelial cells.

retroperitoneal Lying behind the peritoneum.

retrovirus A member of a family of viruses sharing several physicochemical properties, including the type of organization of the RNA genome and an enzyme (known as reverse transcriptase) which makes a DNA copy of the genome (provirus, q.v.) to become incorporated into the chromosomal DNA of the infected host cell.

reverse transcriptase An enzyme, RNA dependent DNA polymerase, encoded by retroviruses. In the viral life cycle, the enzyme carried in the virus particle facilitates the synthesis of a DNA copy of the viral RNA genome. It then makes a second DNA strand complementary to the first, and also degrades the viral RNA (template). Used in laboratory procedures to prepare complementary DNA copies (cDNA) of other RNAs.

reversion (reverted) The process by which a mutation is corrected, by 'back mutation' to the original (wild type) DNA sequence. The reverted cell (or virus, etc.) then has a normal phenotype.

ribosomes Cellular particles at which proteins are synthesized.

risk factors Environmental or inherited influences that increase the chance of cells progressing from a normal to neoplastic phenotype.

ros An oncogene originally found in an avian sarcoma virus. Its product has tyrosine protein kinase (q.v.) activity.

salvage pathway A biochemical pathway in the synthesis of DNA which reutilizes preexisting nucleic acids and their precursors rather than synthesizing them *de novo* from single carbon units.

sarcoma A malignant tumour of mesenchyme.

serum The fluid left after plasma has clotted due to substances released from platelets; some plasma proteins have been removed.

signal transduction Used in reference to the process by which the interactions between a growth factor and its specific receptor at the cell surface generate a signal that is transmitted to the cell nucleus as a stimulus to proliferate.

sis An oncogene originally found in a simian sarcoma virus. The gene is part of the cellular gene encoding platelet derived growth factor (PDGF, q.v.).

ski An oncogene originally found in an avian carcinoma virus. Its product is found in the nucleus of cells.

somatic Refers to cells that are not part of the germ line and so their genetic complement is not passed from parent to offspring.

Southern blotting/hybridization A technique wherein DNA is fractionated according to size by electrophoresis in agarose gels (the DNA may be precut using restriction endonucleases, q.v.), and then the DNA is transferred ('blotted') onto nitrocellulose paper. The DNA is then fixed to the paper by baking and may then be identified by using specific nucleic acid sequences ('probes'; these may be RNA or DNA) of a particular gene or part of a gene ('hybridization'). The double-stranded DNA in the gel is treated with alkali before blotting; this provides single-stranded nucleic acid which can then bind covalently ('anneal') to the probes. The technique allows identification of the size of a gene, a map of restriction enzyme sites, gene amplification, gene deletion, gene rearrangement, etc.

specificity (of antibody or cells) The ability to distinguish between different antigens.

splicing An event that removes specifically the sequences of the noncoding parts of a gene (introns, q.v.) from the initial RNA molecule complementary in sequence to the gene. This is part of the 'processing' of the RNA molecule to its active form (the messenger RNA transcript) used to produce the gene product.

src An oncogene originally found in an avian sarcoma virus. Its product has tyrosine protein kinase (q.v.) activity.

stem cell Precursor cell capable of growing and differentiating in response to a stimulus.

stilboestrol A powerful, synthetic oestrogen.

symbiosis 'Living together': an association of two organisms that confers mutual benefit.

synergism (synergy) Two or more compounds whose effects are additive or more than additive.

syngeneic graft Graft between individuals that have been inbred until their genetic similarity allows acceptance of grafts between members of the strain e.g. between mice of an inbred strain.

targeting The directing of substances such as drugs or toxins to target cells by attaching them to carriers, such as antibodies (q.v.), which bind to the target cell specifically.

T cell T lymphocytes: a group of cells responsible for cell mediated immunity.

testosterone The main male sex hormone, secreted by the testis.

tetraploid Having four times the haploid number of chromosomes.

transcription A base pairing process that copies one nucleic acid into a complementary polynucleotide chain.

transduction The process by which a virus genome recombines with other nucleic acids leading to the capture of new sequences or genes. The new material is 'transduced'.

transfect To introduce foreign DNA into a cell by experimental means so that the DNA integrates into the genome and is expressed in its new host cell. Transfection, the process.

transformation A word used in many ways. In this book, (unless qualified) it means a change of morphological appearance of a cell ('morphological transformation') generally by a virus, chemical carcinogen, physical reagent or even some unidentified ('spontaneous') event.

transforming growth factor (TGF) A factor that can cause a reversible change in normal cell phenotype such that cells grow into colonies in semi-solid media (anchorage independent growth). TGF-β requires EGF to produce this phenotype whereas TGF-α can work alone.

translation A term describing the process whereby the triplet code sequence of a messenger RNA molecule is used to produce a specific order (chain) of amino acids which form a protein.

translocation A chromosomal aberration in which part of one chromosome joins onto another chromosome. A reciprocal translocation refers to the transfer of material between two chromosomes.

transmembrane Something spanning the membrane. Generally in regard to plasma membrane; e.g. a protein found external to, within, and internal to the plasma membrane.

triplet code The code by which a sequence of three nucleic acids (bases) specifies one amino acid. Each triplet thus forms one codon.

triploid Having three times the haploid number of chromosomes.

trisomy The presence of three chromosomes of one type.

truncation Literally, a shortening. In the context of this book, it means that a gene has been shortened by some event and thereby the protein product of the gene is smaller.

tumour promoter An agent capable of providing the second step in two step carcinogenesis systems whereby an initiated (preneoplastic) cell is converted to a neoplastic one (*see* initiation, and promotion). Generally a specific tumour promoter is required for a particular initiating agent.

ultimate metabolite/carcinogen *See* proximate metabolite/carcinogen.

v-*onc* An oncogene identified in a virus (*see* oncogene).

xenograft Graft between individuals of different species.

yes An oncogene originally found in two avian sarcoma viruses. Its product has tyrosine protein kinase (q.v.) activity.

Index

simian sarcoma virus (SSV) 186, 204
  and *sis* 217, 262, 268–9
sis oncogene
  cellular 225
    and platelet derived growth factor
      217–9, 262, 268–70
    associated with Philadelphia
      chromosome 237
    viral 204
ski oncogene
  cellular 220–1, 225
  viral 203
skin tumours 9, 12, 16, 20, 88, 101
  and chemical carcinogens 133, 134,
    135
  and hormones 293
  and immunosuppression 335
  and viruses 188
  Merkel cell tumours 312
  rodent ulcer 357
  treatment 351, 357, 361
SOD, *see* superoxide dismutase
somatic cell mutation 94, 97, 98, 132,
    180, 227, 411
  hypothesis of carcinogenesis 180, 412
somatomedin 257, 261
somatostatin 310, 318, 321
somatostatinoma 318–9
somatotropin 281, 285, 293, 300
sources for chemotherapeutic drugs 365,
    366–7
Southern blotting and hybridization 107,
    213
src oncogene 276
  cellular 214–6, 225
    kinase activity 216, 265
  viral 203
    and Rous sarcoma virus 214, 221
stem cells 3, 4, 57–8, 60, 254
  in bone marrow 40, 43, 58
  leukaemia 59
steroid hormones 88, 280, 282–3, 284,
    300, 301, 304; *see* glucocorticoids;
    mineralocorticoids
  as chemotherapeutic agents 367
  steroid-sensitive cells 57–8
  steroid-sensitive tumours 299–300
stilboestrol 287, 289, 293, 295, 296,
    302
stomach cancer 68, 86, 351, 413, 417
  and immunosuppression 335
  and radiation exposure 160, 161, 162
substance P 309, 321
superoxide dismutase (SOD) 172–3
surgery 353, 354, 358
  and combined therapy 359
SV40 virus 187, 193, 195, 223, 226

T4, *see* interleukin, IL2
T6 46
T9 46, 264
TAF, *see* tumour angiogenesis factor
T-ALL, *see* acute lymphoblastic leukaemia,
    T-ALL
tamoxifen, *see* antioestrogen
target cell 293
  target cell concept 278–9, 280
tautomerism 115, 116, 123, 125
T cells (lymphocytes) 41, 43, 46, 184,
    326–7, 330–3, 336, 386, 406
  cytotoxicity assays 342, 347
  deficiency 49, 187; *see* immunoglobulin
  immunoregulatory function 331, 336,
    341, 343–5, 395
  infections 184, 189, 190
  leukaemia 185, 218
    T cell leukaemia virus 102; *see also*
      human T cell leukaemia virus
  malignancy 187
  receptor 43
    for interleukin 2 53, 255
    for antigen 330
  removal from marrow 61
  surveillance against Epstein Barr virus
    49, 58, 335–6
TCGF, *see* interleukin, IL2
T-CLL, *see* chronic lymphocytic
    leukaemia, thymic
tcl oncogene 209
TdT (terminal deoxynucleotidyl
    transferase) 43, 46
teratocarcinoma 18, 19, 218, 414
teratoma 18, 19, 22
  of testis 368, 371
testis, cancer of 9, 65, 82–5, 88; *see also*
    teratoma
  and hormones 280, 300
  therapy 368, 407
testosterone 279, 280, 296–7
  and prostate 295
thymidine kinase (TK) 149
thyroid 320, 392
  hormone secretion 280, 282, 301, 310
  thyroid hormone releasing hormone
    311
  thyroid stimulating hormone 311
  tumours 15, 16, 88, 302, 320–1
    and bone scan 356
    related to radiation 160, 161
thyrotropin (TT) 280, 281, 320
  releasing hormone (TRH) 280
thyroxine (tetraiodothyroxine) 280, 282–3
  and tumour growth 283, 289, 293
tissue culture 25, 26, 178, 285, 291
TK, *see* thymidine kinase